NETTER'S ATLAS OF NEUROSCIENCE

Second Edition

David L. Felten, MD, PhD
Vice President, Research
Medical Director of the Research Institute
William Beaumont Hospitals
Royal Oak, MI

Associate Dean for Research
Clinical Research Professor
Oakland University William Beaumont School of Medicine
Rochester, MI

Anil N. Shetty, PhD
Chief, MR Physics
Diagnostic Radiology
William Beaumont Hospitals
Royal Oak, MI

Adjunct Assistant Professor of Radiology
Wayne State University School of Medicine
Detroit, MI

Illustrations by
Frank H. Netter, MD

Contributing Illustrators
Carlos A. G. Machado, MD
James A. Perkins, MS, MFA
John A. Craig, MD

SAUNDERS

ELSEVIER

SAUNDERS
ELSEVIER

1600 John F. Kennedy Blvd.
Ste 1800
Philadelphia, PA 19103-2899

NETTER'S ATLAS OF NEUROSCIENCE ISBN: 978-1-4160-5418-4

Notice

Previous edition copyrighted 2003

Library of Congress Cataloging-in-Publication Data
Felten, David L.
    Netter's atlas of neuroscience / David L. Felten, Anil N. Shetty ; illustrations by Frank H. Netter ; contributing
        illustrators, Carlos A.G. Machado, James A. Perkins, John A. Craig. — 2nd ed.
        p. ; cm.
    Includes index.
    Rev. ed. of: Netter's atlas of human neuroscience / David L. Felten, Ralph Józefowicz. 1st ed. c2003.
    ISBN 978-1-4160-5418-4
1. Nervous system—Atlases. I. Shetty, Anil Narsinha. II. Felten, David L. Netter's atlas of human neuroscience.
    III. Title. IV. Title: Atlas of neuroscience.
    [DNLM: 1. Nervous System—anatomy & histology—Atlases. 2. Nervous System Physiological Phenomena—
    Atlases. WL 17 F325n 2010]

    QM451.F44 2010
    612.8022'2—dc22

    2009002530

Acquisitions Editor: Elyse O'Grady
Developmental Editor: Marybeth Thiel
Publishing Services Manager: Linda Van Pelt
Project Manager: Sharon Lee
Design Direction: Louis Forgione
Illustrations Manager: Kari Wszolek
Marketing Manager: Jason Oberacker

Printed in Canada

Last digit is the print number: 9 8 7 6 5 4 3 2 1

About the Authors

DAVID L. FELTEN, MD, PhD is Vice President for Research and Medical Director of the Research Institute at William Beaumont Hospitals in Royal Oak, Michigan. He also is the Associate Dean for Research at Oakland University William Beaumont School of Medicine, a newly created allopathic medical school in Oakland County, Michigan. He previously served as Dean of the School of Graduate Medical Education at Seton Hall University in South Orange, NJ; the Founding Executive Director of the Susan Samueli Center for Integrative Medicine; and Professor of Anatomy and Neurobiology at the University of California, Irvine, School of Medicine; the Founding Director of the Center for Neuroimmunology at Loma Linda University School of Medicine in Loma Linda, CA and the Kilian J. and Caroline F. Schmitt Professor and Chair of the Department of Neurobiology & Anatomy; and Director of the Markey Charitable Trust Institute for Neurobiology of Neurodegenerative Diseases and Aging, at the University of Rochester School of Medicine in Rochester, NY. He received a BS from MIT and an MD and PhD from the University of Pennsylvania. Dr. Felten carried out pioneering studies of autonomic innervation of lymphoid organs and neural-immune signaling that underlies the mechanistic foundations for psychoneuroimmunology and many aspects of integrative medicine.

Dr. Felten is the recipient of numerous honors and awards, including the prestigious John D. and Catherine T. MacArthur Foundation Prize Fellowship, two simultaneous NIH MERIT Awards from the National Institutes of Mental Health and the National Institute on Aging, an Alfred P. Sloan Foundation Fellowship, an Andrew W. Mellon Foundation Fellowship, a Robert Wood Johnson Dean's Senior Teaching Scholar Award, the Norman Cousins Award in Mind-Body Medicine, the Building Bridges of Integration Award from the Traditional Chinese Medicine World Foundation, and numerous teaching awards.

Dr. Felten co-authored the definitive scholarly text in the field of neural-immune interactions, *Psychoneuroimmunology* (Academic Press, 3rd edition, 2001), and was the founding co-editor of the major journal in the field, *Brain, Behavior and Immunity*, with Drs. Robert Ader and Nicholas Cohen of the University of Rochester. Dr. Felten is the author of over 210 peer-reviewed journal articles and reviews, many on links between the nervous system and immune system. His work has been featured on Bill Moyer's PBS series and book, *Healing and the Mind*, on "20/20," BBC's "Worried Sick," and many other programs on U.S., Canadian, Australian, and German National Public Television. He served for over a decade on the National Board of Medical Examiners, including Chair of the Neurosciences Committee for the U.S. Medical Licensure Examination.

Dr. Felten also has an active role in business activities related to medical science. He currently serves as Chairman of the Scientific and Medical Advisory Boards of The Medingen Group and Clerisy Corp. He enjoys fostering clinical translational research and clinical trials that advance the quality and standard of care for challenging clinical diseases, and enjoys bringing new scientific innovations into the practical realm of product development and commercialization.

ANIL N. SHETTY, PhD, is chief of MR Physics in the Department of Radiology at William Beaumont Hospitals in Royal Oak, Michigan. He also is an Adjunct Assistant Professor of Radiology at Wayne State University School of Medicine. Prior to joining William Beaumont Hospitals, Dr. Shetty worked as a scientist in the research and development division of Siemens Medical Solutions. He received his MA and PhD from Kent State University, Kent, Ohio. Subsequently, he received an NIH Fellowship to continue postdoctoral work in magnetic resonance imaging in the Department of Radiology of University of Pennsylvania, Philadelphia, PA. He also held an Assistant Professor of Physics position at Hunter College of City University of New York.

Dr. Shetty has been very active in the field of MRI, with over 50 peer-reviewed publications and 3 patents. He has authored and co-authored chapters in several books. He is the vice president of a start-up company, magneticmoments, LLC, that is developing and marketing one of the intellectual properties for which he holds the key patent. Currently, he spends time in clinical research in cardiovascular and neurovascular areas and teaches residents and fellows at William Beaumont about magnetic resonance imaging.

In memory of Walle J.H. Nauta, MD, PhD, Institute Professor of Neuroscience at the Massachusetts Institute of Technology in Cambridge, MA.

> *A distinguished, brilliant, and pioneering neuroscientist*
> *An outstanding and inspirational teacher*
> *A kind, supportive, insightful, and gracious mentor*
> *An incredible role model and human being*

and

To my wife, Mary (Maida) Felten, PhD

> *A wonderful wife, partner, and friend*
> *My inspiration and motivation*
> *A superb researcher, teacher, scientific innovator, and CEO*
> *A woman who has it all—brains, beauty, kindness, and accomplishment.*

David L. Felten

In memory of Jalil Farah, MD, Chairman of the Department of Radiology (1962–1996), William Beaumont Hospital, Royal Oak, MI.

An outstanding and inspirational teacher and a visionary who had the prudence to start an imaging center dedicated to basic MRI research and development, in addition to routine clinical support. His kind support and encouragement have been a tremendous source of inspiration to me.

and

To Renu, a wonderful wife and a great partner, whose silent sacrifice of nights and weekends allowed me to achieve our goal.

To my children, Nikhil, Rohan, and Tushar: I hope your lives will be enriched by realizing your dreams, as mine has been.

Anil N. Shetty, Ph.D.

Acknowledgments

For decades, Dr. Frank Netter's beautiful and informative artwork has provided the visual basis for understanding anatomy, physiology, and relationships of great importance in medicine. Generations of physicians and health care professionals have "learned from the master" and have carried Dr. Netter's legacy forward through their own knowledge and contributions to patient care. There is no way to compare Dr. Netter's artwork to anything else, because it stands in a class of its own. For many decades, the Netter Collection volume on the Nervous System has been a flagship for the medical profession and for students of neuroscience. It was a great honor to provide the framework, organization, and new information for the updated first edition of *Netter's Atlas of Human Neuroscience* and now, the second edition of *Netter's Atlas of Neuroscience*. The opportunity to make a lasting contribution to the next generations of physicians and health care professionals is perhaps the greatest honor anyone could receive.

I also gratefully acknowledge Walle J.H. Nauta, MD, PhD, whose inspirational teaching of the nervous system at MIT contributed to the organizational framework for this Atlas. Professor Nauta always emphasized the value of an overview; the plates in the beginning of Section II, Regional Neurosciences, on the conceptual organization of sensory, motor, and autonomic systems especially reflect his approach. I am particularly honored to contribute to the updated *Netter Atlas of Neuroscience* because I first learned neurosciences as an undergraduate in Professor Nauta's laboratory at MIT through his personal mentorship, masterful insights, and explanations—using the first Nervous System "green book" volume by Dr. Frank Netter. It is my hope that continuing generations of students can benefit from the legacy of this wonderful teacher and great scientist.

I thank the outstanding artists, Jim Perkins, MS, MFA,. and John Craig, MD, for their clear and beautiful contributions to the first edition of this revised Atlas, now continuing in the second edition. Special thanks go to the outstanding editors at Elsevier: Marybeth Thiel, Senior Developmental Editor, and Elyse O'Grady, Editor, Netter Products. They helped to guide the process of the second edition and gave us the latitude to introduce new components, such as the imaging plates and the clinical correlations. I also would like to acknowledge my friend, colleague, and co-author on this atlas, Dr. Anil Shetty. We spent many delightful hours of conversation and viewing of spectacular 3D images and video sequences of images at Beaumont's Imaging Center. His contributions to this atlas and to the excellence of imaging at Beaumont for our many thousands of patients are deeply appreciated.

And finally, to my wife, Mary—I again thank you for your unwavering support and encouragement to continue this challenging project, and for your patience with the long hours and the clutter of papers and folders you tolerated along the way. Just when you thought the task was completed with the first edition, I launched into the Netter Neurosciences Flash Cards, and now the second edition of this atlas. Your love and support are deeply appreciated.

David L. Felten

First, I offer thanks to David Felten, MD, PhD, for suggesting that I collaborate with him on this project. Second, I have deepest gratitude for the support I received from my esteemed colleagues and predecessors in the Department of Radiology. In particular, I would like to thank Kenneth Matasar, MD, chairman, for being very supportive in my research efforts, and chief of Neuroradiology, Ay-Ming Wang, MD, for supporting me with many explanations of anatomic structures as seen in MRI. I am indebted to Kostaki Bis, MD, for many years of steady collaboration in many research projects; and Ali Shirkhoda, MD, for supporting and encouraging me in many areas of imaging. Finally, I am grateful to my wife, Renu, for her unconditional love, support, and understanding in putting up with my nights and weekends spent working for most of my professional life.

Anil N. Shetty

PREFACE

As in the first edition, *Netter's Atlas of Neuroscience, 2nd Edition,* combines the richness and beauty of Dr. Frank Netter's illustrations with key information about the many regions and systems of the brain, spinal cord, and periphery.

The first edition included cross-sectional illustrations through the spinal cord and brain stem, as well as coronal and axial (horizontal) sections. The second edition builds on the first edition, with several additional illustrations and extensive new imaging utilizing computed tomography (CT), magnetic resonance imaging (MRI), both T1- and T2-weighted, position emission tomography (PET) scanning, functional MRI (fMRI), and diffusion tensor imaging (DTI), which provides pseudocolor images of central axonal commissural, association, and projection pathways. Full-plate MRIs have been included for direct side-by-side comparisons with Dr. John Craig's illustrations of the brain stem cross sections, axial (horizontal) sections, and coronal sections.

More than 200 "clinical boxes" have been added to offer succinct clinical discussions of the functional importance of key topics. These clinical discussions are intended to assist the reader in bridging the anatomy and physiology depicted in each relevant plate to important related clinical issues.

The second edition retains the organization of the first edition (I: Overview; II: regional Neuroscience; III: Systemic Neuroscience), but further breaks these three sections into component chapters for ease of use. Consistent with the first edition, we have provided succinct figure legends to point out some of the major functional aspects of each illustration, particularly as they relate to problems that a clinician may encounter in the assessment of a patient with neurological symptoms. We believe that it is important for an atlas of the depth and clarity of *Netter's Atlas of Neuroscience, 2nd Edition* to let the illustrations provide the focal point for learning, not long and detailed written explanations that constitute a full textbook in itself. However, the figure legends, combined with the excellent illustrations and the additional clinical discussions, provide content for a thorough understanding of the basic components, organization, and functional aspects of the region or system under consideration.

Netter's Atlas of Neuroscience, 2nd Edition provides a comprehensive view of the entire nervous system, including the peripheral nerves and their target tissues, the central nervous system, the ventricular system, the meninges, the cerebral vascular system, developmental neuroscience, and neuroendocrine regulation. We have provided substantial but not exhaustive details and labels so that the reader can understand the basics of human neuroscience, including the neural information usually presented in neuroscience courses, the nervous system components of anatomy courses, and neural components of physiology courses in medical schools.

We are confronted with an era of rapid change in health care and exploding knowledge in all fields of medicine, particularly with the revolution in molecular biology. Medical schools are under enormous pressure to add many new areas of instruction to the undergraduate medical curriculum, including cultural and social aspects, business and economic aspects, robotics, simulation science, nanotechnology, molecular biology (genomics, proteomics, and other new "-omics"), patient-centered medicine, team building and treatment approaches, preventive medicine and wellness, complementary and alternative medicine, and a seemingly endless array of important concepts and ideas that an ideal physician would benefit from knowing. Furthermore, many curricula are under pressure to "decompress" the intensity of teaching, and to incorporate far more problem-based and small-group teaching exercises as a replacement for lectures—to hasten the students into clinical experiences.

In the long run, much of the additional information crammed into the medical curriculum has come at the expense of the basic sciences, particularly anatomy, physiology, histology, and embryology. Yet we believe that there is a fundamental core of knowledge that every physician must know. It is not sufficient for a medical student to learn only 3 of the 12 cranial nerves, their functional importance, and their clinical application as "representative examples" in order to further reduce the length of basic science courses. Although medical students are always anxious to get into clinics and see patients, they need a substantial fund of knowledge to be even marginally competent, particularly if they strive to apply evidence-based practice, instead of rote memory, to patient care. As an additional challenge, many neuroscience courses in medical schools around the country have a cavalcade of researcher specialists and superstars, usually not MDs, presenting lectures that constitute "what I do in research" instead of a consistent, cohesive, and comprehensive body of factual and conceptual information that provides an integrative, patient-centered understanding of the nervous system.

Netter's Atlas of Neuroscience, 2nd Edition provides the fundamental core of knowledge for the neurosciences in a three-part form: overview, regional neuroscience, and systemic neuroscience. This format aims to give the reader an integrated view in a consistent and organized fashion, with additional imaging, clinical discussions, and helpful figure legends.

ORGANIZATION OF NETTER'S ATLAS OF NEUROSCIENCE

In order to provide an optimal learning experience for the student of neuroscience, we have organized this Atlas into three sections: (1) An Overview of the Nervous System; (2) Regional Neuroscience; and (3) Systemic Neuroscience. The Overview is a presentation of the basic components and organization of the nervous system, a "view from 30,000 feet" that is an essential foundation for understanding the details of regional and systemic neurosciences. The Overview includes chapters on neurons and their properties, an introduction to the forebrain, brain stem and cerebellum, spinal cord, meninges, ventricular system, cerebral vasculature, and developmental neuroscience.

The Regional Neuroscience section provides the structural components of the peripheral nervous system; the spinal cord; the brain stem and cerebellum; and the forebrain (diencephalon and telencephalon). We begin in the periphery and move from caudal to rostral with the peripheral nervous system, spinal cord, brain stem and cerebellum, diencephalon, and telencephalon. This detailed regional understanding is necessary to diagnose and understand the consequences of a host of lesions whose localization depends on regional knowledge, such as strokes, local effects of tumors, injuries, specific demyelinating lesions, inflammatory reactions, and many other localized problems. In this section, many of the clinical correlations assist the reader in integrating a knowledge of the vascular supply with the consequences of

infarcts (e.g., brain stem syndromes), which requires a detailed understanding of brain stem anatomy and relationships.

The Systemic Neurosciences section evaluates the sensory systems, motor systems (including cerebellum and basal ganglia, acknowledging that they also are involved in many other spheres of activity besides motor), autonomic-hypothalamic-limbic systems (including neuroendocrine), and higher cortical functions. Within this section, we have organized each sensory system, when appropriate, with a sequential presentation of reflex channels, cerebellar channels, and lemniscal channels, reflecting Professor Nauta's conceptual organization of sensory systems. For the motor systems, we begin with lower motor neurons and then show the various systems of upper motor neurons, followed by the cerebellum and basal ganglia, whose major motor influences are ultimately exerted through regulation of upper motor neuronal systems. For the autonomic-hypothalamic-limbic system, we begin with the autonomic preganglionic and postganglionic organization and then show brain stem and hypothalamic regulation of autonomic outflow, and finally limbic and cortical regulation of the hypothalamus and autonomic outflow. The systemic neurosciences constitute the basis for carrying out and interpreting the neurological examination. We believe that it is necessary for a student of neuroscience to understand both regional organization and systemic organization. Without this dual understanding, clinical evaluation of a patient with a neurological problem would be incomplete.

We have provided extensive imaging plates in this second edition to help the reader visualize the central nervous system in a clinical setting. We selected imaging illustrations that reflect the type of information that a practicing clinician would evaluate in order to make decisions related to a patient with a neurological problem. But we do not believe that obtaining imaging studies should be the initial diagnosing and localizing approach taken by the clinician. The heart and soul of neurological diagnosis remains the neurological history and physical examination, based on a thorough understanding of regional and systemic neuroscience. By the time an imaging study is ordered, the physician should have a very good idea of what to look for.

We have organized the Atlas in this manner for several reasons. We want the reader to appreciate the value of looking at some of these complex neural structures and systems in two or three different contexts, or from two or three different points of view—sometimes as part of an overview, sometimes with a regional emphasis, and sometimes with a view toward understanding the functioning of a specific system spanning the neuraxis. Thoughtful repetition from novel perspectives is a useful tool in acquiring a comfortable working knowledge of the nervous system, which will serve the clinician well in the evaluation and treatment of patients with neurological problems, and will provide the neuroscience researcher and educator with a broader and more comprehensive understanding of the nervous system. With some subject matter, such as that on upper and lower motor neurons and their control, detailed factual information must be understood and mastered as a first step toward understanding clinical aspects of motor disorders. Following such understanding, the clinical aspects fall nicely into place. A "walk on" clinical correlation or a single "clinical correlation atlas plate" simply will not do. We have observed that many courses—in a rush to pare down the basic sciences to a skeletal framework, where "core information" is presented only once (or not at all), often without any functional context—encourage rote memorization rather than true understanding.

In a discipline as complex as the neurosciences, the acquisition of a solid organization and understanding of the major regions and hierarchies of the nervous system is not just a "nice idea" or a luxury—it is essential. The fact that this approach has been stunningly successful for our students (in a course organized and taught for 15 years by both authors of the first edition at the University of Rochester School of Medicine) is an added benefit, but is not why we organized this Atlas—and the University of Rochester Medical Neuroscience course we co-directed—as we

have. A working competence for students in basic and clinical neuroscience, and its value for outstanding patient care, are always the main focus of our efforts. We truly value success in this arena. Knowledgeable and highly competent students are the finest outcome of our teaching that we could ever achieve. We hope that our students will come to appreciate both the beauty and the complexity of the nervous system, and be inspired to contribute to the knowledge and functional application to patients of this greatest biological frontier, which constitutes the substrate for human behavior and our loftiest human endeavors.

David L. Felten, MD, PhD
Anil N. Shetty, PhD

About the Artists

FRANK H. NETTER, MD was born in 1906 in New York City. He studied art at the Art Students League and the National Academy of Design before entering medical school at New York University, where he received his MD degree in 1931. During his student years, Dr. Netter's notebook sketches attracted the attention of the medical faculty and other physicians, allowing him to augment his income by illustrating articles and textbooks. He continued illustrating as a sideline after establishing a surgical practice in 1933, but he ultimately opted to give up his practice in favor of a full-time commitment to art. After service in the United States Army during World War II, Dr. Netter began his long collaboration with the CIBA Pharmaceutical Company (now Novartis Pharmaceuticals). This 45-year partnership resulted in the production of the extraordinary collection of medical art so familiar to physicians and other medical professionals worldwide.

In 2005, Elsevier, Inc. purchased the Netter Collection and all publications from Icon Learning Systems. There are now over 50 publications featuring the art of Dr. Netter available through Elsevier, Inc. (in the United States: www.us.elsevierhealth.com/Netter and outside the US: www.elsevierhealth.com)

Dr. Netter's works are among the finest examples of the use of illustration in the teaching of medical concepts. The 13-book *Netter Collection of Medical Illustrations*, which includes the greater part of the more than 20,000 paintings created by Dr. Netter, became and remains one of the most famous medical works ever published. *The Netter Atlas of Human Anatomy*, first published in 1989, presents the anatomical paintings from the Netter Collection. Now translated into 16 languages, it is the anatomy atlas of choice among medical and health professions students the world over.

The Netter illustrations are appreciated not only for their aesthetic qualities, but, more important, for their intellectual content. As Dr. Netter wrote in 1949, ". . . clarification of a subject is the aim and goal of illustration. No matter how beautifully painted, how delicately and subtly rendered a subject may be, it is of little value as a *medical illustration* if it does not serve to make clear some medical point." Dr. Netter's planning, conception, point of view, and approach are what inform his paintings and what makes them so intellectually valuable.

Frank H. Netter, MD, physician and artist, died in 1991.

Learn more about the physician-artist whose work has inspired the Netter Reference collection: http://www.netterimages.com/artist/netter.htm

CARLOS MACHADO, MD was chosen by Novartis to be Dr. Netter's successor. He continues to be the main artist who contributes to the Netter collection of medical illustrations.

Self-taught in medical illustration, cardiologist Carlos Machado has contributed meticulous updates to some of Dr. Netter's original plates and has created many paintings of his own in the style of Netter as an extension of the Netter collection. Dr. Machado's photorealistic expertise and his keen insight into the physician/patient relationship informs his vivid and unforgettable visual style. His dedication to researching each topic and subject he paints places him among the premier medical illustrators at work today.

Learn more about his background and see more of his art at: http://www.netterimages. com/artist/machado.htm

CONTENTS

Section III: **SYSTEMIC NEUROSCIENCE**

Section I: **OVERVIEW OF THE NERVOUS SYSTEM**

1

NEURONS AND THEIR PROPERTIES

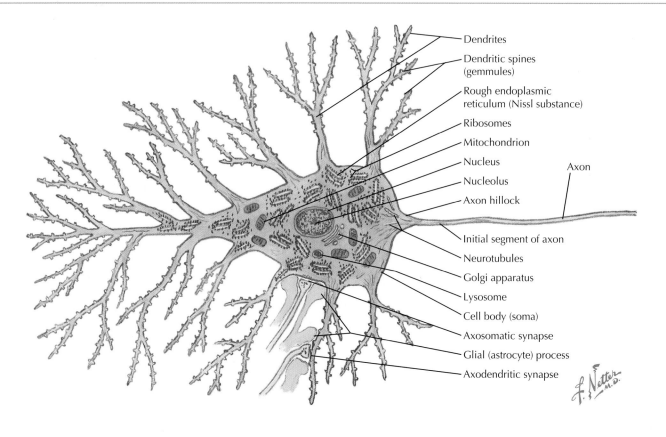

Dendrites
Dendritic spines (gemmules)
Rough endoplasmic reticulum (Nissl substance)
Ribosomes
Mitochondrion
Nucleus
Nucleolus
Axon hillock
Axon
Initial segment of axon
Neurotubules
Golgi apparatus
Lysosome
Cell body (soma)
Axosomatic synapse
Glial (astrocyte) process
Axodendritic synapse

ANATOMICAL PROPERTIES

1.1 NEURONAL STRUCTURE

Neuronal structure reflects the functional characteristics of the individual neuron. Incoming information is projected to a neuron mainly through axonal terminations on the cell body and dendrites. These synapses are isolated and are protected by astrocytic processes. The dendrites usually make up the greatest surface area of the neuron. Some protrusions from dendritic branches (dendritic spines) are sites of specific axodendritic synapses. Each specific neuronal type has a characteristic dendritic branching pattern called the dendritic tree, or dendritic arborizations. The neuronal cell body varies from a few micrometers (μm) in diameter to more than 100 μm. The neuronal cytoplasm contains extensive rough endoplasmic reticulum (rough ER), reflecting the massive amount of protein synthesis necessary to maintain the neuron and its processes. The Golgi apparatus is involved in packaging potential signal molecules for transport and release. Large numbers of mitochondria are necessary to meet the huge energy demands of neurons, particularly those related to the maintenance of ion pumps and membrane potentials. Each neuron has a single (or occasionally no) axon. The cell body tapers to the axon at the axon hillock, followed by the initial segment of the axon, which contains the Na^+ channels, the first site where action potentials are initiated. The axon extends for a variable distance from the cell body (up to 1 m or more). An axon larger than 1 to 2 μm in diameter is insulated by a sheath of myelin provided by oligodendroglia in the central nervous system (CNS) or Schwann cells in the peripheral nervous system (PNS). An axon may branch into more than 500,000 axon terminals, and may terminate in a highly localized and circumscribed zone

(e.g., primary somatosensory axon projections used for fine discriminative touch) or may branch to many disparate regions of the brain (e.g., noradrenergic axonal projections of the locus coeruleus). A neuron whose axon terminates at a distance from its cell body and dendritic tree is called a macroneuron or a Golgi type I neuron; a neuron whose axon terminates locally, close to its cell body and dendritic tree, is called a microneuron, a Golgi type II neuron, a local circuit neuron, or an interneuron. There is no typical neuron because each type of neuron has its own specialization. However, pyramidal cells and lower motor neurons are commonly used to portray a so-called typical neuron.

CLINICAL POINT

Neurons require extraordinary metabolic resources to sustain their functional integrity, particularly that related to the maintenance of membrane potentials for the initiation and propagation of action potentials. Neurons require aerobic metabolism for the generation of adenosine triphosphate (ATP) and have virtually no ATP reserve, so they require continuous delivery of glucose and oxygen, generally in the range of 15% to 20% of the body's resources, which is a disproportionate consumption of resources. During starvation, when glucose availability is limited, the brain can shift gradually to using beta-hydroxybutyrate and acetoacetate as energy sources for neuronal metabolism; however, this is not an instant process and is not available to buffer acute hypoglycemic episodes. An ischemic episode of even 5 minutes, resulting from a heart attack or an ischemic stroke, can lead to permanent damage in some neuronal populations such as pyramidal cells in the CA1 region of the hippocampus. In cases of longer ischemia, widespread neuronal death can occur. Because neurons are postmitotic cells, except for a small subset of interneurons, dead neurons are not replaced. One additional consequence of the postmitotic state of most neurons is that they are not sources of tumor formation. Brain tumors derive mainly from glial cells, ependymal cells, and meningeal cells.

A. Simple axodendritic or axosomatic synapse

Axon

Glial process

Dendrite or cell body

B. Dendritic spine synapse

Axon

Dendrite

Dendritic spine (gemmule)

C. Dendritic crest synapse

Axon

D. Simple synapse plus axoaxonic synapse

E. Combined axoaxonic and axodendritic synapse

F. Varicosities ("boutons en passant")

I. Serial synapse

G. Dendrodendritic synapse

Dendrite

Dendrodendritic synapse

H. Reciprocal synapse

K. Inner plexiform layer of retina

Ganglion cell

Bipolar cell axon

Müller cell (supporting)

Amacrine cell processes

J. Cerebellar glomerulus

Granule cell dendrites

Glial capsule

Golgi cell axon

Golgi cell dendrite

Mossy cell axon

1.2 **TYPES OF SYNAPSES**

A synapse is a site where an arriving action potential, through excitation-secretion coupling involving Ca^{2+} influx, triggers the release of one or more neurotransmitters into the synaptic cleft (typically 20 μm across). The neurotransmitter acts on receptors on the target neuronal membrane, altering the membrane potential from its resting state. These postsynaptic potentials are called graded potentials. Most synapses carrying information toward a target neuron terminate as axodendritic or axosomatic synapses. Specialized synapses, such as reciprocal synapses or complex arrays of synaptic interactions, provide specific regulatory control over the excitability of their target neurons. Dendrodendritic synapses aid in the coordinated firing of groups of related neurons such as the phrenic nucleus neurons that cause contraction of the diaphragm.

CLINICAL POINT

The configurations of the synapses of key neuronal populations in particular regions of the brain and of target cells in the periphery determine the relative influence of that input. At the neuromuscular junction, a sufficient amount of acetylcholine is usually released by an action potential in the motor axon to guarantee that the muscle end plate potential reaches threshold and initiates an action potential. In contrast, the neuronal inputs into reticular formation neurons and many other types of neurons require either temporal or spatial summation to allow the target neuron to reach threshold; this orchestration involves coordinated multisynaptic regulation. In some key neurons such as lower motor neurons (LMNs), input from brain stem upper motor neurons (UMNs) is directed mainly through spinal cord interneurons and requires extensive summation to activate the LMNs; in contrast, direct monosynaptic corticospinal UMNs input into some LMNs, such as those regulating fine finger movements, terminate close to the axon hillock/initial segment; and can directly initiate an action potential in the LMNs. Some complex arrays of synapses among several neuronal elements, such as those seen in structures such as the cerebellum and retina, permit modulation of key neurons by both serial and parallel arrays of connections, providing lateral modulation of neighboring neuronal excitability.

Multipolar (pyramidal) cell of cerebral motor cortex

Associational, commissural, and thalamic endings

Astrocyte

Striated (somatic) muscle

Motor end plate

Multipolar somatic motor cell of nuclei of cranial nerves III, IV, V, VI, VII, IX, X, XI, or XII

Multipolar cell of lower brain motor centers

Oligodendrocyte

Corticospinal (pyramidal) fiber

Axodendritic ending

Axosomatic ending

Axoaxonic ending

Multipolar somatic motor cell of anterior horn of spinal cord

Nissl substance

Astrocyte

Collateral

Renshaw interneuron (feedback)

Myelinated somatic motor fiber of spinal nerve

Myelin sheath

Motor end plate with Schwann cell cap

Striated (voluntary) muscle

Interneurons

Blood vessel

Interneuron

Astrocyte

Multipolar visceral motor (autonomic) cell of spinal cord

Autonomic preganglionic (sympathetic or para-sympathetic) nerve fiber

Myelin sheath

Autonomic postganglionic neuron of sympathetic or parasympathetic ganglion

Satellite cells

Unmyelinated nerve fiber

Schwann cells

Endings on cardiac muscle or nodal cells

Beaded varicosities and endings on smooth muscle and gland cells

Bipolar cell of cranial nerve VIII

Unipolar cell of sensory ganglia of cranial nerves V, VII, IX, or X

Satellite cells

Schwann cell

Myelinated fibers

Free nerve endings (unmyelinated fibers)

Encapsulated ending

Specialized ending

Muscle spindle

Unipolar sensory cell of dorsal spinal root ganglion

Satellite cells

Myelinated afferent fiber of spinal nerve

Myelin sheath

Myelin sheath

Schwann cells

Unmyelinated fibers

Free nerve endings

Encapsulated ending

Muscle spindle

Red:	Motor neurons, preganglionic autonomic neuron
Blue:	Sensory neuron
Purple:	CNS neurons
Gray:	Glial and neurilemmal cells and myelin

Note: Cerebellar cells not shown here

1.3 NEURONAL CELL TYPES

Local interneurons and projection neurons demonstrate characteristic size, dendritic arborizations, and axonal projections. In the CNS (denoted by dashed lines), glial cells (astrocytes, microglia, oligodendroglia) provide support, protection, and maintenance of neurons. Schwann cells and satellite cells provide these functions in the PNS. The primary sensory neurons (blue) provide sensory transduction of incoming energy or stimuli into electrical signals that are carried into the CNS. The neuronal outflow from the CNS is motor (red) to skeletal muscle fibers via neuromuscular junctions, or is autonomic preganglionic (red) to autonomic ganglia, whose neurons innervate cardiac muscle, smooth muscle, secretory glands, metabolic cells, or cells of the immune system. Neurons other than primary sensory neurons, LMNs, and preganglionic autonomic neurons are located in the CNS in the brain (enclosed by upper dashed lines) or spinal cord (enclosed by lower dashed lines).

CLINICAL POINT

Neuronal form and configuration provide evidence of the role of that particular type of neuron. Dorsal root ganglion cells have virtually no synapses on the cell body; the sensory receptor is contiguous with the initial segment of the axon to permit direct activation of the initial segment upon reaching a threshold stimulus. This arrangement provides virtually no opportunity for centrifugal control of the initial sensory input; rather, control and analysis of the sensory input occurs in the CNS. Purkinje neurons in the cerebellum have huge planar dendritic trees, with activation occurring via hundreds of parallel fibers and the background excitability influenced by climbing fiber control. This type of array allows network modulation of Purkinje cell output to UMNs, a control mechanism that permits fine-grained, ongoing adjustments to smooth and coordinated motor activities. Small interneurons in many regions have local and specialized functions that have local circuit connections, whereas large isodendritic neurons of the reticular formation receive widespread, polymodal, nonlocal input, which is important for general arousal of the cerebral cortex and consciousness. Damage to these key neurons may result in coma. LMNs and preganglionic autonomic neurons receive tremendous convergence upon their dendrites and cell bodies to orchestrate the final pattern of activation of these final common pathway neurons through which the peripheral effector tissues are signaled and through which all behavior is achieved.

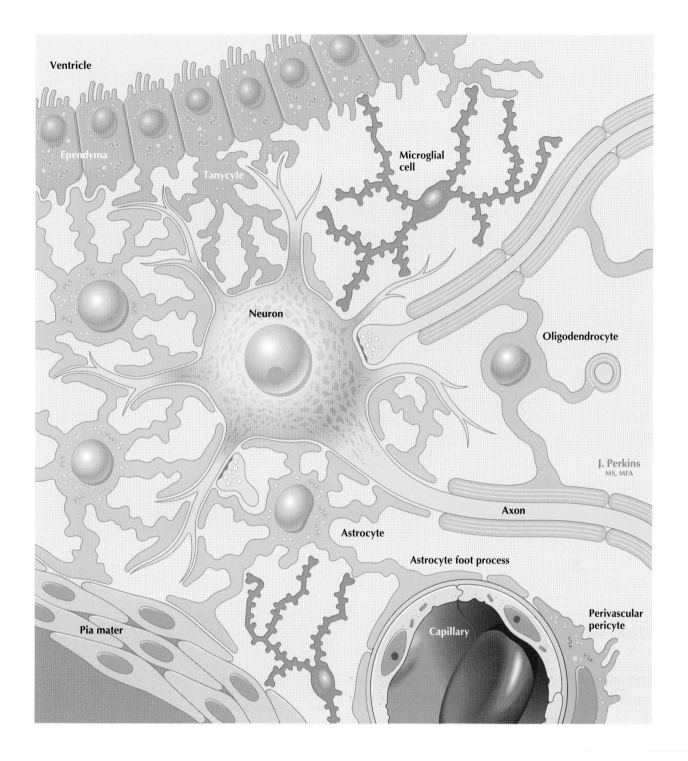

1.4 **GLIAL CELL TYPES**

Astrocytes provide structural isolation of neurons and their synapses and provide ionic (K^+) sequestration, trophic support, and support for growth and signaling functions to neurons. Oligodendroglia provide myelination of axons in the CNS. Microglia are scavenger cells that participate in phagocytosis, inflammatory responses, cytokine and growth factor secretion, and some immune reactivity in the CNS. Perivascular cells participate in similar activities at sites near the blood vessels. Schwann cells provide myelination, ensheathment, trophic support, and actions that contribute to the growth and repair of peripheral neurons. Activated T lymphocytes normally can enter and traverse the CNS for immune surveillance for a period of approximately 24 hours.

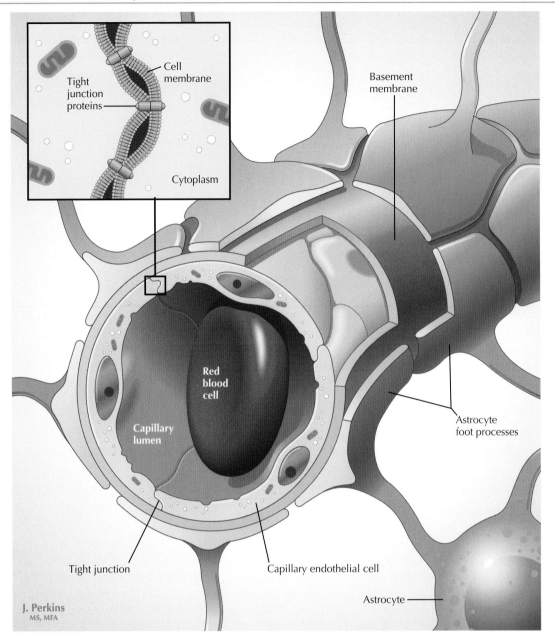

Tight junction proteins

Cell membrane

Cytoplasm

Basement membrane

Red blood cell

Capillary lumen

Astrocyte foot processes

Tight junction

Capillary endothelial cell

Astrocyte

J. Perkins
MS, MFA

1.5 THE BLOOD-BRAIN BARRIER

The blood-brain barrier (BBB) is the cellular interface between the blood and the CNS. It serves to protect the brain from unwanted intrusion by many large molecules and potentially toxic substances and to maintain the interstitial fluid environment to ensure optimal functioning of the neurons and their associated glial cells. The major cellular basis for the BBB consists of the capillary endothelial cells which have an elaborate network of tight junctions; these tight junctions restrict access by many large molecules, including many drugs, to the CNS. Endothelial cells in the CNS also exhibit a low level of pinocytotic activity across the cell, providing selected specific carrier systems for the transport of essential substrates of energy production and amino acid metabolism into the CNS. Astrocytic endfoot processes abut the endothelial cells and their basement membranes; these processes help to transfer important metabolites from the blood to neurons and can influence the expression of some specific gene products in the endothelial cells. These astrocytic processes also can remove excess K^+ and some neurotransmitters from the interstitial fluid.

CLINICAL POINT

The BBB, anatomically consisting mainly of the capillary tight junctions of the vascular endothelial cells, serves to protect the CNS from the intrusion of large molecules and potentially damaging agents from the peripheral circulation. The neurons need protection of their ionic and metabolic environment, which is aided by glial cells and the BBB. There are selected areas (windows on the brain) where the BBB is not present, such as the median eminence, the area postrema, the organum vasculosum of the lamina terminalis, and others, and where specialized cells can sample the peripheral circulation and can initiate corrective brain mechanisms to protect the neuronal environment. The presence of the BBB presents a challenge for pharmacotherapy aimed at the CNS; many antibiotics and other agents will not penetrate the BBB and must be coupled to a carrier molecule that does cross or must be injected intrathecally. In some pathological circumstances, such as the presence of a brain tumor, neuronal degeneration resulting from a neurodegenerative disease, the presence of a high concentration of a solute, or a stroke, the BBB is disrupted extensively, exposing the internal CNS milieu to molecules in the peripheral circulation. Therapeutic strategies now are being tested that will achieve transport of desired pharmacotherapeutic agents across the BBB and will protect the brain from unwanted disruption of the BBB in pathological circumstances.

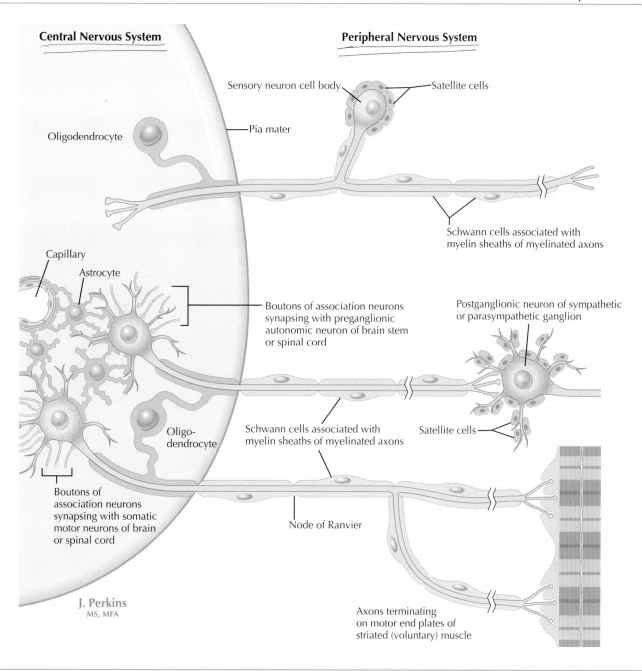

Central Nervous System

Peripheral Nervous System

Sensory neuron cell body

Satellite cells

Oligodendrocyte

Pia mater

Schwann cells associated with
myelin sheaths of myelinated axons

Capillary

Astrocyte

Boutons of association neurons
synapsing with preganglionic
autonomic neuron of brain stem
or spinal cord

Postganglionic neuron of sympathetic
or parasympathetic ganglion

Oligo-
dendrocyte

Schwann cells associated with
myelin sheaths of myelinated axons

Satellite cells

Boutons of
association neurons
synapsing with somatic
motor neurons of brain
or spinal cord

Node of Ranvier

J. Perkins
MS, MFA

Axons terminating
on motor end plates of
striated (voluntary) muscle

1.6 MYELINATION OF CNS AND PNS AXONS

Central myelination of axons is provided by oligodendroglia. Each oligodendroglial cell can myelinate a single segment of several separate central axons. In the PNS, sensory, motor, and preganglionic autonomic axons are myelinated by Schwann cells. A Schwann cell myelinates only a single segment of one axon. Unmyelinated sensory and autonomic postganglionic autonomic axons are ensheathed by a Schwann cell, which provides a single enwrapping arm of cytoplasm around each of several such axons. The space between adjacent myelin segments of an axon is called a node of Ranvier; this site of axon membrane contains sodium channels and allows the reinitiation of action potentials in the course of propagation down the axon, a process called saltatory conduction.

CLINICAL POINT

The integrity of the myelin sheath is essential for proper neuronal function in both the CNS and the PNS. Disruption of the myelin sheath around axons in either system results in the inability of the formerly myelinated axons to carry out their functional activities. In the CNS, the myelin sheath of central axons can be attacked in an autoimmune disease such as multiple sclerosis, resulting in a variety of symptoms, such as blindness, diplopia caused by discoordinated eye movements, loss of sensation, loss of coordination, paresis, and others. This condition may occur episodically, with intermittent remyelination occurring as the result of oligodendroglia proliferation and remyelination. In the PNS, a wide variety of insults, including exposure to toxins and the presence of diabetes or autoimmune Guillain-Barré syndrome, result in peripheral axonal demyelination, which is manifested mainly as sensory loss and paralysis or weakness. Remyelination also can occur around peripheral axons, initiated by the Schwann cells. Clinically, the status of axonal conduction is assessed by examining sensory evoked potentials in the CNS and by conduction velocity studies in the PNS.

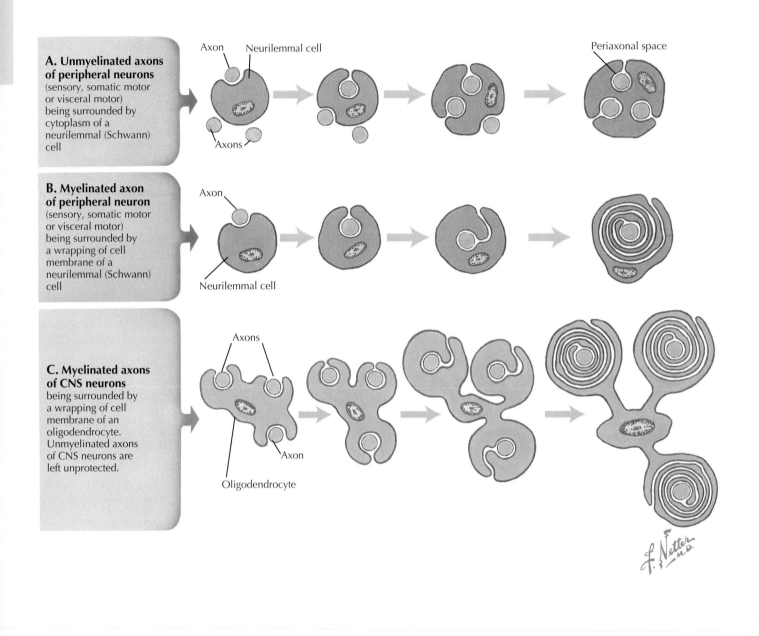

A. Unmyelinated axons of peripheral neurons (sensory, somatic motor or visceral motor) being surrounded by cytoplasm of a neurilemmal (Schwann) cell

Axon   Neurilemmal cell

Periaxonal space

Axons

B. Myelinated axon of peripheral neuron (sensory, somatic motor or visceral motor) being surrounded by a wrapping of cell membrane of a neurilemmal (Schwann) cell

Axon

Neurilemmal cell

C. Myelinated axons of CNS neurons being surrounded by a wrapping of cell membrane of an oligodendrocyte. Unmyelinated axons of CNS neurons are left unprotected.

Axons

Axon

Oligodendrocyte

1.7 DEVELOPMENT OF MYELINATION AND AXON ENSHEATHMENT

Myelination requires a cooperative interaction between the neuron and its myelinating support cell. Unmyelinated peripheral axons are invested with a single layer of Schwann cell cytoplasm. When a peripheral axon at least 1 to 2 μm in diameter triggers myelination, a Schwann cell wraps many layers of tightly packed cell membrane around a single segment of that axon. In the CNS, an oligodendroglia cell extends several arms of cytoplasm, which then wrap multiple layers of tightly packed membrane around a single segment of each of several axons. Although myelination is a process that occurs most intensely during development, Schwann cells may remyelinate peripheral axons following injury, and oligodendroglial cells may proliferate and remyelinate injured or demyelinated central axons in diseases such as multiple sclerosis.

Cell body of an oligodendrocyte (neurilemmal cells play similar role in peripheral nervous system)

Cell membrane of myelinated axon

Mitochondrion in cytoplasm of neuronal axon

Node of Ranvier

Minute masses of cytoplasm trapped between fused layers of cell membrane of oligodendrocyte

Fused layers of cell membrane of oligodendrocyte wrapped around axon of a myelinated neuron of central nervous system (the lipid of lipoprotein constituting fused cell membrane is myelin, which gives myelinated axon a white, glistening appearance)

1.8 HIGH-MAGNIFICATION VIEW OF A CENTRAL MYELIN SHEATH

Fused layers of oligodendroglial cell membrane wrap around a segment of a central axon, preventing ionic flow across the cell membrane for the entire myelinated segment. The node between two adjacent segments is bare axon membrane possessing Na^+ channels. These nodes are sites where action potentials are reinitiated in the conduction of propagated action potentials.

Chemical Neurotransmission

NEUROTRANSMISSION

1.9 CHEMICAL NEUROTRANSMISSION

AMINO ACID SYNAPSE

Amino acids used by a neuron as neurotransmitters are compartmentalized for release as neurotransmitters in synaptic vesicles. The amino acid glutamate (depicted in this diagram) is the most abundant excitatory neurotransmitter in the CNS. Following release from synaptic vesicles, some glutamate binds to postsynaptic receptors. Released glutamate is inactivated by uptake into both pre- and postsynaptic neurons, where the amino acid is incorporated into the Krebs cycle or reused for a variety of functions.

CATECHOLAMINE SYNAPSE

Catecholamines are synthesized from the dietary amino acid tyrosine, which is taken up competitively into the brain by a carrier system. Tyrosine is synthesized into L-dopa by tyrosine hydroxylase (TH), the rate-limiting synthetic enzyme. Additional conversion into dopamine takes place in the cytoplasm via aromatic L-amino acid decarboxylase (ALAAD). Dopamine is taken up into synaptic vesicles and stored for subsequent release. In noradrenergic nerve terminals, dopamine beta-hydroxylase (DBH) further hydroxylates dopamine into norepinephrine in the synaptic vesicles. In adrenergic nerve terminals, norepinephrine is methylated to epinephrine by phenolethanolamine N-methyl transferase. Following release, the catecholamine neurotransmitter binds to appropriate receptors (dopamine and alpha- and beta-adrenergic receptors) on the postsynaptic membrane, altering postsynaptic excitability, second-messenger activation, or both. Catecholamines also can act on presynaptic receptors, modulating the excitability of the presynaptic terminal and influencing subsequent neurotransmitter release. Catecholamines are inactivated by presynaptic reuptake (high-affinity uptake carrier) and, to a lesser extent, by metabolism (monoamine oxidase deamination and catechol-O-methyltransferase) and diffusion.

SEROTONIN SYNAPSE

Serotonin is synthesized from the dietary amino acid tryptophan, taken up competitively into the brain by a carrier system. Tryptophan is synthesized to 5-hydroxytryptophan (5-OH-tryptophan) by tryptophan hydroxylase (TrH), the rate-limiting synthetic enzyme. Conversion of 5-hydroxytryptophan to 5-hydroxytryptamine (5-HT, serotonin) takes place in the cytoplasm by means of ALAAD. Serotonin is stored in synaptic vesicles. Following release, serotonin can bind to receptors on the postsynaptic membrane, altering postsynaptic excitability, second messenger activation, or both. Serotonin also can act on presynaptic receptors (5-HT receptors), modulating the excitability of the presynaptic terminal and influencing subsequent neurotransmitter release. Serotonin is inactivated by presynaptic reuptake (high-affinity uptake carrier) and to a lesser extent by metabolism and diffusion.

PEPTIDE SYNAPSES

Neuropeptides are synthesized from prohormones, large peptides synthesized in the cell body from mRNA. The larger precursor peptide is cleaved posttranslationally to active neuropeptides, which are packaged in synaptic vesicles and transported anterogradely by the process of axoplasmic transport. These vesicles are stored in the nerve terminals until released by appropriate excitation-secretion coupling induced by an action potential. The neuropeptide binds to receptors on the postsynaptic membrane. In the CNS, there is often an anatomic mismatch between the localization of peptidergic nerve terminals and the localization of cells possessing membrane receptors responsive to that neuropeptide, suggesting that the amount of release and the extent of diffusion may be important factors in neuropeptide neurotransmission. Released neuropeptides are inactivated by peptidases.

ACETYLCHOLINE (CHOLINERGIC) SYNAPSE

Acetylcholine (ACh) is synthesized from dietary choline and acetyl coenzyme A (CoA), derived from the metabolism of glucose by the enzyme choline acetyltransferase (ChAT). ACh is stored in synaptic vesicles; following release, it binds to cholinergic receptors (nicotinic or muscarinic) on the postsynaptic membrane, influencing the excitability of the postsynaptic cell. Enzymatic hydrolysis (cleavage) by acetylcholine esterase rapidly inactivates ACh.

CLINICAL POINT

Synthesis of catecholamines in the brain is rate limited by the availability of the precursor amino acid tyrosine; synthesis of serotonin, an indoleamine, is rate limited by the availability of the precursor amino acid tryptophan. Tyrosine and tryptophan compete with other amino acids—phenylalanine, leucine, isoleucine, and valine—for uptake into the brain through a common carrier mechanism. When a good protein source is available in the diet, tyrosine is present in abundance, and robust catecholamine synthesis occurs; when a diet lacks sufficient protein, tryptophan is competitively abundant compared with tyrosine, and serotonin synthesis is favored. This is one mechanism by which the composition of the diet can influence the synthesis of serotonin as opposed to catecholamine and influence mood and affective behavior. During critical periods of development, if low availability of tyrosine occurs because of protein malnourishment, central noradrenergic axons cannot exert their trophic influence on cortical neuronal development such as the visual cortex; stunted dendritic development occurs, and the binocular responsiveness of key cortical neurons is prevented. Thus, nutritional content and balance are important to both proper brain development and ongoing affective behavior.

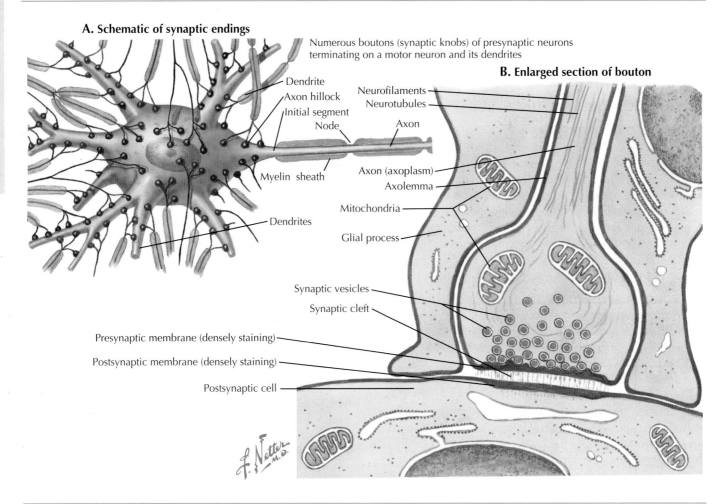

A. Schematic of synaptic endings

Numerous boutons (synaptic knobs) of presynaptic neurons terminating on a motor neuron and its dendrites

B. Enlarged section of bouton

Dendrite
Axon hillock
Initial segment
Node
Myelin sheath
Dendrites

Neurofilaments
Neurotubules
Axon
Axon (axoplasm)
Axolemma
Mitochondria
Glial process

Synaptic vesicles
Synaptic cleft
Presynaptic membrane (densely staining)
Postsynaptic membrane (densely staining)
Postsynaptic cell

1.10 SYNAPTIC MORPHOLOGY

Synapses are specialized sites where neurons communicate with each other and with effector or target cells. (A) A typical neuron that receives numerous synaptic contacts on its cell body and associated dendrites. The contacts are derived from both myelinated and unmyelinated axons. Incoming myelinated axons lose their myelin sheaths, exhibit extensive branching, and terminate as synaptic boutons (terminals) on the target (in this example, motor) neuron. (B) An enlargement of an axosomatic terminal. Chemical neurotransmitters are packaged in synaptic vesicles. When an action potential invades the terminal region, depolarization triggers Ca^{2+} influx into the terminal, causing numerous synaptic vesicles to fuse with the presynaptic membrane, releasing their packets of neurotransmitter into the synaptic cleft. The neurotransmitter can bind to receptors on the postsynaptic membrane, resulting in graded excitatory or inhibitory postsynaptic potentials or in neuromodulatory effects on intracellular signaling systems in the target cell. There is sometimes a mismatch between the site of release of a neurotransmitter and the location of target neurons possessing receptors for the neurotransmitter (can be immediately adjacent or at a distance). Many nerve terminals can release multiple neurotransmitters; the process is regulated by gene activation and by the frequency and duration of axonal activity. Some nerve terminals possess presynaptic receptors for their released neurotransmitters. Activation of these presynaptic receptors regulates neurotransmitter release. Some nerve terminals also possess high-affinity uptake carriers for transport of the neurotransmitters (e.g. dopamine, norepinephrine, serotonin) back into the nerve terminal for repackaging and reuse.

CLINICAL POINT

Synaptic endings, particularly axodendritic and axosomatic endings, terminate abundantly on some neuronal cell types such as LMNs. The distribution of synapses, based on a hierarchy of descending pathways and interneurons, orchestrates the excitability of the target neuron. If one of the major sources of input is disrupted (such as the corticospinal tract in an internal capsule lesion, which may occur in an ischemic stroke) or if damage has occurred to the collective descending UMN pathways (as in a spinal cord injury), the remaining potential sources of input can sprout and occupy regional sites left bare because of the degeneration of the normal complement of synapses. As a result, primary sensory inputs from Ia afferents and other sensory influences, via interneurons, can take on a predominant influence over the excitability of the target motor neurons, leading to a hyperexcitable state. This may account in part for the hypertonic state and hyperreflexic responses to stimulation of primary muscle spindle afferents (muscle stretch reflex) and of flexor reflex afferents (nociceptive stimulation). Recent studies indicate that synaptic growth, plasticity, and remodeling can continue into adulthood and even into old age.

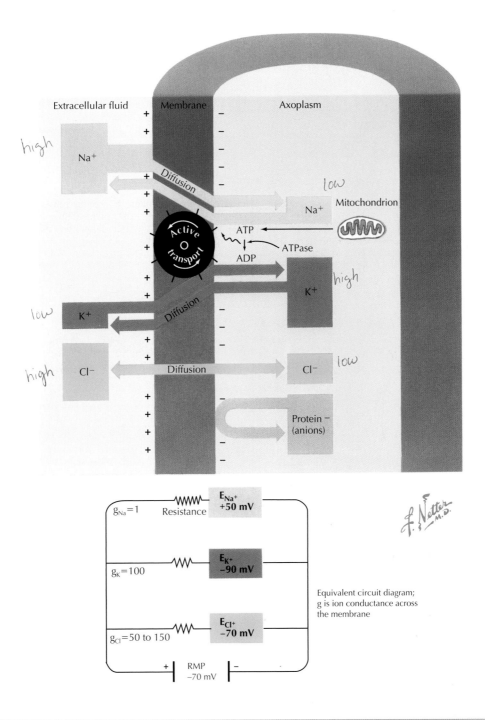

Extracellular fluid

Membrane

Axoplasm

high

Na$^+$

Diffusion

low

Na$^+$

Mitochondrion

ATP

ATPase

ADP

high

K$^+$

low

K$^+$

Diffusion

high

Cl$^-$

Diffusion

Cl$^-$

low

Protein $-$
(anions)

$g_{Na}=1$ Resistance

E_{Na^+}
+50 mV

$g_K=100$

E_{K^+}
−90 mV

$g_{Cl}=50$ to 150

E_{Cl^+}
−70 mV

RMP
−70 mV

Equivalent circuit diagram;
g is ion conductance across
the membrane

ELECTRICAL PROPERTIES

1.11 NEURONAL RESTING POTENTIAL

Cations (+) and anions (−) are distributed unevenly across the neuronal cell membrane because the membrane is differentially permeable to these ions. The uneven distribution depends on the forces of charge separation and diffusion. The permeability of the membrane to ions changes with depolarization (toward 0) or hyperpolarization (away from 0). The typical neuronal resting potential is approximately −90 mV with respect to the extracellular fluid. The extracellular concentrations of Na$^+$

and Cl$^-$ of 145 and 105 mEq/L, respectively, are high compared to the intracellular concentrations of 15 and 8 mEq/L. The extracellular concentration of K$^+$ of 3.5 mEq/L is low compared to the intracellular concentration of 130 mEq/L. The resting potential of neurons is close to the equilibrium potential for K$^+$ (as if the membrane were permeable only to K$^+$). Na$^+$ is actively pumped out of the cell in exchange for inward pumping of K$^+$ by the Na$^+$-K$^+$-ATPase membrane pump. Equivalent circuit diagrams for Na$^+$, K$^+$, and Cl$^-$, calculated using the Nernst equation, are illustrated in the lower diagram.

Chemical Synaptic Transmission

A. Ion movements

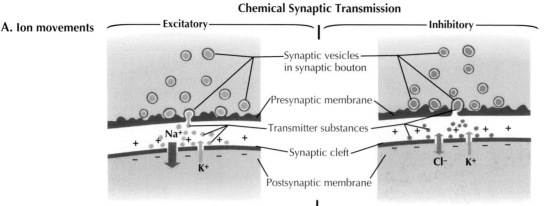

─── Excitatory ───   ─── Inhibitory ───

Synaptic vesicles in synaptic bouton

Presynaptic membrane

Transmitter substances

Synaptic cleft

Postsynaptic membrane

Na⁺   K⁺   Cl⁻   K⁺

When impulse reaches excitatory synaptic bouton, it causes release of a transmitter substance into synaptic cleft. This increases permeability of postsynaptic membrane to K⁺ and Na⁺. More Na⁺ moves into postsynaptic cell than K⁺ moves out, due to greater electrochemical gradient.

At inhibitory synapse, transmitter substance released by an impulse increases permeability of postsynaptic membrane to K⁺ and Cl⁻ but not Na⁺. K⁺ moves out of postsynaptic cell.

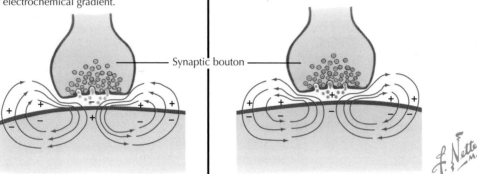

Synaptic bouton

Resultant net ionic current flow is in a direction that tends to depolarize postsynaptic cell. If depolarization reaches firing threshold at the axon hillock, an impulse is generated in postsynaptic cell.

Resultant ionic current flow is in a direction that tends to hyperpolarize postsynaptic cell. This makes depolarization by excitatory synapses more difficult—more depolarization is required to reach threshold.

B. EPSPs, IPSPs, and current flow

EPSP

IPSP

Current flow
Potential change

Current flow and potential change

1.12 GRADED POTENTIALS IN NEURONS

A. Ion movements. Excitatory and inhibitory neurotransmissions are processes by which released neurotransmitter, acting on postsynaptic membrane receptors, elicits a local or regional perturbation in the membrane potential: (1) toward 0 (depolarization, excitatory postsynaptic potential; EPSP) via an inward flow of Na⁺ caused by increased permeability of the membrane to positively charged ions; or (2) away from 0 (hyperpolarization, inhibitory postsynaptic potential; IPSP) via an inward flow of Cl⁻ and a compensatory outward flow of K⁺ caused by increased membrane permeability to Cl⁻. Following the action of neurotransmitters on the postsynaptic membrane, the resultant EPSPs and IPSPs exert local influences that dissipate over time and distance but contribute to the overall excitability and ion distribution in the neuron. It is unusual for a single excitatory input to generate sufficient EPSPs to bring about depolarization of the initial segment of the axon above threshold so that an action potential is fired. However, the influence of multiple EPSPs, integrated over space and time, may sum to collectively reach threshold. IPSPs reduce the ability of EPSPs to bring the postsynaptic membrane to threshold. **B.** EPSPs, IPSPs, and current flow. EPSP- and IPSP-induced changes in postsynaptic current (red) and potential (blue).

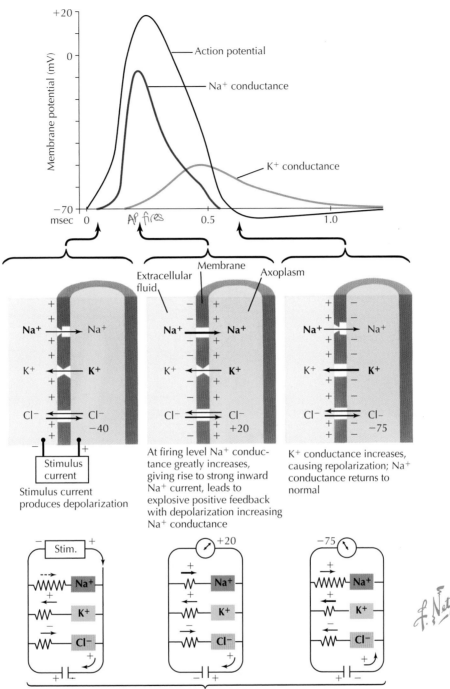

Equivalent circuit diagrams

Graded potentials (previous pg.) can lead to action potentials

1.13 ACTION POTENTIALS

Action potentials (APs) are all-or-nothing, nondecremental, electrical potentials that allow an electrical signal to travel for very long distances (a meter or more) and trigger neurotransmitter release through electrochemical coupling (excitation-secretion coupling). APs are usually initiated at the initial segment of axons when temporal and spatial summation of EPSPs cause sufficient excitation (depolarization) to open Na^+ channels, allowing the membrane to reach threshold. Threshold is the point at which Na^+ influx through these Na^+ channels cannot be countered by efflux of K^+. When threshold is reached, an action potential is fired. As the axon rapidly depolarizes during the rising phase of the AP, the membrane increases its K^+ conductance, which then allows influx of K^+ to counter the rapid depolarization and bring the membrane potential back toward its resting level. Once the action potential has been initiated, it rapidly propagates down the axon by reinitiating itself at each node of Ranvier (myelinated axon) or adjacent patch of membrane (unmyelinated axon) by locally bringing that next zone of axon membrane to threshold.

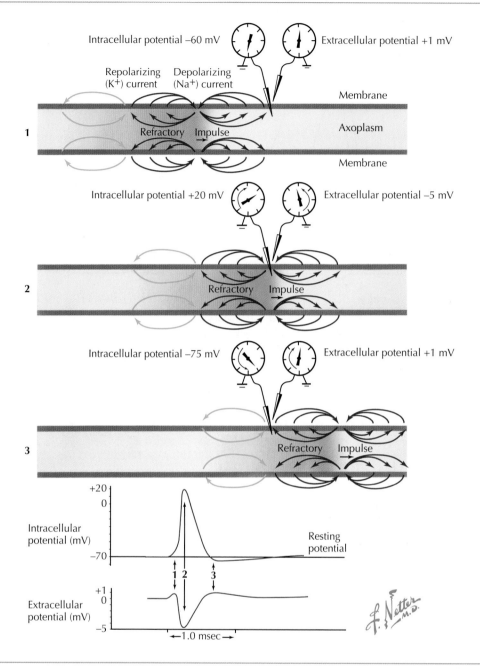

1.14 PROPAGATION OF THE ACTION POTENTIAL

When an AP is initiated at a specific site of the axonal membrane (usually the initial segment), the inward flow of Na⁺ alters the extracellular ion environment, causing a local flow of charge from adjacent regions of the axon. This induces a depolarized state in the adjacent node of Ranvier (myelinated axon) or patch of axonal membrane (unmyelinated axon), bringing that region to threshold and resulting in the reinitiation of the action potential. The presence of myelination along axonal segments results in the reinitiation of the action potential at the next node, thus hastening the velocity of conduction of the AP. The resultant appearance of the AP skipping from node to node down the axon is saltatory conduction.

CLINICAL POINT

An action potential is an explosive reversal of the neuronal membrane potential that takes place because of an increase in Na⁺ conductance induced by depolarization, usually due to the cumulative effects of graded potentials from incoming neurotransmitters; this explosive reversal is followed later by an increase in K⁺ conductance, restoring the membrane back toward the resting potential. This process normally takes place at the initial segment of an axon. The conduction of an AP down a myelinated axon, saltatory conduction, requires the reinitiation of the AP at each bare patch of axonal membrane, a node of Ranvier. The reinitiation of the AP occurs because of a voltage change at the next node brought about by passive current flow from the AP at its present site. If several nodes distal to the site of AP propagation are blocked with a local anesthetic, preventing Na⁺ conductance, then the AP will die, or cease, because the closest fully functional, nonblocked node is too far from the point of AP propagation to reach threshold by means of passive current flow. This mechanism of blocking reinitiation of the action potential at nodes of Ranvier underlies the use of the *-caine* derivatives, as in novocaine and xylocaine, for local anesthesia during surgical and dental procedures.

A. Myelinated fibers

Site where action potential is reinitiated

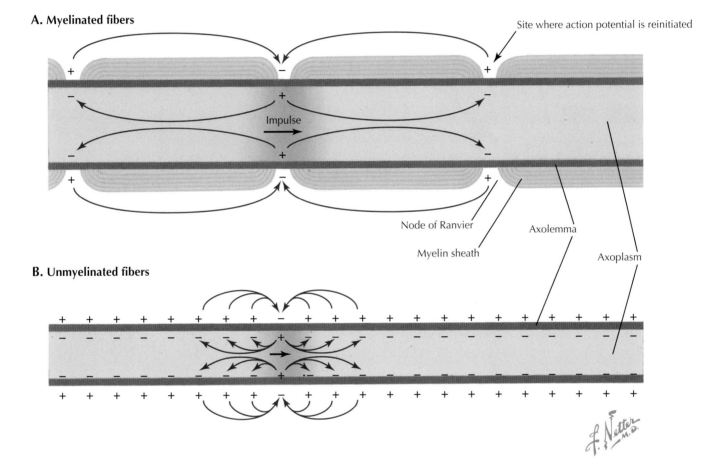

Impulse

Node of Ranvier

Myelin sheath

Axolemma

Axoplasm

B. Unmyelinated fibers

1.15 CONDUCTION VELOCITY

A, The speed of propagation increases with larger axonal diameter and in the presence of a myelin sheath. In myelinated axons the AP is propagated from node to node by saltatory conduction. **B,** The AP travels down the unmyelinated axon by depolarizing adjacent patches of membrane, leading to reinitiation of the action potential.

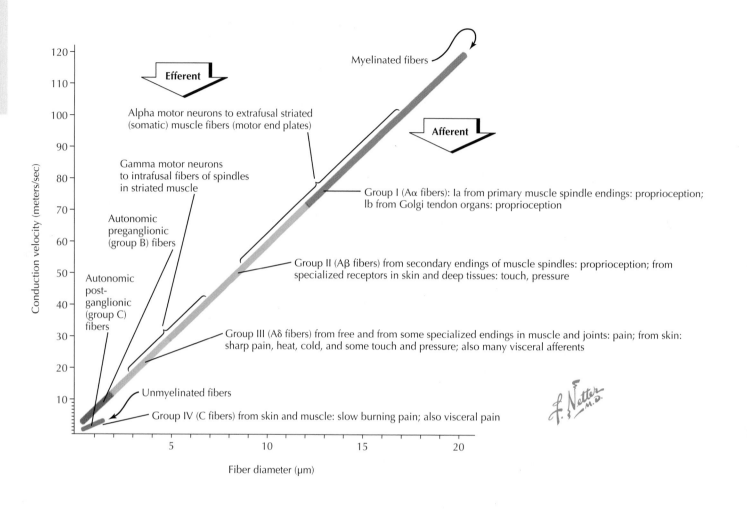

1.16 CLASSIFICATION OF PERIPHERAL NERVE FIBERS BY SIZE AND CONDUCTION VELOCITY

Unmyelinated peripheral nerve fibers (1 to 2 μm in diameter) conduct APs slowly (1 to 2 m/sec) because propagation requires reinitiation of the AP at each adjacent patch of axonal membrane along the entire course of the axon. These peripheral fibers are called group IV fibers. Myelinated peripheral nerve fibers (2 to 20+ μm in diameter) conduct APs rapidly (2 to 120+ m/sec) because propagation is aided by the distant spacing of nodes of Ranvier resulting from the successive internodal myelin sheaths. The larger diameter axons conduct APs the most rapidly. Clinical conduction-velocity studies can document the conduction velocity of successive classes of myelinated peripheral nerve fibers (group I, II, and III fibers), and they provide evidence of normal or altered nerve conduction and possibly function. Conduction velocity is measured by placing a stimulating electrode at a specific site (in the popliteal fossa) where a current can initiate APs in axons in a specific nerve. Recording electrodes are placed at a distant site, where muscle contractions can be measured and where the time delay of conduction of APs in axons can be measured. The classification system of myelinated nerve fibers in the figure is accompanied by descriptions of the functional types of axons included in each group.

CLINICAL POINT

Peripheral axons larger than approximately 2 μm in diameter trigger the process of myelination by adjacent Schwann cells. Peripheral axons of different sizes subserve different functions and are subject to damage by a variety of separate insults. Thus, small-fiber neuropathies, such as leprosy, damage pain, and temperature sensation (via small-diameter axons) can occur without concomitant damage to discriminative touch, LMN function, or Ia afferent reflex activity. In contrast, damage to large-diameter axons, as seen in demyelinating neuropathies, can result in flaccid paralysis with loss of tone and reflexes (motor axons) and loss of fine, discriminative sensation (sensory axons) without loss of autonomic functions or loss of pain and temperature sensation, which are carried in part by small unmyelinated axons.

Electrodiagnostic Studies in Compression Neuropathy

Electromyography (EMG)

Nerve impulse (action potential)

Bipolar recording needle

First dorsal interosseous muscle

EMG detects and records electric activity or potentials within muscle in various phases of voluntary contraction

EMG of dorsal interosseous muscle (ulnar innervation)

Normal — Action potential — Maximal contraction
Needle insertion

Abnormal — Fibrillation — Denervation positive waves — Fasciculation

Compression–induced denervation produces abnormal spontaneous potentials

Nerve conduction studies

Stimulating electrode
Stimulation at elbow
Distance
Stimulation at wrist
Motor (recording electrodes)
Sensory (recording electrodes)

Time — Normal amplitude
Increased threshold
Normal threshold — Decreased amplitude
Normal latency
Increased latency

$$\text{Conduction velocity} = \frac{\text{Difference in elbow and wrist latency}}{\text{Distance between electrodes}}$$

Increased threshold for depolarization, increased latency, and decreased conduction velocity suggest compression neuropathy

Nerve conduction studies evaluate ability of nerve to conduct electrically evoked action potentials. Sensory and motor conduction stimulated and recorded

1.17 ELECTROMYOGRAPHY AND CONDUCTION VELOCITY STUDIES

Electromyography detects and records electrical activity within muscles in various phases of voluntary contraction. These studies are useful for diagnosing myopathies and axonal damage in neuropathies. Nerve conduction velocity studies assess the ability of nerves (especially myelinated nerve fibers) to conduct electrically evoked APs in sensory and motor axons. Conduction velocity studies are particularly helpful in evaluating damage to myelinated axons.

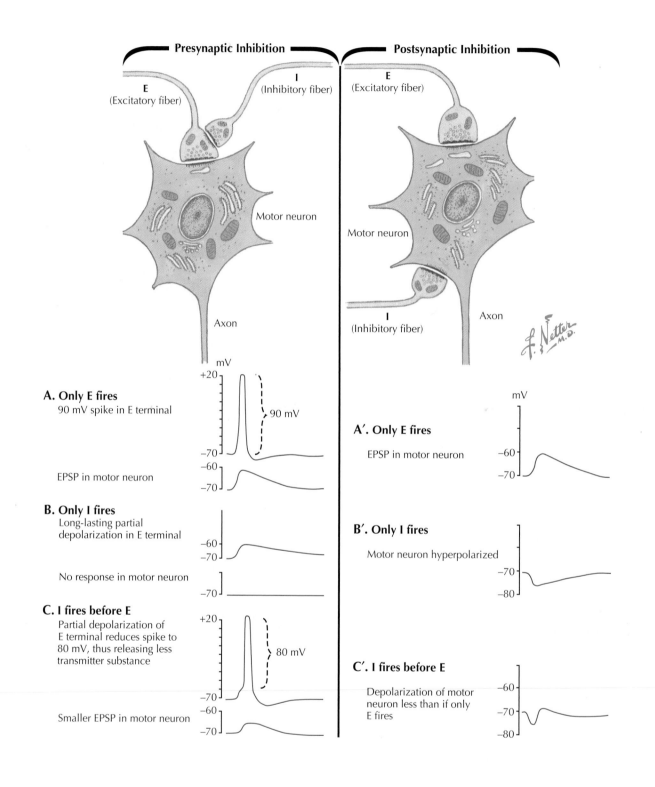

Presynaptic Inhibition

Postsynaptic Inhibition

E
(Excitatory fiber)

I
(Inhibitory fiber)

E
(Excitatory fiber)

Motor neuron

Motor neuron

Axon

I
(Inhibitory fiber)

Axon

mV

A. Only E fires
90 mV spike in E terminal

+20

90 mV

−70

−60
−70

EPSP in motor neuron

A′. Only E fires

EPSP in motor neuron

mV

−60

−70

B. Only I fires
Long-lasting partial
depolarization in E terminal

−60
−70

No response in motor neuron

−70

B′. Only I fires

Motor neuron hyperpolarized

−70

−80

C. I fires before E
Partial depolarization of
E terminal reduces spike to
80 mV, thus releasing less
transmitter substance

+20

80 mV

−70
−60
−70

Smaller EPSP in motor neuron

C′. I fires before E

Depolarization of motor
neuron less than if only
E fires

−60

−70

−80

1.18 PRESYNAPTIC AND POSTSYNAPTIC INHIBITION

Inhibitory synapses modulate neuronal excitability. Presynaptic inhibition (left) and postsynaptic inhibition (right) are shown in relation to a motor neuron. Postsynaptic inhibition causes local hyperpolarization at the postsynaptic site. Presynaptic inhibition involves the depolarization of an excitatory axon terminal, which decreases the amount of Ca^{2+} influx that occurs with depolarization of that excitatory terminal, thus reducing the resultant EPSP at the postsynaptic site.

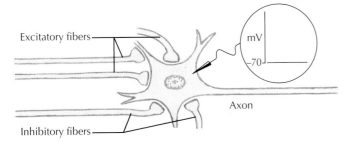

A. Resting state: motor nerve cell shown with synaptic boutons of excitatory and inhibitory nerve fibers ending close to it

B. Partial depolarization: impulse from one excitatory fiber has caused partial (below firing threshold) depolarization of motor neuron

C. Temporal excitatory summation: a series of impulses in one excitatory fiber together produce a suprathreshold depolarization that triggers an action potential

D. Spatial excitatory summation: impulses in two excitatory fibers cause two synaptic depolarizations that together reach firing threshold, triggering an action potential

E. Spatial excitatory summation with inhibition: impulses from two excitatory fibers reach motor neuron but impulses from inhibitory fiber prevent depolarization from reaching threshold

■ Axon(s) activated in each scenario

E. (continued): motor neuron now receives additional excitatory impulses and reaches firing threshold despite a simultaneous inhibitory impulse; additional inhibitory impulses might still prevent firing

1.19 SPATIAL AND TEMPORAL SUMMATION

Neurons receive multiple excitatory and inhibitory inputs. **C,** Temporal summation occurs when a series of subthreshold EPSPs in one excitatory fiber produce an AP in the postsynaptic cell. This occurs because the EPSPs are superimposed on each other temporally before the local region of membrane has completely returned to its resting state. **D,** Spatial summation occurs when subthreshold impulses from two or more synapses trigger an AP because of synergistic interactions. **E,** Both temporal and spatial summation can be modulated by simultaneous inhibitory input. Inhibitory and excitatory neurons use a wide variety of neurotransmitters, whose actions depend on the ion channels opened by the ligand-receptor interactions.

Origin and Spread of Seizures

A. Normal firing pattern of cortical neurons

Normal activation of cortical neurons (P) modulated by excitatory (E) and inhibitory (I) feedback circuits.

Excitatory pathways between cerebral cortex and thalamus modulated by tonic midbrain inhibitory stimuli.

B. Epileptic firing pattern of cortical neurons

Repetitive cortical activation potentiates excitatory transmission and depresses inhibitory transmission, creating self-perpetuating excitatory circuit (burst) and facilitating excitation (recruitment) of neighboring neurons.

Cortical bursts to corpus striatum and thalamus block inhibitory projections and create self-perpetuating feedback circuit.

JOHN A. CRAIG—AD

1.20 NORMAL ELECTRICAL FIRING PATTERNS OF CORTICAL NEURONS AND THE ORIGIN AND SPREAD OF SEIZURES

The collective electrical activity of the cerebral cortex can be monitored by electroencephalography (EEG). Normal cortical electrical activity reflects the summation of excitatory and inhibitory actions, which is modulated through feedback circuits. Thalamic inputs to the cortex can drive electrical excitability; the midbrain can provide inhibitory control over this process. Repetitive cortical activation can dampen inhibition, enhance excitatory feedback circuits, and recruit repetitive excitatory circuitry in adjacent cortical neurons. These self-perpetuating excitatory feedback circuits can initiate and spread seizure activity.

Electrode placement and lead identification

Odd numbers, left side
Even numbers, right side
z locations, midline

EEG in normal awake person, eyes closed

Fp1–F3
β
F3–C3
C3–P3
P3–O1
α
Fp2–F4
β
F4–C4
C4–P4
P4–O2
α

Normal sleep

F3–A1
F4–A2
C3–A1
C4–A2
P3–A1
P4–A2
O1–A1
O2–A2

Sleep spindles

Right temporal tumor

Fp1–F7
F7–T3
T3–T5
T5–O1
Fp2–F8
F8–T4
T4–T6
T6–O2

Right temporal δ activity

Epilepsy

Fp1–F7
F7–T3
T3–T5
T5–O1
Fp2–F8
F8–T4
T4–T6
T6–O2

Left temporal spikes

1.21 ELECTROENCEPHALOGRAPHY

EEG permits the recording of the collective electrical activity of the cerebral cortex as a summation of activity measured as a difference between two recording electrodes. Recording electrodes (leads) are placed on the scalp on at least 16 standard sites, and recordings of potential differences between key electrodes are obtained. The principal wave forms recorded in the EEG are alpha (9 to 10 Hz, occipital location, predominant activity in adults, awake in resting state with eyes closed); beta (20 to 25 Hz, frontal and precentral locations, prominent in wakefulness, seen in light sleep); delta (2 to 2.5 Hz, frontal and central location, not prominent in wakefulness, generalized in deep sleep and coma or toxic states); and theta (5 to 6 Hz, central location, constant and not prominent when awake and active, sometimes generalized when drowsy). Electrode placement is shown in figure B. Examples are provided of a normal EEG taken when client is awake with eyes closed (C), and when sleeping normally (D). Abnormal patterns of activity can be seen in the presence of tumors (E) and in seizures (F); for example, the spike-and-wave appearance in a generalized tonic-clonic seizure (generalized fast repetitive spikes and generalized spikes and slow waves, respectively); and a 3 Hz spike-and-wave EEG in the case of an absence seizure.

2

SKULL AND MENINGES

Frontal bone
Sulcus of superior sagittal sinus
Frontal crest
Sulcus for anterior meningeal vessels
Foramen cecum
Internal surface of orbital part

Ethmoid bone
Crista galli
Cribriform plate

Sphenoid bone
Lesser wing
Anterior clinoid process
Greater wing
Sulcus for middle meningeal
vessels (frontal branches)
Body
Jugum
Prechiasmatic sulcus
Sella turcica
Tuberculum sellae
Hypophyseal fossa
Posterior clinoid process
Dorsum sellae
Groove for internal carotid artery

Temporal bone
Squamous part
Petrous part
Sulcus of lesser petrosal nerve
Sulcus of greater petrosal nerve
Cartilage of auditory tube
Arcuate eminence
Sulcus of superior petrosal sinus
Sulcus of sigmoid sinus

Parietal bone
Sulcus for middle meningeal
vessels (parietal branches)
Mastoid angle

Occipital bone
Basilar part
Sulcus of inferior petrosal sinus
Sulci for posterior meningeal vessels
Condyle
Sulcus of transverse sinus
Sulcus of occipital sinus
Internal occipital crest
Internal occipital protuberance
Sulcus of superior sagittal sinus

Anterior cranial fossa

Middle cranial fossa

Posterior cranial fossa

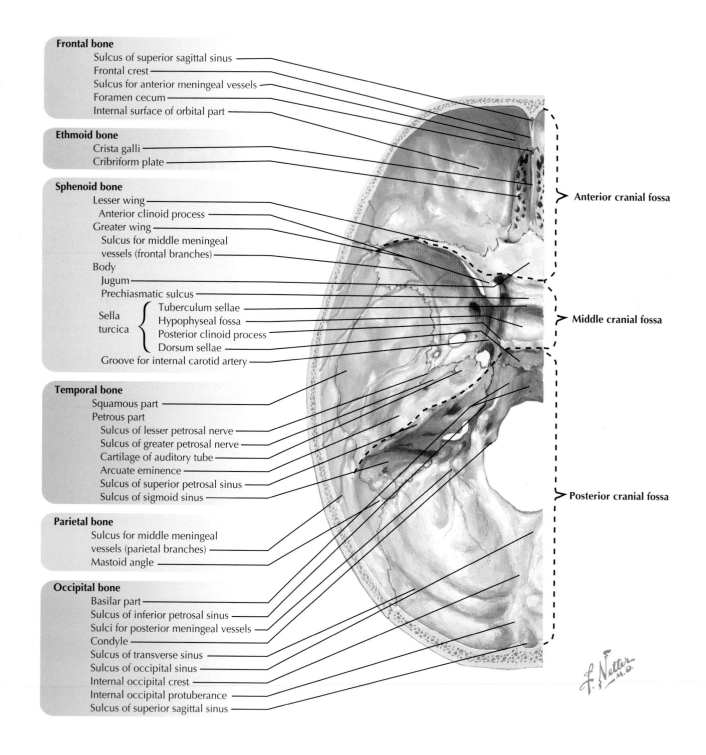

2.1 INTERIOR VIEW OF THE BASE OF THE ADULT SKULL

The anterior, middle, and posterior cranial fossae house the anterior frontal lobe, temporal lobe, and cerebellum and brain stem, respectively. The fossae are separated from each other by bony structures and dural membranes. A swelling of the brain or the presence of mass lesions can selectively exert pressure within an individual fossa. The perforated cribriform plate allows the olfactory nerves to penetrate into the olfactory bulb, a site where head trauma can result in the tearing of the penetrating olfactory nerve fibers.

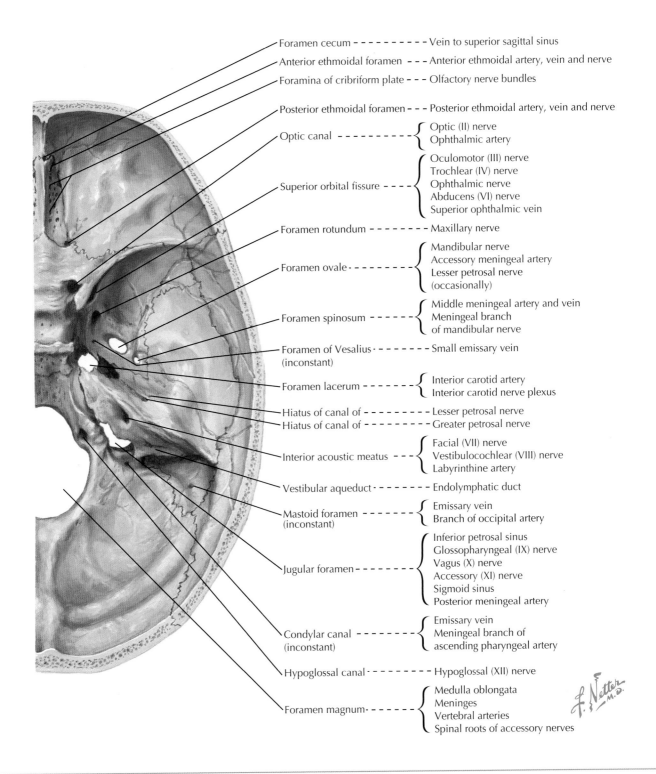

Foramen cecum – – – – – – – Vein to superior sagittal sinus

Anterior ethmoidal foramen – – – Anterior ethmoidal artery, vein and nerve

Foramina of cribriform plate – – – Olfactory nerve bundles

Posterior ethmoidal foramen – – – Posterior ethmoidal artery, vein and nerve

Optic canal – – – – – – – – {
Optic (II) nerve
Ophthalmic artery

Superior orbital fissure – – – – {
Oculomotor (III) nerve
Trochlear (IV) nerve
Ophthalmic nerve
Abducens (VI) nerve
Superior ophthalmic vein

Foramen rotundum – – – – – – – Maxillary nerve

Foramen ovale – – – – – – – – {
Mandibular nerve
Accessory meningeal artery
Lesser petrosal nerve
(occasionally)

Foramen spinosum – – – – – – {
Middle meningeal artery and vein
Meningeal branch
of mandibular nerve

Foramen of Vesalius – – – – – – – Small emissary vein
(inconstant)

Foramen lacerum – – – – – – – {
Interior carotid artery
Interior carotid nerve plexus

Hiatus of canal of – – – – – – – Lesser petrosal nerve
Hiatus of canal of – – – – – – – Greater petrosal nerve

Interior acoustic meatus – – – {
Facial (VII) nerve
Vestibulocochlear (VIII) nerve
Labyrinthine artery

Vestibular aqueduct – – – – – – Endolymphatic duct

Mastoid foramen – – – – – – – {
Emissary vein
(inconstant)   Branch of occipital artery

Jugular foramen – – – – – – – {
Inferior petrosal sinus
Glossopharyngeal (IX) nerve
Vagus (X) nerve
Accessory (XI) nerve
Sigmoid sinus
Posterior meningeal artery

Condylar canal – – – – – – – {
Emissary vein
(inconstant)   Meningeal branch of
ascending pharyngeal artery

Hypoglossal canal – – – – – – – Hypoglossal (XII) nerve

Foramen magnum – – – – – – {
Medulla oblongata
Meninges
Vertebral arteries
Spinal roots of accessory nerves

2.2 FORAMINA IN THE BASE OF THE ADULT SKULL

The foramina in the base of the skull allow major nerves and blood vessels to course through the skull through each opening. Pressure, traction, and masses can damage structures traversing these small spaces that snugly confine the structures.

CLINICAL POINT

The foramina of the skull are narrow openings that allow the passage of nerves and blood vessels. Under normal circumstances, there is enough room for comfortable passage of these structures without traction or pressure. However, with the presence of a tumor at a foramen, the passing structures can be compressed or damaged. A tumor at the internal acoustic meatus can result in ipsilateral facial and vestibuloacoustic nerve damage, and a tumor at the jugular foramen can result in damage to the glossopharyngeal, vagus, and spinal accessory nerves.

Temporal bone
Sphenoid bone
Temporal fossa
Zygomatic arch
Condylar process of mandible
Mandibular notch
Coronoid process of mandible
Lateral pterygoid plate (*broken line*)
Hamulus of medial pterygoid plate (*broken line*)
Pterygomandibular raphe (*broken line*)

Mandible { Ramus
Angle
Body

Stylohyoid ligament

Hyoid bone { Body
Lesser horn
Greater horn

Spine of sphenoid bone
Foramen spinosum
Foramen ovale

Epiglottis
Thyroid cartilage
Cricoid cartilage
Trachea

Mastoid process
External acoustic meatus
Atlas (C1)
Styloid process
Axis (C2)
Stylomandibular ligament
C3 vertebra

C7 vertebra

T1 vertebra

1st rib

Sphenopalatine foramen
Pterygopalatine fossa
Choanae (posterior nares)
Lateral plate }
Medial plate } of pterygoid process
Hamulus }
Pyramidal process of palatine bone

Tuberosity of maxilla
Infratemporal fossa
Alveolar process of maxilla

f. Netter m.d.

2.3 **BONY FRAMEWORK OF THE HEAD AND NECK**

The skull provides bony protection for the brain. The spine, consisting of vertebrae and their intervertebral disks, provides bony protection for the spinal cord. The spine and skull articulate at the foramen magnum, where the C1 vertebral body (the atlas) abuts the occipital bone.

2.4 SCHEMATIC OF THE MENINGES AND THEIR RELATIONSHIPS TO THE BRAIN AND SKULL

The meninges provide protection and support for neural tissue in the central nervous system. The innermost membrane, the pia mater, adheres to every contour of neural tissue, including sulci, folia, and other infoldings. It adheres tightly to glial endfoot processes of astrocytes; this association is called the pial-glial membrane. The arachnoid mater, a fine, lacy membrane external to the pia, extends across the neural sulci and foldings. The space between these two membranes is the subarachnoid space, a space into which the cerebrospinal fluid flows, providing buoyancy and protection for the brain. Arteries and veins run through the subarachnoid space to and from the central nervous system. The rupture of an arterial aneurysm in a cerebral artery results in a subarachnoid hemorrhage. The dura mater, usually adherent to the inner arachnoid, is a tough protective outer membrane. It splits into two layers in some locations to provide channels for the venous blood, the venous sinuses. The arachnoid granulations, one-way valves, extend from the subarachnoid space into the venous sinuses, especially the superior sagittal sinus, allowing cerebrospinal fluid to drain into the venous blood and return

to the heart. Blockage of these arachnoid granulations (e.g., in acute purulent meningitis) can result in increased intracranial pressure. Cerebral arteries and veins traverse the subarachnoid space. The veins, called bridging veins, drain into the dural sinuses. As they enter the sinus, these bridging veins are subject to tearing in cases of head trauma. If there is atrophy in the brain, as occurs with age, these veins may tear with relatively minor head trauma; in younger adults, more severe head trauma is needed to tear these bridging veins. Such tearing permits venous blood to accumulate in the subdural space as it dissects the inner dura from the arachnoid. This process may be gradual (chronic subdural hematoma) in older individuals or may be abrupt (acute subdural hematoma) with severe head trauma. A subdural hematoma, especially when it occurs acutely, may be life-threatening as the result of increased intracranial pressure caused by accompanying edema and by the accumulation of the blood in the hematoma itself. The dura is closely adherent to the inner table of the skull. A skull fracture may tear a branch of the middle meningeal artery, permitting arterial blood to dissect the dura from the skull, resulting in an epidural hematoma.

Temporal Fossa Hematoma

Shift of normal midline structures

Compression of posterior cerebral artery

Skull fracture crossing middle meningeal artery

Shift of brain stem to opposite side may reverse lateralization of signs by tentorial pressure on contralateral pathways

Herniation of temporal lobe under tentorium cerebelli

Herniation of cerebellar tonsil

Compression of corticospinal and associated pathways, resulting in contralateral hemiparesis, deep tendon hyperreflexia, and Babinski's sign

Compression of oculomotor (III) nerve leading to ipsilateral pupil dilatation and third cranial nerve palsy

Subfrontal Hematoma

Frontal trauma: headache, poor cerebration, intermittent disorientation, anisocoria

Posterior Fossa Hematoma

Occipital trauma and/or fracture: headache, meningismus, cerebellar and cranial nerve signs, Cushing's triad

Acute Subdural Hematoma

Section showing acute subdural hematoma on right side and subdural hematoma associated with temporal lobe intracerebral hematoma ("burst" temporal lobe) on left

2.5 HEMATOMAS

Epidural hematomas occur with trauma or skull fractures that tear meningeal arteries (especially middle meningeal artery branches). Blood from the tear dissects the outer layer of the dura from the skull, forming a space-occupying mass in what was normally only a potential space. The hematoma may compress adjacent brain tissue, producing localized signs, and may also cause herniation of distant brain regions across the free edge of the tentorium cerebelli (a transtentorial herniation) or across the falx cerebri (a subfalcial herniation). Such herniation may produce changes in consciousness, breathing, and blood pressure and altered motor, pupillary, and other

neurological signs. It may be fatal. Severe head trauma in an adult may tear bridging veins that lead from the brain through the subarachnoid space and into the dural sinuses, especially the superior sagittal sinus. The subsequent venous bleeding dissects the arachnoid membrane from the inner layer of the dura, and the blood accumulates as a subdural hematoma. The subdural space is normally only a potential space. Some of the proteins and other solutes in the hematoma attract edema, adding fluid accumulation to the hematoma and further exacerbating the space-occupying nature of the bleed. A subdural hematoma also may be associated with a bleeding directly into the brain, an intracerebral hematoma.

3

BRAIN

Central sulcus
Precentral gyrus
Precentral sulcus
Frontal (F), frontoparietal (FP) and temporal (T) opercula
Superior frontal gyrus
Superior frontal sulcus
Middle frontal gyrus
Inferior frontal sulcus
Inferior frontal gyrus
Frontal pole
Lateral (sylvian) fissure { Anterior ramus / Ascending ramus / Posterior ramus
Temporal pole
Superior temporal gyrus
Superior temporal sulcus
Middle temporal gyrus
Inferior temporal sulcus

Superior (superomedial) margin of cerebrum
Postcentral gyrus
Postcentral sulcus
Supramarginal gyrus
Superior parietal lobule
Intraparietal sulcus
Inferior parietal lobule
Angular gyrus
Parietooccipital sulcus
Transverse occipital sulcus
Calcarine fissure
Occipital pole
Lunate sulcus (inconstant)
Preoccipital notch
Inferior (inferolateral) margin of cerebrum
Inferior temporal gyrus

FP
F
T

Parietal lobe
Frontal lobe
Occipital lobe
Temporal lobe

Forebrain

Central sulcus of insula
Circular sulcus of insula
Insula { Short gyri / Limen / Long gyrus

3.1 SURFACE ANATOMY OF THE FOREBRAIN: LATERAL VIEW

The convolutions of the cerebral cortex allow a large expanse of cortex to be compactly folded into a small volume, an adaptation particularly prominent in primates. Major dependable landmarks separate the forebrain into lobes; the lateral (sylvian) fissure separates the temporal lobe below from the parietal and frontal lobes above, and the central sulcus separates the parietal and frontal lobes from each other. Several of the named gyri are associated with specific functional activities, such as the precentral gyrus (motor cortex) and the postcentral gyrus (primary sensory cortex). Some gyri, such as the superior, middle, and inferior frontal and temporal gyri, serve as anatomical landmarks of the cerebral cortex. The insula, the fifth lobe of the cerebral cortex, is deep to the outer cortex and can be seen by opening the lateral fissure.

CLINICAL POINT

Some functional characteristics of the cerebral cortex, such as long-term memory and some cognitive capabilities, cannot be localized easily to a particular gyrus or region of cortex. However, other functional capabilities are regionally localized. For example, the inferior frontal gyrus on the left contains the neuronal machinery for expressive language capabilities; the occipital pole, particularly along the upper and lower banks of the calcarine fissure, are specialized for visual processing from the retino-geniculo-calcarine system. Some very discrete lesions in further processing sites such as vision-related regions of the temporal lobe can result in specific deficits, such as agnosia for the recognition of faces or the inability to distinguish animate objects. This knowledge provides some clues about how feature extraction in sensory systems might be achieved in neuronal networks.

outer { 1. Frontal / 2. Temporal / 3. Parietal / 4. Occipital
inner { 5. Insula

Lobes of cerebral cortex

Central sulcus

Supplemental motor cortex

Primary motor cortex

Superior parietal lobule

Frontal eye fields

Premotor cortex

Primary somatosensory cortex

Wernicke's area

Broca's area

Primary trigeminal region of

Secondary somatosensory cortex

motor cortex

somatosensory cortex

Visual association areas of cortex

Primary Auditory cortex

Multisensory association areas of cortex

Primary visual cortex

Lateral fissure

3.2 LATERAL VIEW OF THE FOREBRAIN: FUNCTIONAL REGIONS

Some circumscribed regions of the cerebral hemisphere are associated with specific functional activities, including the motor cortex, the supplemental and premotor cortices, the frontal eye fields, the primary sensory cortex, and other association regions of the sensory cortex. Part of the auditory cortex is visible at the inferior edge of the lateral fissure (the transverse temporal gyrus of Heschl). Part of the visual cortex is visible at the occipital pole. Language areas of the left hemisphere include Broca's area (expressive language) and Wernicke's area (receptive language). Damage to these cortical regions results in loss of specific functional capabilities. There is some overlap between functional areas and named gyri (e.g., the motor cortex and the precentral gyrus), but there is no absolute concordance.

CLINICAL POINT

Some specific regions (gyri) of the cerebral cortex, such as the precentral gyrus (primary motor cortex) and the postcentral gyrus (primary somatosensory cortex), demonstrate topographic organization. Thus, information from the contralateral hand and arm are localized laterally, the body is represented more medially, and the lower extremity is represented along the midline and over the edge into the paracentral lobule. The face and head are represented in far lateral regions, just above the lateral fissure. This has important functional implications; damage to selected regions such as the midline territory, which is supplied with blood from the anterior cerebral artery, results in somatosensory loss and paresis in the contralateral lower extremity, while sparing the upper extremity.

HAL

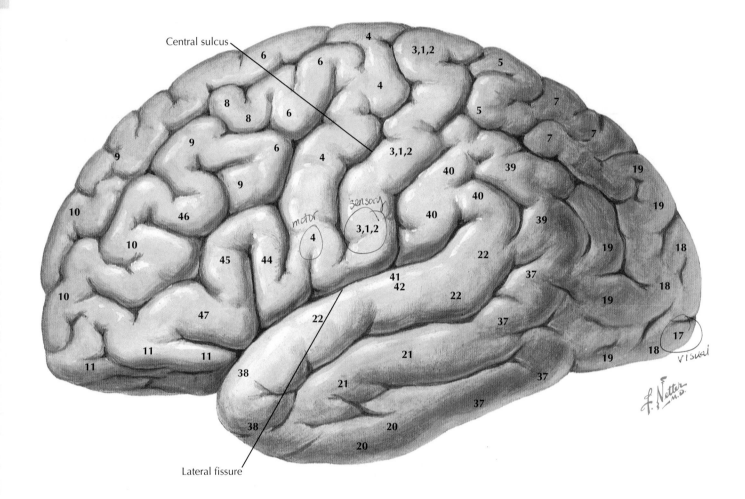

Central sulcus

Lateral fissure

3.3 LATERAL VIEW OF THE FOREBRAIN: BRODMANN'S AREAS

Brodmann's areas of the cerebral cortex have unique architectural characteristics in terms of the thickness and layering of the cerebral cortex; this knowledge is based on histological observations originally made by Korbinian Brodmann in 1909.

His numbering of cortical areas is still used as a shorthand for describing the functional regions of the cortex, particularly those related to sensory functions. Some overlap exists among functional areas. For example, the motor cortex is area 4; the primary sensory cortex includes areas 3, 1, and 2; and the primary visual cortex is area 17.

Cingulate gyrus
Cingulate sulcus
Medial frontal gyrus
Sulcus of corpus callosum
Fornix
Septum pellucidum
Interventricular foramen (of Monro)
Interthalamic adhesion
Thalamus
Anterior commissure
Hypothalamic sulcus
Subcallosal (parolfactory) area
Paraterminal gyrus
Gyrus rectus
Lamina terminalis
Optic recess
Optic chiasm
Tuber cinereum
(median eminence)
Mammillary body
Pituitary gland (anterior and posterior)
Midbrain
Pons
Medulla oblongata
Cerebral aqueduct (of Sylvius)

Precentral sulcus
Central (rolandic) sulcus
Paracentral lobule
Corpus callosum
Precuneus
Superior sagittal sinus
Choroid plexus of 3rd ventricle
Parieto-occipital sulcus
Stria medullaris of thalamus
Cuneus
Calcarine cortex (upper bank)
Habenular commissure
Calcarine sulcus
Lingual gyrus
Calcarine cortex (lower bank)
Pineal gland
Straight sinus (in tentorium cerebelli)
Great cerebral vein (of Galen)
Posterior (epithalamic) commissure
Superior and inferior colliculi
Cerebellum
Superior medullary velum
4th ventricle and choroid plexus
Inferior medullary velum

cerebral cortex
corpus callosum
thalamus, fornix, subcortical forebrain

3.4 ANATOMY OF THE MEDIAL (MIDSAGITTAL) SURFACE OF THE BRAIN IN SITU

The entire extent of the neuraxis, from the spinomedullary junction through the brain stem, diencephalon, and telencephalon, is visible in a midsagittal section. The corpus callosum, a major commissural fiber bundle interconnecting the two hemispheres, is a landmark separating the cerebral cortex above from the thalamus, fornix, and subcortical forebrain below. The ventricular system, including the interventricular foramen (of Munro); the third ventricle (diencephalon); the cerebral aqueduct (midbrain); and the fourth ventricle (pons and medulla), is visible in a midsagittal view. This subarachnoid fluid system provides internal and external protection to the brain and also may serve as a fluid transport system for important regulatory molecules. The thalamus serves as a gateway to the cortex. The hypothalamic proximity to the median eminence (tuber cinereum) and the pituitary gland

reflects the important role of the hypothalamus in regulating neuroendocrine function. A midsagittal view also reveals the midbrain colliculi, sometimes called the visual (superior) and auditory (inferior) tecta.

CLINICAL POINT

The right and left hemispheres are interconnected by commissural fiber bundles. The largest is the corpus callosum, which interconnects all lobes with their counterparts. The anterior commissure interconnects regions of the temporal lobes. When these commissural fiber bundles are disconnected (split brain), the hemispheres do not know what their counterparts are doing, and inputs to one hemisphere cannot produce an appropriate response from the opposite hemisphere. With a split brain, only a more generalized recognition of mood states occurs between the two hemispheres, presumably communicated through interconnections between lower structures, such as the diencephalon and brain stem.

Note: the fornix is the associated axonal fiber tract of the hippocampus

Cingulate gyrus

Mammillothalamic fasciculus

Mammillary body

Uncus

Optic (III) nerve

Olfactory tract

Collateral sulcus

Rhinal sulcus

Medial occipitotemporal gyrus

Occipitotemporal sulcus

Lateral occipitotemporal gyrus

Genu
Rostrum
Body
Splenium
} of corpus callosum

Cuneus

Calcarine sulcus

Lingual gyrus

Body
Crus
Column
} of fornix

Fimbria of hippocampus

Dentate gyrus

Parahippocampal gyrus

CC Body

CC Splenium

3.5 ANATOMY OF THE MEDIAL (MIDSAGITTAL) SURFACE OF THE BRAIN, WITH BRAIN STEM REMOVED

When the brain stem is removed, a midsagittal view reveals the C-shaped course of the fornix, extending from the hippocampal formation in the temporal lobe to the septum and hypothalamus. Temporal lobe structures, such as the parahippocampal cortex, the dentate gyrus and fimbria of the hippocampus, and the uncus (olfactory cortex) also are visible. In the hypothalamus, the caudal mammillary bodies and the interconnecting pathway to the thalamus, the mammillothalamic tract, are revealed.

Primary motor cortex
Precentral sulcus
Limbic cingulate cortex
Paracentral lobule
Supplemental motor cortex
Somatosensory association cortex
Parietal
Frontal
Limbic
Corpus callosum
Occipital
Visual association cortex
Thalamus
Primary visual cortex
Calcarine fissure
Pituitary gland
Pons
Cerebellum
Medulla oblongata

A. Lobes and functional areas

motor
primary sensory
6   4   3
8   1 2   7
9   24   31   7
32 33   23   19
10   18   *primary + associative visual*
32   17
12   25   18 17

B. Brodmann's areas

f. Netter M.D.

3.6 MEDIAL SURFACE OF THE BRAIN

A. Lobes and functional areas. The cingulate cortex is labeled the limbic lobe, reflecting its association with other limbic forebrain structures and with hypothalamic control of the autonomic nervous system. Functional areas of the cortex, particularly those involved with vision, are best seen on a midsagittal view. The sensory and motor cortices associated with the lower extremities are located medially and are supplied with blood by the anterior cerebral artery. This region is selectively vulnerable to specific vascular (anterior cerebral artery infarct) and mass (parasagittal meningioma) lesions that result in contralateral motor and sensory deficits of the lower extremity. **B.** Brodmann's areas of the cerebral cortex are labeled on this midsagittal view of the brain. The major regions are the primary (17) and associative (18, 19) visual cortices, and the continuation of areas 4 (motor) and areas 3, 1, and 2 (primary sensory) onto the paracentral lobule in the midline.

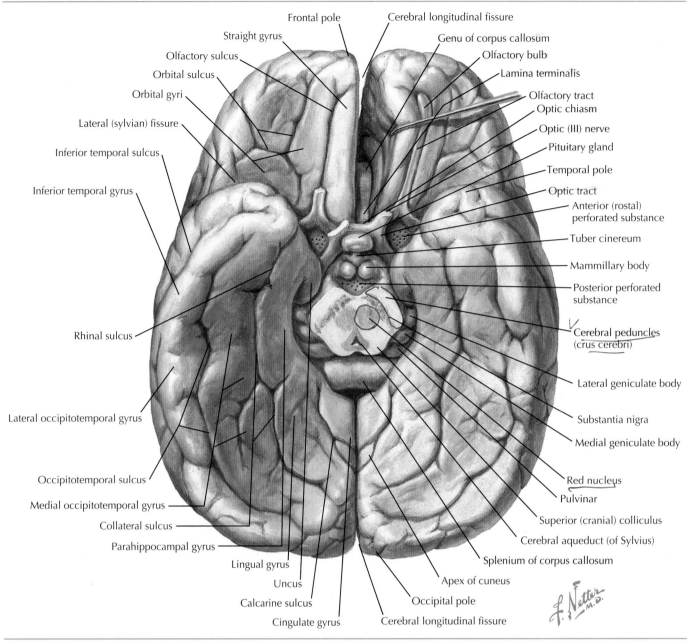

Frontal pole
Cerebral longitudinal fissure
Straight gyrus
Genu of corpus callosum
Olfactory sulcus
Olfactory bulb
Orbital sulcus
Lamina terminalis
Orbital gyri
Olfactory tract
Lateral (sylvian) fissure
Optic chiasm
Inferior temporal sulcus
Optic (III) nerve
Pituitary gland
Inferior temporal gyrus
Temporal pole
Optic tract
Anterior (rostal) perforated substance
Tuber cinereum
Mammillary body
Posterior perforated substance
Rhinal sulcus
Cerebral peduncles (crus cerebri)
Lateral geniculate body
Lateral occipitotemporal gyrus
Substantia nigra
Medial geniculate body
Occipitotemporal sulcus
Red nucleus
Medial occipitotemporal gyrus
Pulvinar
Collateral sulcus
Superior (cranial) colliculus
Parahippocampal gyrus
Cerebral aqueduct (of Sylvius)
Splenium of corpus callosum
Lingual gyrus
Uncus
Apex of cuneus
Calcarine sulcus
Occipital pole
Cingulate gyrus
Cerebral longitudinal fissure

3.7 ANATOMY OF THE BASAL SURFACE OF THE BRAIN, WITH THE BRAIN STEM AND CEREBELLUM REMOVED

Removal of the brain stem and cerebellum by a cut through the midbrain exposes the underlying cerebral cortex, the base of the diencephalon, and the basal forebrain. Basal hypothalamic landmarks, from caudal to rostral, include the mammillary bodies, tuber cinereum, pituitary gland, and optic chiasm. The proximity of the pituitary to the optic chiasm is important because bitemporal hemianopsia can result from optic chiasm fiber damage, often an early sign of a pituitary tumor. The genu and splenium of the corpus callosum are revealed in this view. In the cross-section of the midbrain, the superior colliculus, cerebral aqueduct, periaqueductal gray, red nucleus, substantia nigra, and cerebral peduncles are shown.

amygdala, and other limbic regions. This is the only sensory system with direct access to forebrain structures without prior screening through the diencephalon. This reflects the evolutionary importance of olfaction to functions vital for survival, such as detection of food, defense, and reproduction. Olfactory damage can alter emotional behavior. In addition, complex partial seizures involving the temporal lobe frequently are accompanied by an olfactory aura. Changes in olfactory function and gene expression may be among the earliest signs of Alzheimer's.

The optic nerve, chiasm, and tract can be seen extending toward the lateral geniculate body (nucleus), the pulvinar, and the superior colliculus. Optic nerve damage can result in ipsilateral blindness; optic chiasm damage can result in bitemporal visual field deficits; and optic tract damage can result in contralateral hemianopsia. Additional visual input from the optic tract enters the hypothalamus and ends in the suprachiasmatic nucleus. This visual input conveys information of total light flux and exposure, permitting visual influence over diurnal rhythms such as the cortisol rhythm. Disruption of this diurnal input can produce altered production of hormones such as melatonin, and metabolic consequences such as the propensity for abdominal obesity resulting from disruption of the diurnal cortisol rhythm.

CLINICAL POINT

The olfactory bulb and tract send connections directly into limbic forebrain structures, such as the uncus (the primary olfactory cortex),

Brodmann's Areas

Structures

right side of brain

left side of brain

Temporal pole

10

10

11

11

38

34

28

20

20

36

37

19

18

17

Olfactory bulb

Executive anticipatory cortical function

Olfactory tract

Optic chiasm

Optic nerve (II) (cut)

Hypophysis (pituitary gland)

Optic tract

Olfactory cortex

Mammillary body

Multisensory association areas

Visual association cortex

Primary visual cortex

3.8 BASAL SURFACE OF THE BRAIN: FUNCTIONAL AREAS AND BRODMANN'S AREAS

This view provides information about the medial temporal lobe on the left side of the brain, especially cortical regions associated with the hippocampal formation, the amygdaloid nuclei, and the olfactory system. On the right side of the brain, Brodmann's areas are noted.

CT

A. Coronal view

Coronal

Superior sagittal sinus

Skull

Cortical gyrus

Subarachnoid space

Lateral ventricle

Thalamus

Third ventricle

Sagittal

Cortical gyri

Subarachnoid space

Skull

Parietal lobe
Corpus callosum
Frontal lobe
Lateral ventricle
Occipital lobe
Thalamus
Midbrain
Pons
Cerebellum
Medulla
Cisterna magna

B. Sagittal view

3.9 **BRAIN IMAGING: COMPUTED TOMOGRAPHY SCANS, CORONAL AND SAGITTAL**

A and **B,** Computed tomography (CT) is an x-ray–based imaging approach that is used to view the brain, particularly when looking for differences in tissue density such as the presence of blood. The use of spiral (helical) scanners can quickly provide access to views of slices through the brain at the desired thickness. CT delineates soft tissue, fluid, and bone and can be used with contrast to image blood vessels or to reveal the presence of a tumor caused by a disrupted blood-brain barrier that allows leakage of the contrast agent into the surrounding extracellular space of the brain.

A. Axial view

MRI

T1

Axial

- Cortical gyrus
- Insular cortex
- Cortical white matter
- Genu, corpus callosum
- Frontal pole, lateral ventricle
- Head of caudate nucleus
- Putamen
- Columns, fornix
- Globus pallidus
- Internal capsule
- Thalamus
- Hippocampal formation
- Temporal pole, lateral ventricle
- Optic radiations

Sagittal

- Cingulate cortex
- Corpus callosum
- Lateral ventricle
- Fornix
- Thalamus
- Colliculi
- Midbrain
- Hypothalamus
- Pons
- Cerebellum
- Medulla
- Cisterna magna
- Subarachnoid space
- Spinal cord

B. Sagittal view

3.10 BRAIN IMAGING: MAGNETIC RESONANCE IMAGING, AXIAL AND SAGITTAL T1-WEIGHTED IMAGES

A, axial view. **B,** sagittal view. Magnetic resonance imaging (MRI) uses short bursts (radiofrequency pulses) of electromagnetic waves that are sent into the magnet and are absorbed by protons in the tissues of the patient in the scanner. The pulses cause alignment of the protons as the result of raised energy levels; that is followed by a relaxation phase in which the protons return to a lower energy level. During the relaxation process, a detector records the emitted energy, and a computer provides a uniform image of the scanned tissue. The intervals (milliseconds) between the pulses (repetition time, TR) and the intervals between the collection times of the emitted energy (echo time, TE) provide various contrast information, which are indicated by contrast weighting. Short TR and TE intervals result in T1-weighted images, whereas longer TR and TE intervals result in T2-weighted images. The T1-weighted images are particularly useful for viewing normal brain structures and are particularly useful for viewing the brain stem and the cervical and thoracic spinal cord. The T2-weighted images are particularly useful for revealing pathology, such as infarcts, tumors, edema, and demyelination. A contrast agent such as gadolinium can be used to delineate a tumor because of its ability to leak across the blood-brain barrier.

T2 also good for imaging ventricular systems + cisterns for CSF

MRI
T2

A. Axial view

- Subarachnoid space
- Cortical gyrus
- Cortical white matter
- Insular cortex
- Genu, corpus callosum
- Head, caudate nucleus
- Frontal pole, lateral ventricle
- Putamen
- Columns, fornix
- Internal capsule
- Thalamus
- Hippocampal formation
- Temporal pole, lateral ventricle
- Optic radiations
- Cingulate cortex
- Corpus callosum
- Site of lateral ventricle
- Fornix
- Thalamus
- Subarachnoid space
- Colliculi
- Midbrain
- Pons
- Cerebellum
- Medulla
- Cisterna magna
- Subarachnoid space
- Spinal cord

B. Sagittal view

3.11 BRAIN IMAGING: MAGNETIC RESONANCE IMAGING, AXIAL AND SAGITTAL T2-WEIGHTED IMAGES

A, axial view. **B,** sagittal view. T2-weighted images are particularly useful for imaging the ventricular system and the cisterns of cerebrospinal fluid.

3.12 POSITRON EMISSION TOMOGRAPHY SCANNING

Positron emission tomography (PET) scanning is designed to assess the distribution of tracers labeled with positron-emitting nuclides, such as carbon-11 (^{11}C), nitrogen-13 (^{13}N), oxygen-15 (^{15}O), and fluorine-18 (^{18}F). Fluorodeoxyglucose (FDG), a glucose analogue labeled with ^{18}F, can cross the blood-brain barrier. The metabolic products of FDG become immobile and trapped where the molecule is first used, thereby permitting FDG to be used to map glucose uptake in the brain. This is a valuable tool for investigating subtle physiological processes related to neurological diseases. The distribution of FDG can be localized and reconstructed using standard tomographic techniques that show the tracer distribution throughout the body or brain. In this example of axial, sagittal, and coronal views, the transmission measurement and correction was performed immediately following PET acquisition using a 16-slice CT unit. The PET and CT images were automatically fused by anatomical coregistration software (shown as colored images).

Basal ganglia- four masses of gray matter lying deep in cerebral hemispheres. (Masses include: caudate, lentiform, amygdaloid, + claustrum) or (caudate nucleus, putamen, and globus pallidus)

Schematic illustration showing interrelationship of thalamus, lentiform nucleus, caudate nucleus, and amygdaloid body (viewed from side).

3.13 HORIZONTAL BRAIN SECTIONS SHOWING THE BASAL GANGLIA

Two levels of horizontal sections through the forebrain reveal the major anatomical features and the relationships among the basal ganglia, the internal capsule, and the thalamus (schematically shown in the lower illustration). The caudate nucleus is a C-shaped structure that sweeps from the frontal lobe into the temporal lobe; a horizontal section passes through this nucleus in two distinct places (head and tail). The anterior limb, genu, and posterior limb of the internal capsule contain major connections into and out of the cerebral cortex. The head and body of the caudate are medial to the anterior limb, whereas the thalamus is medial to the posterior limb. These relationships are important for understanding imaging studies and for understanding the involvement of specific functional systems in vascular lesions or strokes. The internal and external segments of the globus pallidus are located medial to the putamen. The external capsule, claustrum, extreme capsule, and insular cortex, from medial to lateral, are located lateral to the putamen. The fornix, also a C-shaped bundle, is sectioned in two sites, the crus and the column.

CLINICAL POINT

The basal ganglia (caudate nucleus, putamen, and globus pallidus) form characteristic anatomical relationships with the internal capsule. The head and body of the caudate nucleus are found medial to the anterior limb; the thalamus is found medial to the posterior limb; and the globus pallidus and putamen are found lateral to the anterior and posterior limbs. Basal ganglia disorders are characterized by movement disorders, although emotional and cognitive symptoms also are seen. Some movement disorders involve actual degeneration of basal ganglia and related structures; these disorders include Huntington's chorea and degeneration of the head of the caudate nucleus as well as Parkinson's disease and degeneration of the dopaminergic pars compacta of substantia nigra.

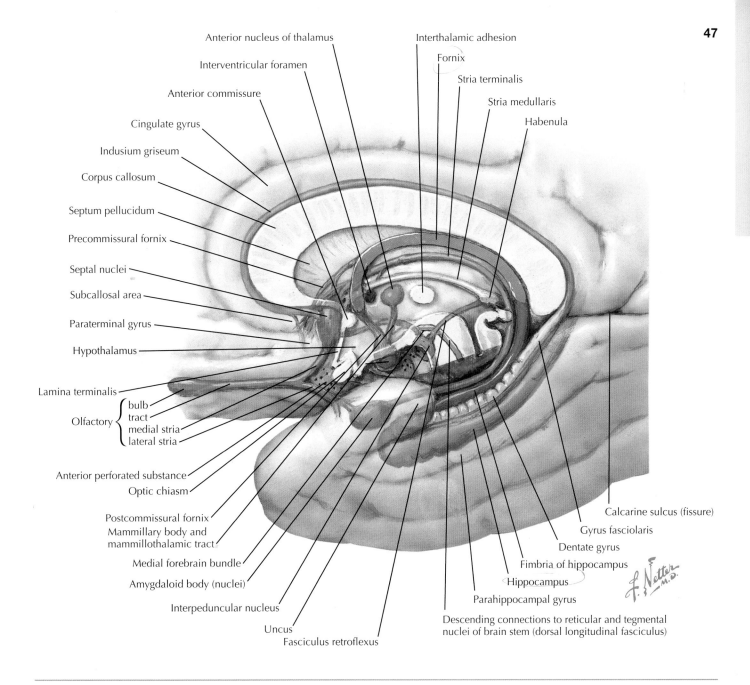

Anterior nucleus of thalamus
Interventricular foramen
Anterior commissure
Cingulate gyrus
Indusium griseum
Corpus callosum
Septum pellucidum
Precommissural fornix
Septal nuclei
Subcallosal area
Paraterminal gyrus
Hypothalamus
Lamina terminalis
Olfactory { bulb, tract, medial stria, lateral stria }
Anterior perforated substance
Optic chiasm
Postcommissural fornix
Mammillary body and mammillothalamic tract
Medial forebrain bundle
Amygdaloid body (nuclei)
Interpeduncular nucleus
Uncus
Fasciculus retroflexus

Interthalamic adhesion
Fornix
Stria terminalis
Stria medullaris
Habenula

Calcarine sulcus (fissure)
Gyrus fasciolaris
Dentate gyrus
Fimbria of hippocampus
Hippocampus
Parahippocampal gyrus
Descending connections to reticular and tegmental nuclei of brain stem (dorsal longitudinal fasciculus)

3.14 MAJOR LIMBIC FOREBRAIN STRUCTURES

The term *limbic* is derived from *limbus,* meaning ring. Many of these structures and their pathways in the limbic system form a ring around the diencephalons. They are involved in emotional behavior and individualized interpretations of external and internal stimuli. The hippocampal formation and its major pathway, the fornix, curve into the anterior pole of the diencephalon, forming precommissural (to the septum) and postcommissural (to the hypothalamus) connections in relation to the anterior commissure. The amygdaloid nuclei give rise to several pathways; one, the stria terminalis, extends in a C-shaped course around the diencephalon into the hypothalamic and basal forebrain. The olfactory tract communicates directly with several limbic forebrain areas; it is the only sensory system to entirely bypass the thalamus and terminate directly in cortical and subcortical zones of the telencephalon. Connections from the septal nuclei to the habenula (stria medullaris thalami) connect the limbic forebrain to the brain stem. The amygdaloid nuclei and hippocampus (shaded) are deep to the cortex.

CLINICAL POINT

Many of the limbic forebrain structures are connected with the hypothalamus by C-shaped structures, such as the hippocampus and the fornix, and with the amygdala and the stria terminalis. The amygdala has additional direct connections into the hypothalamus via the ventral amygdalofugal pathway. The amygdaloid nuclei receive multimodal sensory information from cortical regions and provide contexts for this input, particularly emotions related to fear responses. Bilateral amygdaloid damage results in the loss of the fear response and also in failure to recognize facial responses of fear in others.

The hippocampal formation processes abundant information from the temporal lobe, subiculum, and entorhinal cortex and sends connections through the fornix to the hypothalamus and septal nuclei, with subsequent connections through the thalamus to the cingulate cortex. These structures are part of the so-called Papez circuit. The hippocampal formation is particularly vulnerable to ischemia; damage bilaterally, resulting in the inability to consolidate new information into long-term memory. A common pattern may be observed in older persons who forget who has talked with them minutes before or forget what they had for breakfast (or even whether they had breakfast) but can recall details from the past that have some degree of accuracy.

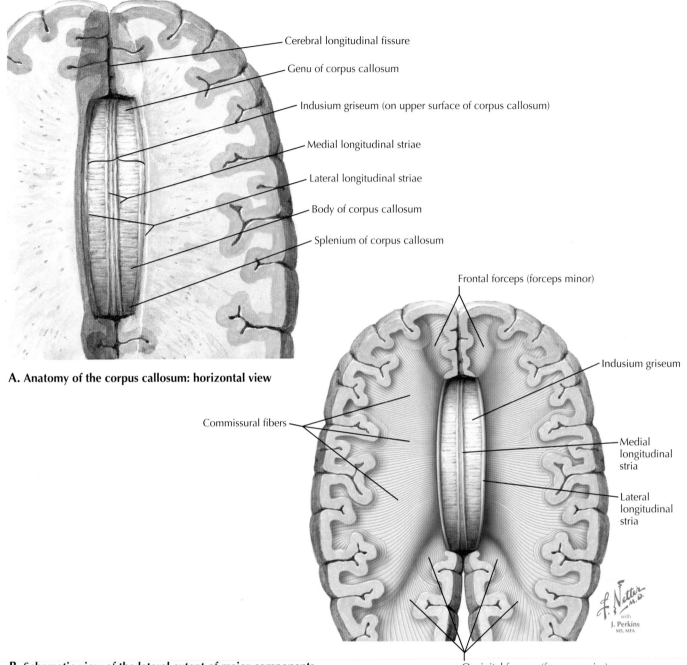

A. Anatomy of the corpus callosum: horizontal view

B. Schematic view of the lateral extent of major components

3.15 CORPUS CALLOSUM

A, Anatomy of the corpus callosum, horizontal view. The corpus callosum, the major fiber commissure between the hemispheres, is a conspicuous landmark in imaging studies. It is viewed from above after dissection of tissue just dorsal to its upper surface. Horizontal cuts taken deeper (more ventrally) section the genu anteriorly and the splenium posteriorly (see Fig. 3.13). **B,** Schematic view of the lateral extent of major components. Many of the commissural fibers of the corpus callosum, particularly the forceps of commissural fibers that interconnect frontal areas with each other and occipital areas with each other, extend rostrally and caudally, respectively, after crossing the midline. These interconnections allow communication between the hemispheres for coordinated activity of these two "separate" hemispheres.

Lateral fibers
of corpus
callosum

Genu

Cortical
association
fibers

Splenium

A. Axial view

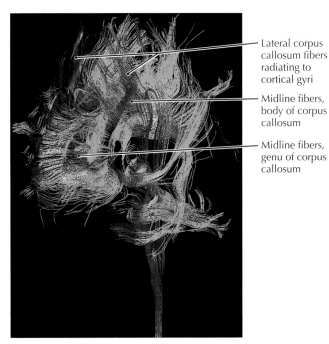

Lateral corpus
callosum fibers
radiating to
cortical gyri

Midline fibers,
body of corpus
callosum

Midline fibers,
genu of corpus
callosum

B. Oblique sagittal view

Forceps minor

Genu

Body

Lateral fibers
of corpus callosum

Splenium

Forceps major

C. Axial view

3.16 COLOR IMAGING OF THE CORPUS CALLOSUM BY DIFFUSION TENSOR IMAGING

A-C, Diffusion-weighted imaging (DWI), also called diffusion tensor imaging (DTI), provides unique information about tissue viability, architecture, and cellular function. In many tissues, restricted water diffusion is isotropic or independent of direction. In structured tissues, such as cerebral white matter and peripheral nerves, diffusion is anisotropic because of cellular arrangements. By using diffusion sensitivity that projects in multiple directions, such diffusion can be evaluated in the form of a tensor. Tensor field calculations for six or more diffusion-weighted measurements are based on an analytical solution of the Stejskal and Tanner diffusion equation system. Diffusion tensor imaging permits reconstruction of axonal tracts in brain and spinal cord; the three-dimensional architecture of the white matter tracts can be traced based on eigenvectors of the diffusion tensor. To discriminate fiber bundles that radiate in different directions, a color scheme is adopted in which green represents eigenvectors pointing in anteroposterior directions; red represents eigenvectors radiating in left-right directions; and blue represents eigenvectors pointing in the superoinferior direction. In these images of the corpus callosum, components of this major commissural bundle are represented in red.

A. Dissection of the Hippocampal Formation and Fornix

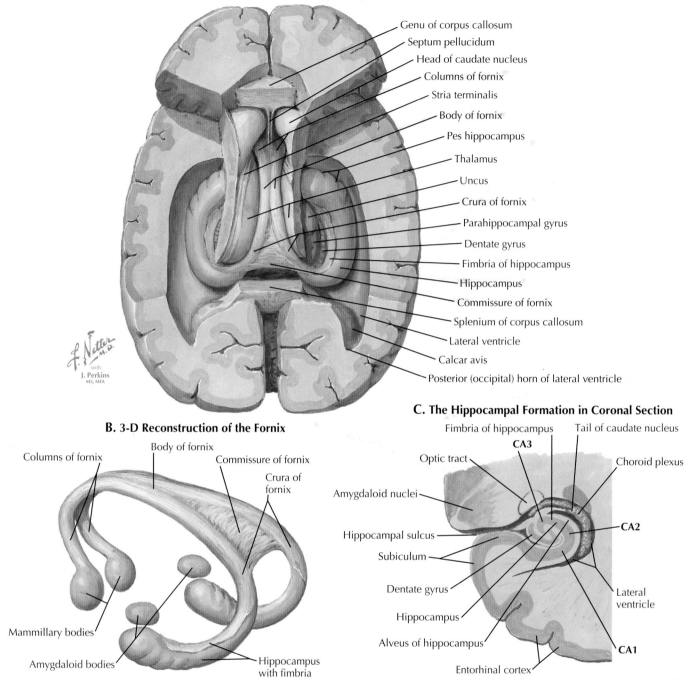

Genu of corpus callosum
Septum pellucidum
Head of caudate nucleus
Columns of fornix
Stria terminalis
Body of fornix
Pes hippocampus
Thalamus
Uncus
Crura of fornix
Parahippocampal gyrus
Dentate gyrus
Fimbria of hippocampus
Hippocampus
Commissure of fornix
Splenium of corpus callosum
Lateral ventricle
Calcar avis
Posterior (occipital) horn of lateral ventricle

B. 3-D Reconstruction of the Fornix

Columns of fornix
Body of fornix
Commissure of fornix
Crura of fornix
Mammillary bodies
Amygdaloid bodies
Hippocampus with fimbria

C. The Hippocampal Formation in Coronal Section

Fimbria of hippocampus
CA3
Tail of caudate nucleus
Optic tract
Choroid plexus
Amygdaloid nuclei
Hippocampal sulcus
CA2
Subiculum
Dentate gyrus
Lateral ventricle
Hippocampus
Alveus of hippocampus
CA1
Entorhinal cortex

3.17 HIPPOCAMPAL FORMATION AND FORNIX

In this dissection, the cortex, white matter, and corpus callosum have been removed. The lateral ventricles have been opened, and the head of the caudate nucleus and the thalamus have been dissected away quite close to the midline, allowing a downward view of the full extent of the hippocampal formation, including the dentate gyrus and the associated fornix. This view reveals the relationship between the hippocampus proper and the dentate gyrus. The two limbs of the fornix sweep upward medially, eventually running side by side at their most dorsal position, just beneath the corpus callosum. The full extent of this arching, C-shaped bundle is shown in the left lower image. The hippocampal formation occupies a large portion of the temporal pole of the lateral ventricle. The dentate gyrus is adjacent to subcomponents of the cornu ammonis (CA) regions of the hippocampus proper (the CA1 and CA3 regions, the subiculum, and the entorhinal cortex). Pyramidal neurons in the CA1 region are particularly sensitive to ischemic damage, and their counterparts in the CA3 region are sensitive to damage from high levels of corticosteroids (cortisol). Damage to pyramidal cells in both regions that has been caused by ischemia or high levels of corticosteroids is synergistic.

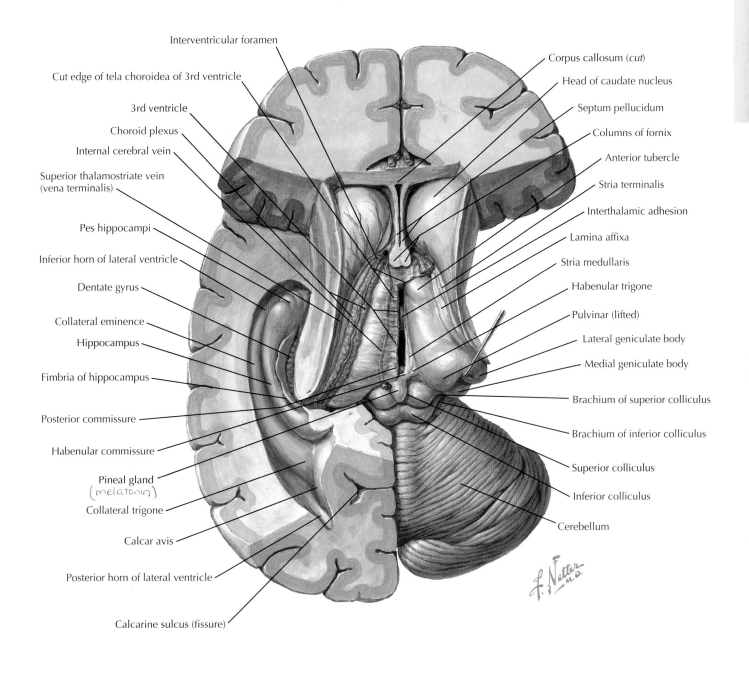

Interventricular foramen

Cut edge of tela choroidea of 3rd ventricle

3rd ventricle

Choroid plexus

Internal cerebral vein

Superior thalamostriate vein
(vena terminalis)

Pes hippocampi

Inferior horn of lateral ventricle

Dentate gyrus

Collateral eminence

Hippocampus

Fimbria of hippocampus

Posterior commissure

Habenular commissure

Pineal gland
(melatonin)

Collateral trigone

Calcar avis

Posterior horn of lateral ventricle

Calcarine sulcus (fissure)

Corpus callosum (cut)

Head of caudate nucleus

Septum pellucidum

Columns of fornix

Anterior tubercle

Stria terminalis

Interthalamic adhesion

Lamina affixa

Stria medullaris

Habenular trigone

Pulvinar (lifted)

Lateral geniculate body

Medial geniculate body

Brachium of superior colliculus

Brachium of inferior colliculus

Superior colliculus

Inferior colliculus

Cerebellum

3.18 THALAMIC ANATOMY

The thalamus is viewed from above. The entire right side of the brain, just lateral to the thalamus, has been removed, the head of the caudate nucleus has been sectioned, the corpus callosum and all tissue dorsal to the thalamus have been removed, and the third ventricle has been opened from its dorsal surface. The pineal gland is present in the midline, just caudal to the third ventricle; it produces melatonin, a hormone that helps regulate circadian rhythms, sleep, and immune responses.

The superior and inferior colliculi are shown, depicting the dorsal surface of the midbrain. On the left, the temporal horn of the lateral ventricle, with the hippocampal formation, has been exposed to show the relationship of these structures to the thalamus. The terminal vein and choroid plexus accompany the stria terminalis along the lateral margin of the thalamus. The stria medullaris runs along the medial surface of the dorsal thalamus.

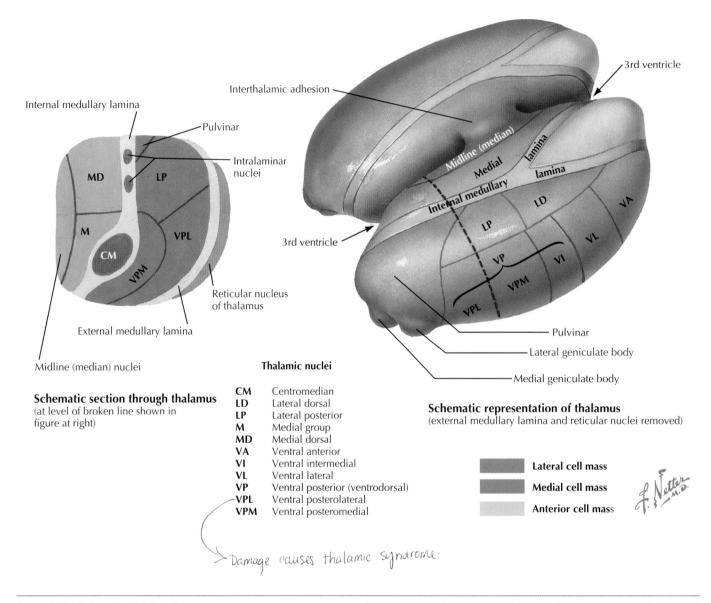

Internal medullary lamina

Interthalamic adhesion

3rd ventricle

Pulvinar

Intralaminar nuclei

MD

LP

M

VPL

CM

VPM

External medullary lamina

3rd ventricle

Midline (median)

Medial

Internal medullary

lamina

lamina

LD

VA

LP

VL

VP

VI

VPM

VPL

Reticular nucleus of thalamus

Pulvinar

Lateral geniculate body

Medial geniculate body

Midline (median) nuclei

Schematic section through thalamus
(at level of broken line shown in figure at right)

Thalamic nuclei

CM	Centromedian
LD	Lateral dorsal
LP	Lateral posterior
M	Medial group
MD	Medial dorsal
VA	Ventral anterior
VI	Ventral intermedial
VL	Ventral lateral
VP	Ventral posterior (ventrodorsal)
VPL	Ventral posterolateral
VPM	Ventral posteromedial

Damage causes thalamic syndrome

Schematic representation of thalamus
(external medullary lamina and reticular nuclei removed)

Lateral cell mass

Medial cell mass

Anterior cell mass

3.19 THALAMIC NUCLEI

The thalamus is subdivided into nuclear groups (medial, lateral, and anterior) that are separated by medullary (white matter) lamina. Many of these thalamic nuclei are "specific" thalamic nuclei that are reciprocally connected with discrete regions of the cerebral cortex. Some nuclei, such as those embedded within the internal medullary lamina (intralaminar nuclei such as the centromedian and parafascicular nuclei) and the outer, lateral shell nucleus (reticular nucleus of the thalamus), have very diffuse, nonspecific associations with the cerebral cortex.

CLINICAL POINT

Thalamic syndrome (posterolateral thalamic syndrome, or De-jerine-Roussy syndrome) results from obstruction of the thalamo-geniculate arterial supply to the region of the thalamus where the ventroposterolateral nucleus is located. Initially, all sensation is lost in the contralateral body, epicritic more completely than protopathic. Commonly, severe spontaneous pain occurs contralaterally, described as stabbing, burning, or tearing pain; it is diffuse and persistent. Even light stimulation can evoke such pain (hyperpathia), and other sensory stimuli or emotionally charged situations can result in these painful sensations. Even when the threshold for pain and temperature sensation (protopathic sensations) is elevated, the thalamic pain may be present; it is called analgesic dolorosa. If the vascular lesion includes the subthalamic nucleus or associated basal ganglia circuitry, the patient may also experience hemiballismus (or choreoform or athetoid) movements in addition to the sensory deficits.

4

BRAIN STEM AND CEREBELLUM

posterior view

Posterolateral View

Pulvinar

Pineal gland

Brachia of superior and inferior colliculi

Superior colliculi

Inferior colliculi

Superior medullary velum

Medial eminence

Rhomboid fossa of 4th ventricle

Facial colliculus

Cuneate tubercle

Gracile tubercle

Dorsal roots of 1st spinal nerve (C1)

Fasciculus cuneatus

Fasciculus gracilis

Thalamus

Optic tract

Lateral geniculate body

Medial geniculate body

Cerebral peduncle

Trochlear (IV) nerve

Pons   *CN 5*

Trigeminal (V) nerve   *@ mid pon*

Superior cerebellar peduncle

Middle cerebellar peduncle

Vestibulocochlear (VIII) nerve

Facial (VII) nerve

Inferior cerebellar peduncle

Vestibular area

Olive

Hypoglossal (XII) nerve

Glossopharyngeal (IX) and vagus (X) nerves

Hypoglossal trigone

Vagal trigone

Accessory (XI) nerve

FG FC

4.1 BRAIN STEM SURFACE ANATOMY: POSTEROLATERAL VIEW

The entire telencephalon, most of the diencephalon, and the cerebellum are removed to reveal the dorsal surface of the brain stem. The three cerebellar peduncles (superior, middle, and inferior) are sectioned and the cerebellum removed. The dorsal roots provide input into the spinal cord, and the cranial nerves provide input into and receive output from the brain stem. The fourth nerve (trochlear) is the only cranial nerve to exit dorsally from the brain stem. The tubercles and trigones on the floor of the fourth ventricle are named for nuclei just beneath them. The superior and inferior colliculi form the dorsal surface of the midbrain, and the medial and lateral geniculate nuclei (associated with auditory and visual processing, respectively) are shown at the caudalmost region of the diencephalon.

CLINICAL POINT

The facial colliculus is an elevation on the floor of the fourth ventricle in the pons under which is located the abducens nucleus (cranial nerve VI) and the axons of the facial nerve nucleus (VII), which arc around the abducens nucleus. A tumor or other lesion on one side of the floor of the fourth ventricle may induce symptoms related to cranial nerves VI and VII, including ipsilateral paralysis of lateral gaze (lateral rectus) and medial gaze (resulting from damage to nerve VI's interneurons, which ascend to the nucleus of CN III via the medial longitudinal fasciculus) as well as ipsilateral facial palsy.

The cerebellar peduncles convey the cerebellar afferent and efferent fibers. The superior peduncle conveys the major efferents to the red nucleus and thalamus (especially the ventrolateral nucleus), whereas the inferior peduncle conveys the major efferents to the vestibular and reticular nuclei. The middle peduncle conveys the cortico-ponto-cerebellar fibers. Afferents enter the cerebellum especially through the inferior peduncle but also through the superior peduncle. Damage to the lateral hemisphere of the cerebellum or its associated peduncles can result in ipsilateral symptoms, including limb ataxia, mild hypotonia, dysmetria (misjudgment of distance), decomposition of movement (especially movement involving several joints), intention tremor (with movement), dysdiadochokinesia (inability to perform rapid alternating movements), and inability to dampen movements appropriately (rebound phenomena).

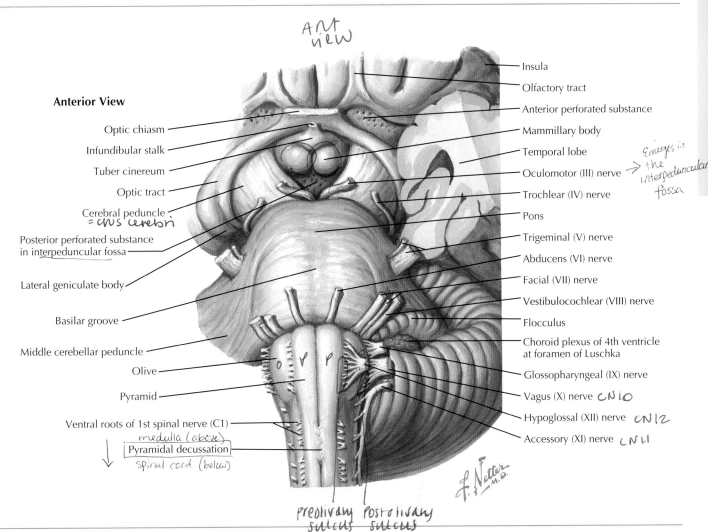

Anterior View

ANT view *(handwritten)*

Optic chiasm
Infundibular stalk
Tuber cinereum
Optic tract
Cerebral peduncle
= cns cerebri *(handwritten)*
Posterior perforated substance in interpeduncular fossa
Lateral geniculate body
Basilar groove
Middle cerebellar peduncle
Olive
Pyramid
Ventral roots of 1st spinal nerve (C1)
medulla (above) *(handwritten)*
Pyramidal decussation
spinal cord (below) *(handwritten)*

Insula
Olfactory tract
Anterior perforated substance
Mammillary body
Temporal lobe
Oculomotor (III) nerve — Emerges in the interpeduncular fossa *(handwritten)*
Trochlear (IV) nerve
Pons
Trigeminal (V) nerve
Abducens (VI) nerve
Facial (VII) nerve
Vestibulocochlear (VIII) nerve
Flocculus
Choroid plexus of 4th ventricle at foramen of Luschka
Glossopharyngeal (IX) nerve
Vagus (X) nerve CN 10 *(handwritten)*
Hypoglossal (XII) nerve CN 12 *(handwritten)*
Accessory (XI) nerve CN 11 *(handwritten)*

preolivary postolivary sulcus sulcus *(handwritten)*

4.2 BRAIN STEM SURFACE ANATOMY: ANTERIOR VIEW

The left temporal lobe is dissected to show the anterior (ventral) surface of the brain stem. The cerebral peduncles, direct caudal extensions of the posterior limb of the internal capsules, carry corticospinal and corticobulbar fibers from the internal capsule to the spinal cord and brain stem, respectively. The decussation of the pyramids marks the boundary between the caudal medulla and the cervical spinal cord. Cranial nerve XI (accessory) is associated with the lateral margin of the upper cervical spinal cord. Cranial nerves XII (hypoglossal), X (vagus), and IX (glossopharyngeal) emerge from the ventrolateral margin of the medulla. Cranial nerves VI (abducens), VII (facial), and VIII (vestibulocochlear) emerge from the boundary between the medulla and the pons. Cranial nerve V (trigeminal) emerges from the lateral margin of the upper pons. Cranial nerve III (oculomotor) emerges from the interpeduncular fossa in the medial portion of the caudal midbrain. The optic nerve, chiasm, and tract (cranial nerve II) and the olfactory tract (cranial nerve I) are not peripheral nerves; they are central nervous system tracts that were mistakenly called cranial nerves by anatomists in centuries past.

CLINICAL POINT

The oculomotor nerve (III) emerges from the ventral surface of the brain stem in the interpeduncular fossa, at the medial edge of the cerebral peduncle. In conditions of increased intracranial pressure in the anterior and middle cranial fossa, such as that caused by a tumor, edema from injury, or other space-occupying lesions, the brain stem can herniate through the tentorium cerebelli, a rigid wing of dura. The resultant transtentorial herniation can compress the third nerve on one side (ipsilateral fixed and dilatated pupil resulting from parasympathetic disruption and paralysis of medial gaze resulting from motor fiber disruption) and compress the cerebral peduncle on that same side, resulting in contralateral hemiparesis.

The medullary pyramids contain the descending corticospinal tract fibers from the ipsilateral cerebral cortex, particularly from the motor and premotor cortex. The major crossing of the corticospinal tract takes place in the decussation of the pyramids (80%), producing the crossed, descending, lateral corticospinal tract in the spinal cord. An infarct in the upper reaches of the anterior spinal artery or the paramedian branches of the vertebral artery can result in damage to the ipsilateral pyramid (contralateral hemiparesis); to the ipsilateral medial lemniscus (contralateral loss of epicritic somatosensory sensations such as fine, discriminative touch, vibratory sensation, and joint position sense); and the ipsilateral hypoglossal nerve (cranial nerve XII; paralysis of the ipsilateral tongue, which deviates toward the weak side when protruded). This condition is called Dejerine's syndrome. The hemiparesis is not spastic and is characterized by mild loss of tone, loss of fine hand movements, and a plantar extensor response (Babinski's sign). It appears that isolated damage to the pyramids does not result in spasticity. Damage to other descending systems, from either the motor-related cortices or the upper motor neurons, must accompany pyramidal tract damage to produce spasticity. Thus, the term *pyramidal tract syndrome,* when used to describe spastic hemiplegia, is a misnomer and is anatomically incorrect.

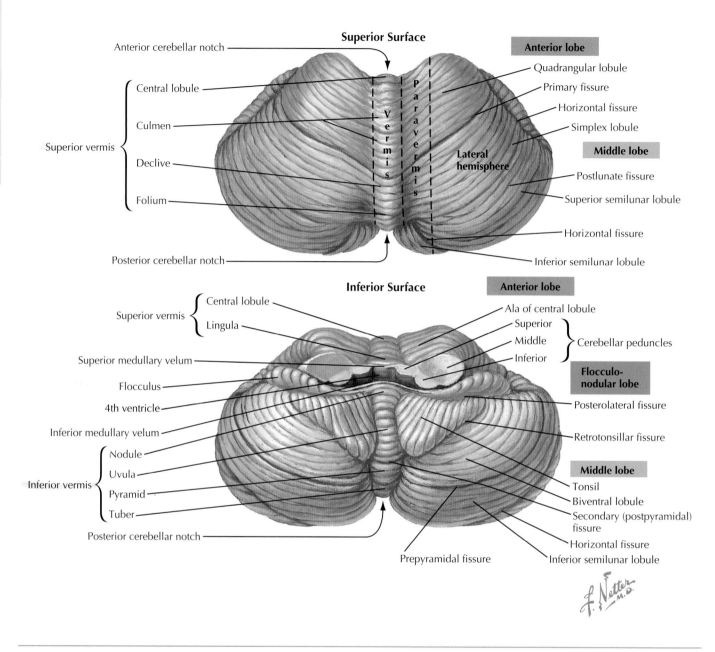

Superior Surface

Anterior cerebellar notch

Central lobule

Culmen

Superior vermis

Declive

Folium

Posterior cerebellar notch

Vermis

Paravermis

Lateral
hemisphere

Anterior lobe

Quadrangular lobule

Primary fissure

Horizontal fissure

Simplex lobule

Middle lobe

Postlunate fissure

Superior semilunar lobule

Horizontal fissure

Inferior semilunar lobule

Inferior Surface

Superior vermis

Central lobule

Lingula

Superior medullary velum

Flocculus

4th ventricle

Inferior medullary velum

Inferior vermis

Nodule

Uvula

Pyramid

Tuber

Posterior cerebellar notch

Prepyramidal fissure

Anterior lobe

Ala of central lobule

Superior

Middle

Inferior

Cerebellar peduncles

**Flocculo-
nodular lobe**

Posterolateral fissure

Retrotonsillar fissure

Middle lobe

Tonsil

Biventral lobule

Secondary (postpyramidal)
fissure

Horizontal fissure

Inferior semilunar lobule

4.3 CEREBELLAR ANATOMY: EXTERNAL FEATURES

These color-coded illustrations show the superior (dorsal) surface and the inferior (ventral) surface of the cerebellum. The cerebellar peduncles are cut to provide this view. The ventral surface of the cerebellum is the roof of the fourth ventricle. The anterior, middle, and flocculo-nodular lobes of the cerebellum are traditional anatomic subdivisions with well-described syndromes derived from lesions. The vermis, paravermis, and lateral hemispheres are cerebellar cortical zones that have specific projection relationships with deep cerebellar nuclei (vermis with fastigial nucleus and lateral vestibular nucleus; paravermis with globose and emboliform nuclei; lateral hemispheres with dentate nucleus) which, in turn, provide neuronal feedback to specific upper motor neuronal systems that regulate specific types of motor responses. These relationships are key to understanding how the major upper motor neuronal systems are coordinated for specific functional tasks.

CLINICAL POINT

The anterior lobe of the cerebellum (paleocerebellum) receives extensive input from the proprioceptors of the body, particularly the limbs, via the spinocerebellar tracts. This region is particularly important for coordination of the lower limbs. The anterior cerebellum also helps to regulate tone in the limbs via connections to the lateral vestibular nucleus. In some alcoholic patients, the anterior lobe of the cerebellum shows selective cortical degeneration. The patient shows a wide-based stance and gait with some ataxia but little involvement of dysarthria or oculomotor dysfunction. The gait tends to be stiff-legged, probably reflecting disinhibition of the extensor-dominant lateral vestibular nucleus. Typically, heel to shin testing is not severely impaired when the patient is tested while lying down. Few treatment options are available.

Section in Plane of Superior Cerebellar Peduncle

Decussation of superior cerebellar peduncles

Cerebral peduncle

Medial longitudinal fasciculus

4th ventricle

Superior medullary velum

Superior cerebellar peduncle

Fastigial nucleus

Globose nuclei

Lingula

Dentate nucleus

Cerebellar cortex

Emboliform nucleus

Vermis

4.4 CEREBELLAR ANATOMY: INTERNAL FEATURES

The major internal subdivisions of the cerebellum are shown in this transverse section. The outer zone, the cerebellar cortex (three-layered), is infolded to form numerous folia. Deep to the folia is the white matter, carrying afferent and efferent fibers associated with the cerebellar cortex. Deep to the white matter are the deep cerebellar nuclei, cell groups that receive most of the output from the cerebellar cortex via Purkinje cell axon projections. The deep cerebellar nuclei also receive collaterals from mossy fiber and climbing fiber inputs to the cerebellum. These direct afferent inputs to the deep nuclei provide a coarse adjustment for their output to upper motor neurons, whereas the loop of afferent input through the cerebellar cortex back to the deep nuclei provides fine adjustments for their output to upper motor neurons. The cerebellar peduncles are interior to the deep nuclei; these massive fiber bundles interconnect the cerebellum with the brain stem and the thalamus.

5

SPINAL CORD

Anterior View

Atlas (C1)
Axis (C2)
C7
T1
T12
L1
L5
Sacrum (S1–5)
Coccyx

Left Lateral View

Atlas (C1)
Axis (C2)
C7
T1
Intervertebral disc
Body
T12
L1
Spinous process
Transverse process
Lamina
Pedicle
L5
Sacrum (S1–5)
Coccyx

Posterior View

5.1 SPINAL COLUMN: BONY ANATOMY

Anterior, lateral, and posterior views of the bony spinal column show the relationships of the intervertebral discs with the vertebral bodies. The discs' proximity to the intervertebral foramina provides an anatomical substrate for understanding the possible impingement of a herniated nucleus pulposus on spinal roots. Such impingement can cause excruciating, radiating pain if dorsal roots are involved and can cause loss of motor control of affected muscles if ventral roots are involved. In the adult, the spinal cord extends caudally only as far as the L1 vertebral body, leaving the lumbar cistern (the subarachnoid space) accessible for withdrawal of cerebrospinal fluid.

Anteroposterior Radiograph

Lateral Radiograph

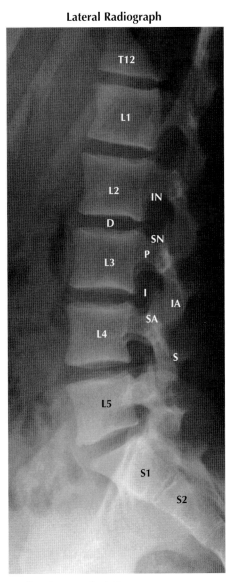

B	Body of L3 vertebra
IA	Inferior articular process of L1 vertebra
L	Lamina of L4 vertebra
P	Pedicle of L3 vertebra
S	Spinous process of L4 vertebra
SA	Superior articular process of L1 vertebra
SF	Sacral foramen
T	Transverse process of L3 vertebra

D	Intervertebral disc space
I	Intervertebral foramen
IA	Inferior articular process of L3 vertebra
IN	Inferior vertebral notch of L2 vertebra
P	Pedicle of L3 vertebra
S	Spinous process of L3 vertebra
SA	Superior articular process of L4 vertebra
SN	Superior vertebral notch of L3 vertebra
Note:	The vertebral bodies are numbered

5.2 LUMBAR VERTEBRAE: RADIOGRAPHY

These lumbar radiographs show the lumbar spine in an anteroposterior view and a lateral view. The vertebral bodies, with their spinous and transverse processes, are visible, and the spaces occupied by the intervertebral discs are uniform and symmetrical in a normal radiograph. A herniated disc may show a disruption of that symmetry. However, the presence of lumbar radiculopathy and a herniated disc is not always accompanied by radiographic abnormalities.

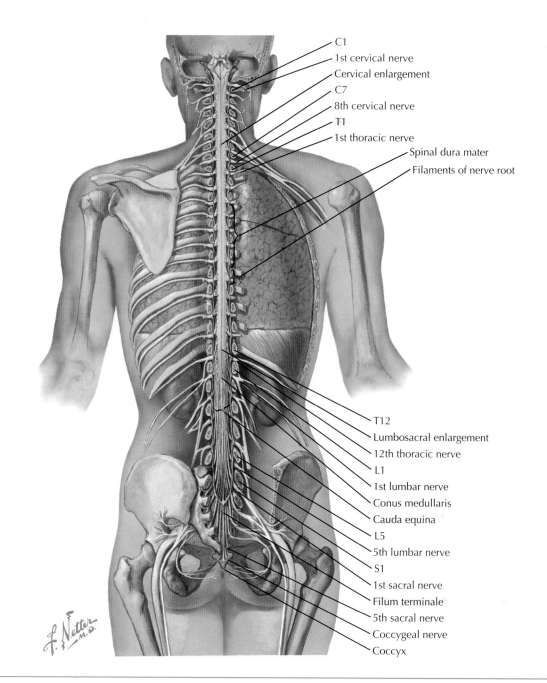

C1
1st cervical nerve
Cervical enlargement
C7
8th cervical nerve
T1
1st thoracic nerve
Spinal dura mater
Filaments of nerve root
T12
Lumbosacral enlargement
12th thoracic nerve
L1
1st lumbar nerve
Conus medullaris
Cauda equina
L5
5th lumbar nerve
S1
1st sacral nerve
Filum terminale
5th sacral nerve
Coccygeal nerve
Coccyx

5.3 SPINAL CORD: GROSS ANATOMY IN SITU

The posterior portions of the vertebrae have been removed to show the posterior (dorsal) surface of the spinal cord. Cervical and lumbosacral enlargements of the spinal cord reflect innervation of the limbs. The spinal cord extends rostrally through the foramen magnum, continuous with the medulla. The conus medullaris is located under the L1 vertebral body. The longitudinal growth of the spinal column exceeds that of the spinal cord, causing the spinal cord to end considerably more rostrally in the adult than in the newborn. The associated nerve roots traverse a considerable distance through the subarachnoid space, particularly more caudally in the lumbar cistern, to reach the appropriate intervertebral foramina of exit. In the lumbar cistern, this collection of nerve roots is called the cauda equina (horse's tail). The lumbar cistern is a large reservoir from which cerebrospinal fluid can be withdrawn.

The filum terminale helps to anchor the spinal cord caudally to the coccyx.

CLINICAL POINT

In the adult, the spinal cord ends at the level of the L1 vertebral body, and the roots extend caudally in the cauda equine to exit in the appropriate intervertebral foramina. As a consequence, a large lumbar cistern is filled with cerebrospinal fluid (CSF); from this cistern, samples can be drawn in a spinal tap with little risk for neurological damage by the needle. Analysis of CSF is a vitally important part of neurological assessment in many conditions, such as infections, bleeds, inflammatory conditions, some degenerative conditions, and other disorders. The CSF is commonly analyzed for color and appearance, viscosity, cytology, and the presence of red and white blood cells, protein, and glucose. It should be noted that in some conditions in which intracranial pressure is elevated, withdrawal of CSF from the lumbar cistern may encourage brain stem herniation through the foramen magnum.

Posterior View

Rami communicantes

Dura mater

Dorsal root

Dorsal root (spinal) ganglion

Arachnoid

Mesothelial septum in posterior median sulcus

Subarachnoid space

Pia mater (overlying spinal cord)

Filaments of dorsal root

Denticulate ligament

Anterior View

Gray matter

Lateral funiculus

Spinal cord with meninges stripped away

Filaments of dorsal root

White matter

Dorsal root

Dorsal root (spinal) ganglion

Spinal nerve

Ventral root

Filaments of ventral root

Anterior median fissure

Anterior funiculus

5.4 THE SPINAL CORD: ITS MENINGES AND SPINAL ROOTS

The upper illustration is a posterior (dorsal) view of the spinal cord showing both intact and reflected meninges. The pia adheres to every contour of the spinal cord surface. The arachnoid extends over these contours and adheres to the overlying dura, a very tough, fibrous, and protective membrane. These meninges extend outward to the nerve roots. The denticulate ligaments are fibrous structures that help to anchor the spinal cord in place. The posterior spinal arteries supply the dorsal spinal cord with blood and run just medial to the dorsal root entry zone. The lower illustration shows an anterior (ventral) view of the spinal cord with the meninges stripped away. Both the dorsal and the ventral roots consist of a convergence of rootlets that provide a continuous dorsal and ventral array of rootlets along the entire longitudinal extent of the spinal cord.

CLINICAL POINT

Groups of contiguous dorsal and ventral spinal rootlets converge to form the major dorsal and ventral roots associated with each level of the spinal cord. Herniation of an intervertebral disc, usually resulting from a flexion injury, may cause the nucleus pulposus to extrude in a posterolateral direction and impinge on a dorsal root. The L5–S1 and L4–L5 discs are most commonly involved in the lower extremities, and the C6–C7, C5–C6, and C4–C5 in the upper extremities. Sharp, radiating pain in the territory of the nerve root is the most common symptom. In some disc herniations, a specific muscle-stretch reflex may be absent or diminished. When there is compression of a dorsal root, there will not be a corresponding nerve root territory in which anesthesia is present, unlike in a branch lesion of the trigeminal nerve; the dorsal roots send sensory axons to at least three dermatomal segments and have sufficient overlap that an isolated root lesion is unlikely to produce complete anesthesia in that territory. Compression of a ventral root because of disc herniation is less common than that of a dorsal root; it may be accompanied by significant weakness in the muscles supplied by that ventral root.

A. Section through thoracic vertebra

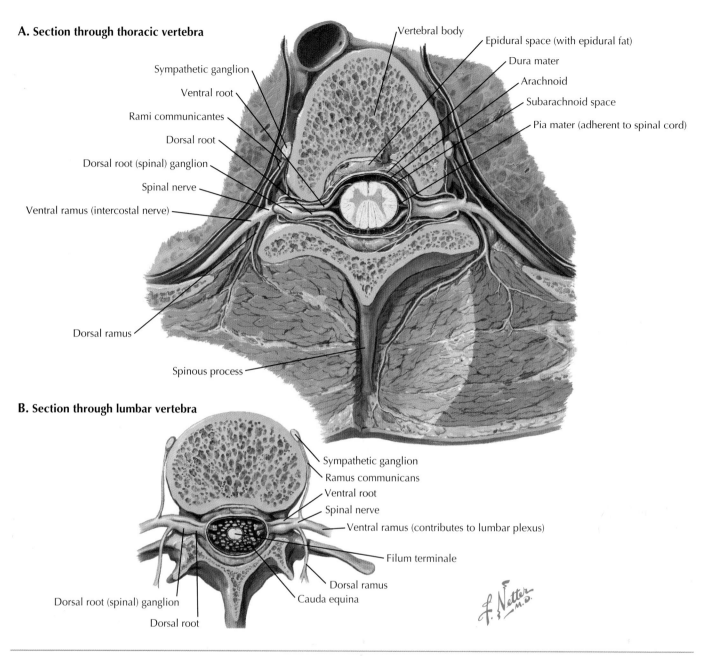

Vertebral body

Epidural space (with epidural fat)

Dura mater

Arachnoid

Subarachnoid space

Pia mater (adherent to spinal cord)

Sympathetic ganglion

Ventral root

Rami communicantes

Dorsal root

Dorsal root (spinal) ganglion

Spinal nerve

Ventral ramus (intercostal nerve)

Dorsal ramus

Spinous process

B. Section through lumbar vertebra

Sympathetic ganglion

Ramus communicans

Ventral root

Spinal nerve

Ventral ramus (contributes to lumbar plexus)

Filum terminale

Dorsal ramus

Cauda equina

Dorsal root (spinal) ganglion

Dorsal root

5.5 SPINAL CORD: CROSS-SECTIONAL ANATOMY IN SITU

A, The spinal cord in the spinal canal is surrounded by meninges. Dorsal and ventral roots course through the intervertebral foramina. The epidural space, with its associated fat, is sometimes used for the infusion of anesthetics. Arteries and veins are associated with the spinal nerves and nerve roots. Some segmental arteries provide crucial anastomotic channels for blood flow from the aorta to augment flow from the anterior and posterior spinal arterial systems, which cannot sustain the entire spinal cord; surgical procedures affecting blood flow through the aorta may affect the spinal cord. The sympathetic chain ganglia (paravertebral), important for fight-or-flight responses, lie adjacent to the vertebral body ventrally. The dorsal and ventral rami of the spinal nerves provide innervation to specific regions. The spinous process of the vertebral body extends dorsally, where it can be palpated by physical exam. **B,** The subarachnoid space of a lumbar vertebra, containing the filum terminale and roots of the cauda equina.

CLINICAL POINT

The dorsal and ventral roots travel through the adjacent subarachnoid space and join to form the peripheral nerves. These nerve roots and resultant nerves are sometimes the targets of acute, autoimmune, inflammatory demyelinating conditions (polyradiculoneuropathy), called Guillain-Barré syndrome (GBS). GBS is an acute, progressive, symmetrical weakness that progresses from distal to proximal in the limbs and may result in total paralysis of all musculature, including respiratory musculature, occurring over the course of hours to days. The weakness is often accompanied by paresthesias in the distal extremities. GBS is commonly preceded by an infectious process, such as *Campylobacter jejuni* enteritis, Epstein-Barr syndrome, or cytomegaloviral infections, or by *Mycoplasma pneumoniae*, which presumably triggers the autoimmune attack on peripheral myelin. Most patients recover through a remyelinating process, which may take a year or more, although at least 10% are left with severe deficits, and a small percent of individuals die.

A. Sections through spinal cord at various levels

C5   T2   T8   L1   L3   S1   S3

B. Principal fiber tracts of spinal cord (composite)

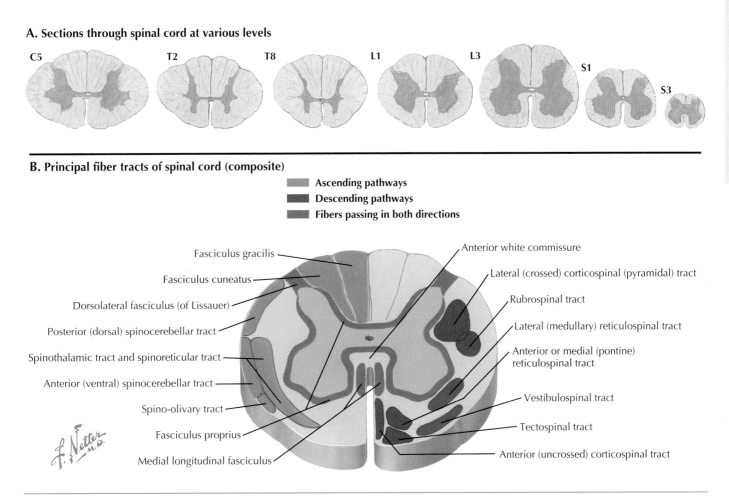

Ascending pathways
Descending pathways
Fibers passing in both directions

Fasciculus gracilis

Fasciculus cuneatus

Dorsolateral fasciculus (of Lissauer)

Posterior (dorsal) spinocerebellar tract

Spinothalamic tract and spinoreticular tract

Anterior (ventral) spinocerebellar tract

Spino-olivary tract

Fasciculus proprius

Medial longitudinal fasciculus

Anterior white commissure

Lateral (crossed) corticospinal (pyramidal) tract

Rubrospinal tract

Lateral (medullary) reticulospinal tract

Anterior or medial (pontine) reticulospinal tract

Vestibulospinal tract

Tectospinal tract

Anterior (uncrossed) corticospinal tract

5.6 SPINAL CORD: WHITE AND GRAY MATTER

A, Seven representative spinal cord levels. The images depict their relative sizes and the variability in the amount of gray matter at each level. Levels associated with the limbs have greater amounts of gray matter. White matter increases in absolute amount from caudal to rostral, reflecting the level-by-level addition of ascending tracts and the termination of descending tracts. B, The gray matter consists of dorsal and ventral horns, and in the T1–L2 segments, there is an inter-mediolateral cell column (lateral horn) where preganglionic sympathetic neurons reside. The white matter is subdivided into dorsal, lateral, and ventral funiculi, each containing multiple tracts (fasciculi, bundles). The tracts conveying pain and temperature information rostrally travel in the anterolateral funiculus, the spinothalamic/spinoreticular system. Fine discriminative sensation is conveyed through the dorsal funiculus. The major descending upper motor neuronal tract, the corticospinal tract, travels mainly in the lateral funiculus, with a component present in the medial part of the anterior funiculus. Dorsal root entry zones and ventral root exit zones are present at each cross-sectional level.

necessary for the afferent and efferent innervation of the limbs. The lower motor neurons (LMNs) in these enlargements are particularly vulnerable to poliovirus. Acute poliomyelitis results in the death of some LMNs, with resultant denervation of corresponding muscles, atrophy, flaccid paralysis, and loss of tone and reflexes. Remaining LMNs that survive the viral infection may sprout axons to reoccupy the sites on skeletal muscles left denuded by death of their original LMNs. These remaining LMNs then possess larger motor units (in-nervate more muscle fibers per cell body); this extra burden may account for some of the later degeneration and weakness seen in post-polio syndrome many decades after the acute disease. Polio is unusual in the United States and Western countries but still occurs in some developing nations.

The ascending and descending tracts are clustered in specific zones of the dorsal (posterior), lateral, and ventral (anterior) funiculi. Some regions of these funiculi are selectively vulnerable to vitamin B_{12} (cobalamin) deficiency; impairment of methylmalonyl-CoA mutase results in damage to myelinated fibers. Pernicious anemia may pre-cede neurological symptoms by months or years. Damage involves the dorsal funiculi and components of the lateral funiculi. Dorsal column damage is accompanied by paresthesias of the feet and legs and often of the hands and arms, with sensory ataxia and broad-based gait; by loss of vibratory sensation, joint position sense, and fine dis-criminatory touch; and by Romberg's sign. Lateral funiculus damage is accompanied by spastic paraparesis with increased tone and muscle stretch reflexes and plantar extensor responses. Early recognition of this condition and treatment with B_{12} can lead to rapid reversal and recovery.

CLINICAL POINT

The spinal cord levels show considerable variation in the size of the dorsal and ventral horns. The cervical and lumbosacral enlargements reflect the large number of sensory, intermediate, and motor neurons

6

VENTRICLES AND THE CEREBROSPINAL FLUID

Ventricles of Brain

Right lateral ventricle

Anterior (frontal) horn

Body

Inferior (temporal) horn

Posterior (occipital) horn

Left lateral ventricle

Cerebral aqueduct (of Sylvius)

4th ventricle

Left lateral aperture (foramen of Luschka)

Left lateral recess

Median aperture (foramen of Magendie)

Left interventricular foramen (of Monro)

3rd ventricle

Optic recess

Interthalamic adhesion

Infundibular recess

Pineal recess

Suprapineal recess

CSF Composition

	CSF	Blood plasma
Na$^+$ (mEq/L)	140–145	135–147
K$^+$ (mEq/L)	3	3.5–5.0
Cl$^-$ (mEq/L)	115–120	95–105
HCO$_3^-$ (mEq/L)	20	22–28
Glucose (mg/dL)	50–75	70–110
Protein (g/dL)	0.05–0.07	6.0–7.8
pH	7.3	7.35–7.45

6.1 VENTRICULAR ANATOMY

The lateral ventricles are C-shaped, reflecting their association with the developing telencephalon as it sweeps upward, back, and then down and forward as the temporal lobe. The position of the lateral ventricles in relation to the head and body of the caudate nucleus is an important radiological landmark in a variety of conditions, such as hydrocephalus, caudate atrophy in Huntington's disease, and shifting of the midline with a tumor. Cerebrospinal fluid (CSF) flows through the interventricular foramen of Monro into the narrow third ventricle, then into the cerebral aqueduct and the fourth ventricle. Blockage of flow in the aqueduct can precipitate internal hydrocephalus, with swelling of the ventricles rostral to the site of blockage. The escape sites where CSF can flow into expanded regions of the subarachnoid space called cisterns are the medial foramen of Magendie and the lateral foramina of Luschka. These foramina are additional sites where blockage of CSF flow can occur. The choroid plexus, extending into the ventricles, produces the CSF.

Corpus callosum
Right lateral ventricle
Body of caudate nucleus
Choroid plexus of lateral ventricle
Stria terminalis
Right thalamostriate vein
Body of fornix
Tela choroidea of 3rd ventricle
Choroid plexus of 3rd ventricle
Thalamus
Putamen _ _ _ _ _ _ _ _ _ _ _ _ _ _ _
Globus pallidus
(internal [i] and external [e] segments)
} Lentiform nucleus *of basal ganglia (gray matter)*
Internal capsule
3rd ventricle
Hypothalamus
Tail of caudate nucleus
Optic tract
Choroid plexus of lateral ventricle
Inferior (temporal) horn of lateral ventricle
Fimbria of hippocampus
Hippocampus
Dentate gyrus
Subiculum
Parahippocampal cortex
Entorhinal cortex

Coronal section of
brain (posterior view;
arrow in left
interventricular foramen)

Ependyma   Pia mater

6.2 VENTRICULAR ANATOMY IN CORONAL FOREBRAIN SECTION

A coronal section through the diencephalon shows the bodies of the lateral ventricles, the narrow interventricular foramina of Munro, and the midline third ventricle. The flow of CSF is from the lateral ventricles into the third ventricle. The choroid plexus protrudes into both the lateral and third ventricles and produces CSF. The temporal (inferior) pole of the lateral ventricle and its associated choroid plexus is shown in the temporal lobe.

Posterior View

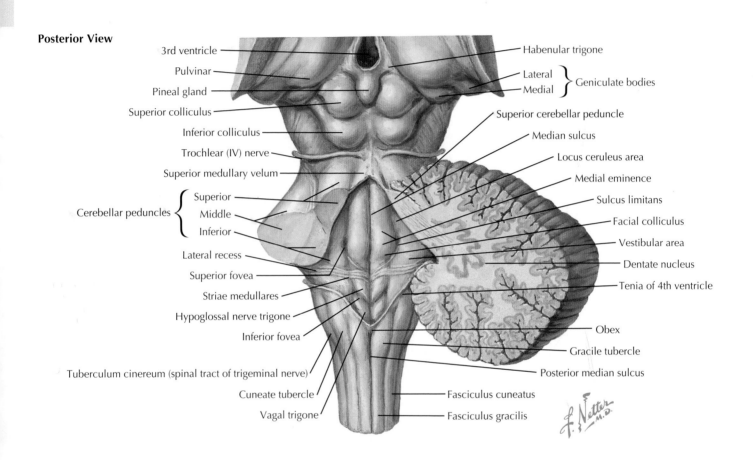

3rd ventricle

Pulvinar

Pineal gland

Superior colliculus

Inferior colliculus

Trochlear (IV) nerve

Superior medullary velum

Cerebellar peduncles { Superior
Middle
Inferior

Lateral recess

Superior fovea

Striae medullares

Hypoglossal nerve trigone

Inferior fovea

Tuberculum cinereum (spinal tract of trigeminal nerve)

Cuneate tubercle

Vagal trigone

Habenular trigone

Lateral
Medial } Geniculate bodies

Superior cerebellar peduncle

Median sulcus

Locus ceruleus area

Medial eminence

Sulcus limitans

Facial colliculus

Vestibular area

Dentate nucleus

Tenia of 4th ventricle

Obex

Gracile tubercle

Posterior median sulcus

Fasciculus cuneatus

Fasciculus gracilis

6.3 ANATOMY OF THE FOURTH VENTRICLE: POSTERIOR VIEW WITH CEREBELLUM REMOVED

The rhomboid-shaped fourth ventricle extends through the pons and medulla. The foramina of Magendie and Luschka must remain patent for proper flow of the CSF into the cisterns. Bilaterally symmetrical protrusions, depressions, and sulci on the floor of the fourth ventricle define the underlying anatomy of brain stem regions, such as the hypoglossal, vagal, and vestibular areas. Vital brain stem centers for cardiovascular, respiratory, and metabolic functions just below the floor of the fourth ventricle can be damaged by tumors in the region. The lateral margins of the fourth ventricle are embraced by the huge cerebellar peduncles interconnecting the cerebellum with the brain stem and diencephalon. These anatomical relationships are important when interpreting imaging studies in the compact brain stem regions where the diagnosis of tumors and vascular lesions is challenging.

Median Sagittal Section

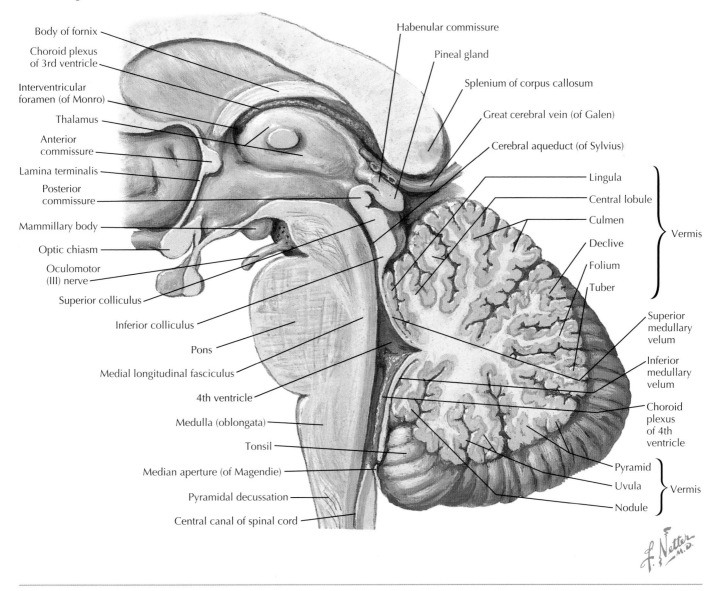

Body of fornix

Choroid plexus of 3rd ventricle

Interventricular foramen (of Monro)

Thalamus

Anterior commissure

Lamina terminalis

Posterior commissure

Mammillary body

Optic chiasm

Oculomotor (III) nerve

Superior colliculus

Inferior colliculus

Pons

Medial longitudinal fasciculus

4th ventricle

Medulla (oblongata)

Tonsil

Median aperture (of Magendie)

Pyramidal decussation

Central canal of spinal cord

Habenular commissure

Pineal gland

Splenium of corpus callosum

Great cerebral vein (of Galen)

Cerebral aqueduct (of Sylvius)

Lingula

Central lobule

Culmen

Declive

Folium

Tuber

Vermis

Superior medullary velum

Inferior medullary velum

Choroid plexus of 4th ventricle

Pyramid

Uvula

Nodule

Vermis

6.4 ANATOMY OF THE FOURTH VENTRICLE: LATERAL VIEW

In a midsagittal section, the rhomboid shape of the fourth ventricle is shown. Rostrally, the narrow cerebral aqueduct leads into the fourth ventricle; caudally, the foramen of Magendie provides for escape of CSF into a cistern of the subarachnoid space. CSF normally does not flow through the central canal of the spinal cord. The dorsal surface of the brain stem is on the floor of the fourth ventricle; the cerebral peduncles form the lateral boundaries; and the medullary velum and cerebellum form the roof of the fourth ventricle. The choroid plexus is present in the fourth ventricle. In the diencephalon, the shallow depression of the third ventricle and the interventricular foramen of Munro are shown.

CLINICAL POINT

The choroid plexus is the site of production of CSF in the lateral, third, and fourth ventricles. Even subtle changes in equilibrium between CSF production and absorption can result in altered intraventricular pressure and intracranial pressure. Hydrocephalus is most commonly caused by obstruction of outflow (internal hydrocephalus) or failure of appropriate absorption into the venous sinuses (external hydrocephalus). Occasionally, alterations in CSF production by the choroid plexus may occur. Inflammation of the choroid plexus or a papilloma can lead to hypersecretion hydrocephalus. In contrast, damage to the choroid plexus by radiation, trauma, or meningitis or secondary to lumbar puncture may result in diminished CSF production (hypoliquorrhea), with resultant long-lasting and persistent headache that is responsive to change in posture.

The CSF escapes from the ventricular system from the medial foramen of Magendie and the lateral foramina of Luschka of the fourth ventricle. These apertures must remain unobstructed in order to allow CSF to escape into the subarachnoid space, bathe the CNS, and then be absorbed into the venous sinuses through the arachnoid granulations. The foramen of Magendie is the most important of these apertures; it may become obstructed by tonsillar herniation into the foramen magnum as the result of Arnold-Chiari malformation; by a cerebellar tumor; or by an intraventricular tumor that obstructs the lower portion of the fourth ventricle. Such an obstruction at this lower level results in expansion of the entire ventricular system, including the fourth, third, and lateral ventricles.

MRI
_____
(T2)

A. Axial view

Subarachnoid space

Frontal pole, lateral ventricle

Interventricular foramen of Monro

Third ventricle

Temporal pole, lateral ventricle

Subarachnoid space

Frontal pole, lateral ventricle

Interventricular foramen of Monro

Third ventricle

Temporal pole, lateral ventricle

Cisterns around brain stem

B. Coronal view

6.5 MAGNETIC RESONANCE IMAGING OF THE VENTRICLES: AXIAL AND CORONAL VIEWS

A and **B,** These T2-weighted magnetic resonance images of the brain in axial and coronal sections demonstrate major components of the ventricular system (in white) and some cisternal structures. Both the frontal and temporal poles of the lateral ventricles are visible. Figure 3.11 also illustrates a T2-weighted midsagittal image, revealing the midsagittal ventricular system and related cisterns.

Bridging veins

Supracallosal cistern

Dura mater

Arachnoid

Choroid plexus of lateral ventricle

Superior sagittal sinus

Subarachnoid space

Arachnoid granulations

Chiasmatic cistern

Choroid plexus of 3rd ventricle

Interpeduncular cistern

Cerebral aqueduct (of Sylvius)

Prepontine cistern

Lateral aperture (foramen of Luschka)

Choroid plexus of 4th ventricle

Dura mater

Arachnoid

Subarachnoid space

Cistern of great cerebral vein

Cerebellomedullary cistern (cisterna magna)

Median aperture (foramen of Magendie)

Blockage or obstruction of flow of CSF ⟹ internal hydrocephalus (ventricular enlargement)

Disruption of drainage of CSF into venous drainage via arachnoid granulations ⟹ external hydrocephalus

6.6 CIRCULATION OF THE CEREBROSPINAL FLUID

CSF flows internally through the ventricles, from lateral ventricles to the third ventricle to the cerebral aqueduct to the fourth ventricle. The CSF passes through several points where blockage or obstruction could precipitate internal hydrocephalus and increased intracranial pressure. CSF flow from the fourth ventricle into the cisterns of the subarachnoid space, surrounding the brain and spinal cord, provides the external protective cushioning and buoyancy to protect underlying central nervous system tissue from minor trauma. Some cisterns such as the lumbar cistern provide sites for withdrawal of CSF (lumbar puncture). The CSF is absorbed from the subarachnoid space into the venous drainage through the arachnoid granulations by a process driven by the pressure of flow through these one-way valves. Disruption of this drainage results in external hydrocephalus. Thus, production, flow, and absorption of CSF must be in precise balance. The flow of the CSF in the ventricles also can act as a fluid-delivery system for downstream influences of specific mediators (e.g., prostaglandins, interleukins) and represents an internal paracrine communication channel for some structures close to the ventricles.

7

VASCULATURE

Arachnoid granulations

Opening of superior cerebral vein

Venous lacuna

Superior sagittal sinus

Dura mater

Parietal (posterior) and frontal (anterior) branches of middle meningeal artery

Middle meningeal artery

Anterior meningeal artery (from anterior ethmoidal artery)

Mastoid branch of occipital artery

Anterior and posterior meningeal branches of vertebral artery

Mastoid branch of occipital artery

Meningeal branches of ascending pharyngeal artery

Tentorial branch (cut) and dorsal meningeal branch of meningohypophyseal trunk

Middle and accessory meningeal arteries

Meningeal branch of posterior ethmoidal artery

Anterior meningeal artery (from anterior ethmoidal artery)

Internal carotid artery and its meningohypophyseal trunk (in phantom)

Middle meningeal artery

Accessory meningeal artery

Superficial temporal artery

Maxillary artery

Posterior auricular artery

Occipital artery

External carotid artery

ARTERIAL SYSTEM

7.1 MENINGEAL ARTERIES: RELATIONSHIP TO SKULL AND DURA

Meningeal arteries are found in the outer portion of the dura; they supply it with blood. They also help to supply blood to adjacent skull and have some anastomoses with cerebral arteries. The skull has grooves, or sulci, for the meningeal vessels. This relationship reflects an important functional consequence of skull fractures. Fractures can rip a meningeal artery (usually the middle meningeal artery) and allow arterial blood to accumulate above the dura. Such an epidural hematoma is a space-occupying mass and can produce increased intracranial pressure and risk for herniation of the brain, particularly across the free edge of the tentorium cerebelli. Even very fine fractures can have this dangerous consequence.

Left middle meningeal artery

Right and left posterior cerebral arteries

Right and left superior cerebellar arteries

Basilar artery

Mastoid branch of left occipital artery

Left interior auditory (labyrinthine) artery

Posterior meningeal branch of left ascending pharyngeal artery

Right and left anterior inferior cerebellar arteries

Right and left posterior inferior cerebellar arteries

Posterior meningeal branches of right and left vertebral arteries

Anterior meningeal branch of right vertebral artery

Right posterior auricular artery

Right occipital artery

Right interior carotid artery

Right ascending pharyngeal artery

Right carotid sinus

Right vertebral artery

Transverse process of C6

Right deep cervical artery

Right thyrocervical trunk

Right costocervical trunk

Right subclavian artery

Right and left middle cerebral arteries

Right and left anterior cerebral arteries

Anterior communicating artery

Right ophthalmic artery

Right posterior communicating artery

Cavernous sinus

Right deep temporal artery

Right maxillary artery

Right middle meningeal artery

Right superficial temporal artery

Right exterior carotid artery

Right facial artery

Right lingual artery

Carotid body

Right superior laryngeal artery

Right superior thyroid artery

Thyroid cartilage

Right common carotid artery

Right inferior thyroid artery

Right interior thoracic artery

Brachiocephalic trunk

7.2 ARTERIAL SUPPLY TO THE BRAIN AND MENINGES

The internal carotid artery (ICA) and the vertebral artery ascend through the neck and enter the skull to supply the brain with blood. The tortuous bends and sites of branching (such as the bifurcation of the common carotid artery into the internal and external carotids) produce turbulence of blood flow and are sites where atherosclerosis can occur. The bifurcation of the common carotid is particularly vulnerable to plaque formation and occlusion, threatening the major anterior part of the brain with ischemia, which would result in a stroke. The ICA passes through the cavernous sinus, a site where carotid-cavernous fistulae can occur, resulting in damage to the extra-ocular and trigeminal cranial nerves, which also pass through this sinus. Studies of blood flow through these arteries are important diagnostic tools. Magnetic resonance arteriography and Doppler flow studies have, for most purposes, replaced the older dye studies for performing cerebral angiography.

CLINICAL POINT

The paired carotid arteries and vertebral arteries supply the brain and part of the spinal cord with blood. The carotids supply the anterior circulation, including most of the forebrain except for the occipital lobe and inferior surface of the temporal lobe. The bifurcation of the common carotid artery is a common site of plaque formation in atherosclerosis, leading to gradual occlusion of blood flow to the forebrain on the ipsilateral side. Early warnings can be seen in the form of transient ischemic attacks, forerunners of a full-blown stroke. The best treatment is prevention, with exercise, proper diet and weight control, careful regulation of lipid levels and other contributing factors such as inflammatory mediators. In cases in which severe and symptomatic occlusion has occurred as the result of atherosclerotic plaque, carotid endarterectomy can be performed to remove the plaque and attempt to open up more robust flow to the anterior circulation. Carefully performed controlled studies have established criteria that determine which patients can best benefit from this surgical procedure as opposed to more conservative medical treatment. Current studies are investigating the use of carotid stents to enhance blood flow to the brain.

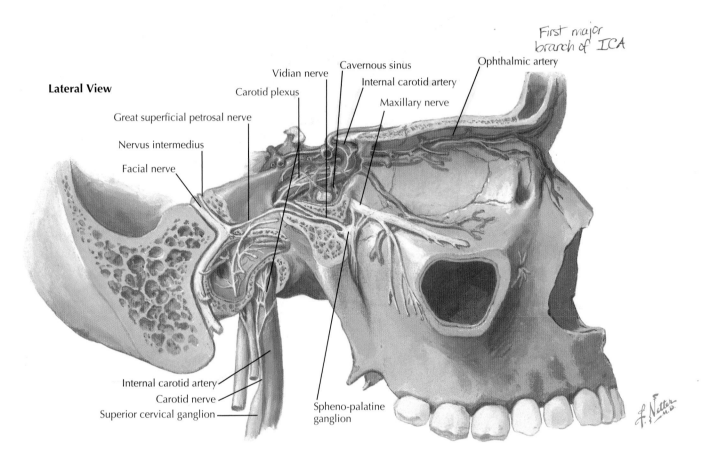

Lateral View

First major branch of ICA

Vidian nerve

Cavernous sinus

Ophthalmic artery

Internal carotid artery

Carotid plexus

Maxillary nerve

Great superficial petrosal nerve

Nervus intermedius

Facial nerve

Internal carotid artery

Carotid nerve

Superior cervical ganglion

Spheno-palatine ganglion

7.3 INTERNAL CAROTID AND OPHTHALMIC ARTERY COURSE

The ophthalmic artery is the first major branch of the ICA. It supplies the eyeball, ocular muscles, and adjacent structures. This artery is commonly involved in the first phases of clinical recognition of cerebrovascular disease. Because of its position as the first branch of the ICA, emboli from atherosclerotic arteries that are found at sites such as the bifurcation of the common carotid artery travel through the ophthalmic artery, resulting in a transient ischemic attack with the symptom of fleeting blindness in the affected eye.

Anterior communicating artery

Anterior cerebral artery

Recurrent artery (of Heubner)

Internal carotid artery

Medial and lateral lenticulostriate arteries

Middle cerebral artery

Lateral orbitofrontal artery

Ascending frontal (candelabra) branch

Anterior choroidal artery

Posterior communicating artery

Posterior cerebral artery

(SCA) Superior cerebellar artery

Basilar artery and pontine branches

Internal auditory (labyrinthine) artery

(AICA) Anterior inferior cerebellar artery

Vertebral artery

Anterior spinal artery

(PICA) Posterior inferior cerebellar artery

Posterior spinal artery

Circle of Willis

7.4 **ARTERIAL DISTRIBUTION TO THE BRAIN: BASAL VIEW**

The anterior circulation (middle and anterior cerebral arteries; MCAs, ACAs) and the posterior circulation (the vertebrobasilar system and its end branch, the posterior cerebral artery; PCA) and their major branches are shown. The right temporal pole is removed to show the course of the MCA through the lateral fissure. The circle of Willis (the paired ACAs, MCAs, and PCAs and the anterior and two posterior communicating arteries) surrounds the basal hypothalamic area. The circle of Willis appears to allow free flow of blood around the anterior and posterior circulation of both sides, but usually it is not sufficiently patent to allow bypass of an occluded zone.

CLINICAL POINT

The vertebrobasilar system supplies the posterior circulation of the brain, including most of the brain stem, part of the diencephalons, and the occipital and inferior temporal lobes of the forebrain. The paired PCAs are the end arteries of the vertebrobasilar system. An infarct in the PCAs (top of the basilar infarct) results in damage to the ipsilateral occipital lobe, including both the upper and lower banks of the calcarine fissure. Functionally, this infarct results in contralateral blindness, called contralateral homonymous hemianopia. There may be macular sparing if the MCA has some anastomoses with the posterior cerebral circulation.

Anterior communicating artery

Recurrent artery (of Heubner)

Anterior cerebral artery

Middle cerebral artery

Posterior communicating artery

Anterior choroidal artery

Optic tract

Cerebral peduncle

Lateral geniculate body

Posterior medial choroidal artery

Posterior lateral choroidal artery

Choroid plexus of lateral ventricle

Medial geniculate body

Pulvinar

Lateral ventricle

7.5 ARTERIAL DISTRIBUTION TO THE BRAIN: CUTAWAY BASAL VIEW SHOWING THE CIRCLE OF WILLIS

The circle of Willis and the course of the choroidal arteries are shown. The arteries supplying the brain are end arteries and do not have sufficient anastomotic channels with other arteries to sustain blood flow in the face of disruption. The occlusion of an artery supplying a specific territory of the brain results in functional damage that affects the performance of structures deprived of adequate blood flow.

CLINICAL POINT

Obstruction of the MCA near its origin is relatively unusual compared with obstruction or infarcts in selected branches, but it demonstrates the full range of blood supply of this critical artery. Obstruction near the origin usually results from embolization, not from atherosclerotic or thrombotic lesions. It causes contralateral hemiplegia (resolving to spastic), contralateral central facial palsy (lower face), contralateral hemianesthesia, contralateral homonymous hemianopia, and global aphasia if the left hemisphere is involved. Additional problems with anosognosia (inability to recognize a physical disability), contralateral neglect, and spatial disorientation may occur.

Frontal View with Hemispheres Retracted, Tilted for a View of the Ventral Brain Stem

Corpus callosum

Medial and lateral
lenticulostriate arteries

Lateral orbitofrontal artery

Ascending frontal
(candelabra) branch

Anterior and posterior
parietal branches

Precentral
(prerolandic)
and central
(rolandic)
branches

Angular branch

Temporal branches
(posterior, middle,
anterior)

**Middle cerebral
artery** and branches,
deep in lateral
cerebral (sylvian) fissure

Anterior commu-
nicating artery

Posterior commu-
nicating artery

Superior cerebellar artery

Anterior inferior cerebellar artery

Posterior spinal artery

End branch infarcts of MCA affect contralateral upper extremity

Paracentral artery

Frontal branches

Pericallosal artery

Callosomarginal artery

Frontopolar artery

**Anterior cerebral
arteries** ACA stroke
affects contralateral
lower limb

Medial orbito-
frontal artery

Recurrent artery
(of Heubner)

Interior carotid
artery

Anterior choroidal
artery

**Posterior cerebral
artery**

Basilar artery

Interior auditory
(labyrinthine) artery

Vertebral artery

Posterior inferior cerebellar artery

Anterior spinal artery

f. Netter M.D.

7.6 ARTERIAL DISTRIBUTION TO THE BRAIN: FRONTAL VIEW WITH HEMISPHERES RETRACTED

With the hemispheres retracted, the course of the ACAs and their distribution along the midline are visible. This artery supplies blood to the medial zones of the sensory and motor cortex, which are associated with the contralateral lower extremity; an ACA stroke thus affects the contralateral lower limb. With the lateral fissure opened up, the MCA is seen to course laterally and to give branches to the entire convexity of the hemisphere. End-branch infarcts of the MCA affect the contralateral upper extremity and, if on the left, also affect language function. More proximal MCA infarcts affecting the MCA distribution to the internal capsule can cause full contralateral hemiplegia with drooping of the contralateral lower face; this results from damage to corticospinal and other corticomotor fibers traveling in the posterior limb of the internal capsule and damage to corticobulbar fibers traveling in the genu of the internal capsule.

CLINICAL POINT

The ACA branches from the internal carotid as it splits from the middle cerebral artery. It supplies a medial strip of the forebrain with blood. ACA occlusion is usually caused by embolization, although an anterior communicating artery aneurysm, vasospasm resulting from a subarachnoid hemorrhage, or subfalcial herniation can occlude this artery. If the ACA is occluded distal to the recurrent artery of Heubner, it results in contralateral spastic paresis and sensory loss in the lower extremity. A more proximal lesion involving the recurrent artery of Heubner may involve the upper body and limb as well. In addition, there may be internal sphincter weakness of the urinary bladder, frontal release signs, and conjugate deviation of the eyes toward the side of the lesion (damage to frontal eye fields with unopposed deviation from the intact side).

Coronal Section through the Head of the Caudate Nucleus

Frontal horn of lateral ventricle

Corpus striatum (head of the caudate and putamen)

Medial and lateral lenticulostriate arteries

Limen of insula

Insula

Precentral (prerolandic), central (rolandic) and parietal branches

Lateral cerebral (sylvian) fissure

Temporal branches

Temporal lobe

Middle cerebral artery

Interior carotid artery

Falx cerebri

Callosomarginal arteries and Pericallosal arteries (branches of anterior cerebral arteries)

Body of corpus callosum

Internal capsule (anterior limb)

Septum pellucidum

Rostrum of corpus callosum

Anterior cerebral arteries

Recurrent artery (of Heubner)

Anterior communicating artery

Optic chiasm

F. Netter M.D. with J. Perkins MS, MFA

7.7 ARTERIAL DISTRIBUTION TO THE BRAIN: CORONAL FOREBRAIN SECTION

The MCA is the major continuation of the ICA. The MCA travels through the lateral fissure, supplying branches both to deep structures and to the convexity of the cerebral cortex. The lenticulostriate arteries, sometimes called the arteries of stroke, are thin branches of the MCA that penetrate into the basal ganglia and internal capsule regions of the forebrain. A stroke in this territory produces a classic contralateral hemiplegia (spastic) with aphasia, often worse in the upper extremity.

Diagnosis of Stroke

Ischemic ⟵ **Stroke** ⟶ Hemorrhagic

Thrombosis

Infarct

Clot in carotid artery extends directly to middle cerebral artery

Embolism

Infarct

Clot fragment carried from heart or more proximal artery

Hypoxia

Infarcts

Hypotension and poor cerebral perfusion: border zone infarcts, no vascular occlusion

Subarachnoid hemorrhage (ruptured aneurysm)

Intracerebral hemorrhage (hypertensive)

7.8 TYPES OF STROKES

There are two types of strokes, ischemic and hemorrhagic. The ischemic strokes include thrombotic strokes, embolic strokes, and hypoxic strokes. The hemorrhagic strokes include subarachnoid hemorrhages (ruptured aneurysm) and intracerebral hemorrhages (hypertensive or bleeds associated with anticoagulant medication).

Anterior cerebral artery

Middle cerebral artery

Posterior communicating artery

Caroticotympanic branch of
internal carotid artery

Posterior cerebral artery

Superior cerebellar artery

Anterior tympanic artery

Middle meningeal artery

Maxillary artery

Basilar artery

Anterior inferior cerebellar artery

Posterior inferior cerebellar artery

External carotid artery

Internal carotid artery

Superior thyroid artery

Common carotid artery

Vertebral artery

Ascending cervical artery

Inferior thyroid artery

Thyrocervical trunk

Subclavian artery

Brachiocephalic trunk

Anterior communicating artery

Ophthalmic artery

Supraorbital artery

Supratrochlear artery

Lacrimal artery

Dorsal nasal artery

Middle meningeal artery

Angular artery

Superficial temporal artery

Posterior auricular artery

Facial artery

Occipital artery

Lingual artery

Ascending pharyngeal artery

Anterior spinal artery

Spinal segmental medullary branches

Vertebral artery

Common carotid artery

Deep cervical artery

Transverse cervical artery

Suprascapular artery

Supreme intercostal artery

Costocervical trunk

Subclavian artery

Internal thoracic artery

Aorta { Arch / Descending / Ascending

Anastomoses

1 Right–Left

2 Carotid–Vertebral

3 Internal carotid–External carotid

4 Subclavian–Carotid

5 Subclavian–Vertebral

7.9 SCHEMATIC OF ARTERIES TO THE BRAIN

This schematic diagram shows the entire layout of the arterial blood supply to the brain, including anastomoses. The circle of Willis is present in the upper central portion of this schematic.

The relative separation of the anterior (MCA, ACA) and posterior (vertebrobasilar system, PCA) circulation is evident in this diagram.

Vessels Dissected Out: Inferior View

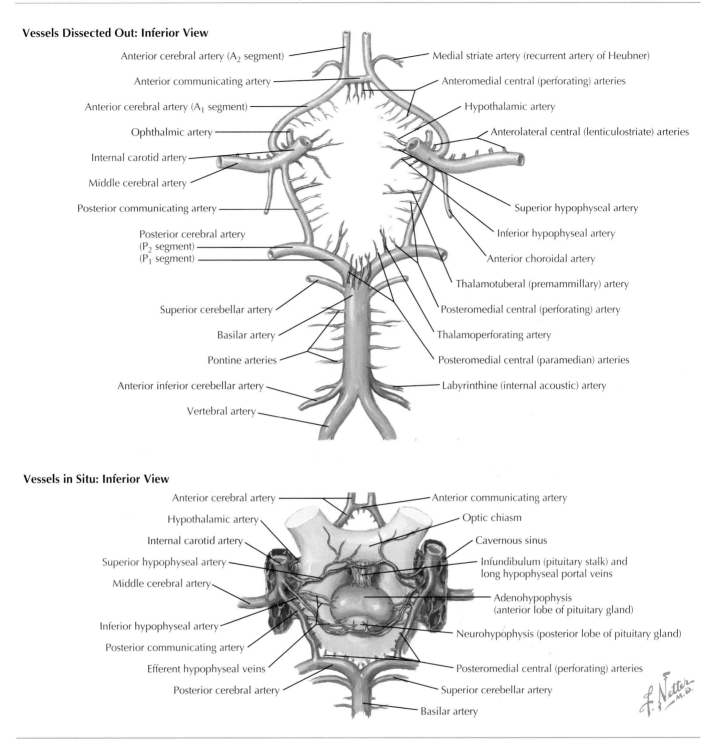

Anterior cerebral artery (A₂ segment)

Anterior communicating artery

Anterior cerebral artery (A₁ segment)

Ophthalmic artery

Internal carotid artery

Middle cerebral artery

Posterior communicating artery

Posterior cerebral artery
(P₂ segment)
(P₁ segment)

Superior cerebellar artery

Basilar artery

Pontine arteries

Anterior inferior cerebellar artery

Vertebral artery

Medial striate artery (recurrent artery of Heubner)

Anteromedial central (perforating) arteries

Hypothalamic artery

Anterolateral central (lenticulostriate) arteries

Superior hypophyseal artery

Inferior hypophyseal artery

Anterior choroidal artery

Thalamotuberal (premammillary) artery

Posteromedial central (perforating) artery

Thalamoperforating artery

Posteromedial central (paramedian) arteries

Labyrinthine (internal acoustic) artery

Vessels in Situ: Inferior View

Anterior cerebral artery

Hypothalamic artery

Internal carotid artery

Superior hypophyseal artery

Middle cerebral artery

Inferior hypophyseal artery

Posterior communicating artery

Efferent hypophyseal veins

Posterior cerebral artery

Anterior communicating artery

Optic chiasm

Cavernous sinus

Infundibulum (pituitary stalk) and
long hypophyseal portal veins

Adenohypophysis
(anterior lobe of pituitary gland)

Neurohypophysis (posterior lobe of pituitary gland)

Posteromedial central (perforating) arteries

Superior cerebellar artery

Basilar artery

7.10 CIRCLE OF WILLIS: SCHEMATIC ILLUSTRATION AND VESSELS IN SITU

The circle of Willis surrounds the optic tracts, pituitary stalk, and basal hypothalamus. It includes the three sets of paired cerebral arteries plus the anterior communicating artery, interconnecting the ACAs, and the posterior communicating arteries, interconnecting the MCAs and PCAs. The free flow of arterial blood through the communicating arteries usually is insufficient to perfuse the brain adequately in the face of an occlusion to a major cerebral artery; the circle of Willis is fully patent and functional for free flow through the communicating arteries in only approximately 20% of individuals. The circle of Willis is the most common site of cerebral aneurysms.

CLINICAL POINT

Saccular, or berry, aneurysms account for more than 80% of all intracranial aneurysms; they are outpouchings of cerebral arteries that probably form over a relatively short period of time (days to weeks). The most likely site of these berry aneurysms is at the junctions of arteries in the circle of Willis. Rupture of the aneurysm results in arterial bleeding into the cerebrospinal fluid (subarachnoid hemorrhage), which produces an acute, excruciating headache, nausea, vomiting, signs of meningeal irritation, and sometimes loss of consciousness. A sudden subarachnoid hemorrhage may be immediately fatal. Autopsy studies show that most cerebral aneurysms never rupture. Untreated ruptured aneurysms have approximately a one third likelihood of rebleeding within 2 months, sometimes with fatal results; other sequelae are cerebral infarction and vasospasm of the affected vessel. Treatment sometimes involves clipping the aneurysm or occluding it with coils or balloons.

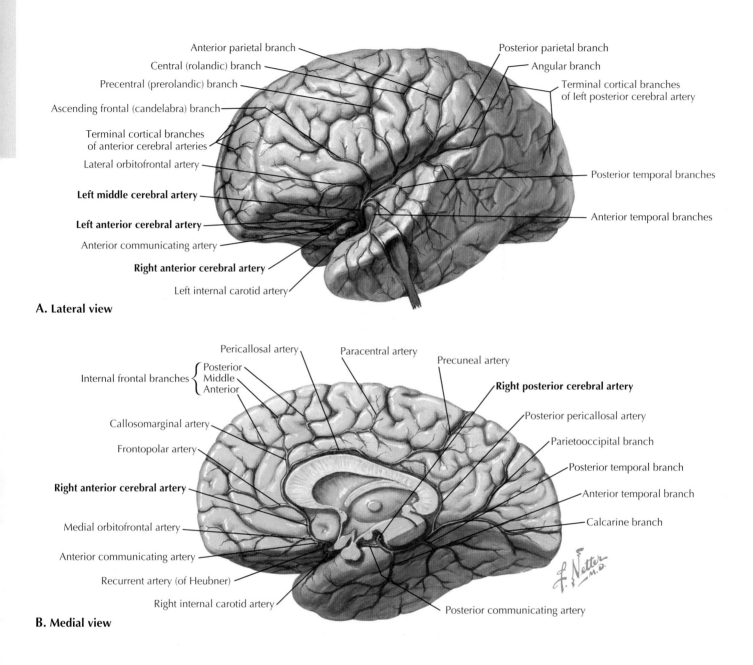

Anterior parietal branch
Central (rolandic) branch
Precentral (prerolandic) branch
Ascending frontal (candelabra) branch
Terminal cortical branches of anterior cerebral arteries
Lateral orbitofrontal artery
Left middle cerebral artery
Left anterior cerebral artery
Anterior communicating artery
Right anterior cerebral artery
Left internal carotid artery

Posterior parietal branch
Angular branch
Terminal cortical branches of left posterior cerebral artery
Posterior temporal branches
Anterior temporal branches

A. Lateral view

Pericallosal artery
Internal frontal branches {Posterior, Middle, Anterior}
Callosomarginal artery
Frontopolar artery
Right anterior cerebral artery
Medial orbitofrontal artery
Anterior communicating artery
Recurrent artery (of Heubner)
Right internal carotid artery

Paracentral artery
Precuneal artery
Right posterior cerebral artery
Posterior pericallosal artery
Parietooccipital branch
Posterior temporal branch
Anterior temporal branch
Calcarine branch
Posterior communicating artery

B. Medial view

7.11 ARTERIAL DISTRIBUTION TO THE BRAIN: LATERAL AND MEDIAL VIEWS

A. The MCA sends named branches along the surface of the hemispheric convexity into the frontal and parietal lobes and into the anterior and middle regions of the temporal lobes. Occlusion disrupts sensory and motor functions in the contralateral body, especially the upper extremity, or in the entire contralateral body if the internal capsule is affected. B. The ACA distributes to the midline region of the frontal and parietal lobes. Occlusion disrupts sensory and motor functions in the contralateral lower extremity. The PCA distributes to the occipital lobe and the inferior surface of the temporal lobe. Occlusion disrupts mainly visual functions in the contralateral visual field.

CLINICAL POINT

The MCA is a continuation of the ICA, extending through the lateral fissure to supply branches to the convexity of the hemisphere, as well as penetrating branches. Cerebrovascular "strokes" appear in several forms. Approximately one third are atherosclerotic/sclerotic strokes (usually preceded by a transient ischemic attack); about one third are embolic strokes; close to 20% are lacunar (small distal) infarcts; 10% are cerebral hemorrhages; and a small percent are ruptured aneurysms or arteriovenous malformations. Lacunar infarcts are small infarcts (between 3 to 4 μm and 2 cm in diameter) in small penetrating vessels supplying the putamen, caudate, internal capsule, thalamus, pons, and cerebral white matter. They occur most commonly as atherosclerosis-related infarcts, particularly in the presence of hypertension or diabetes. Symptoms are determined by which region of the brain is involved; they can include weakness, hemiplegia, contralateral loss of sensation, ataxia, and other symptoms.

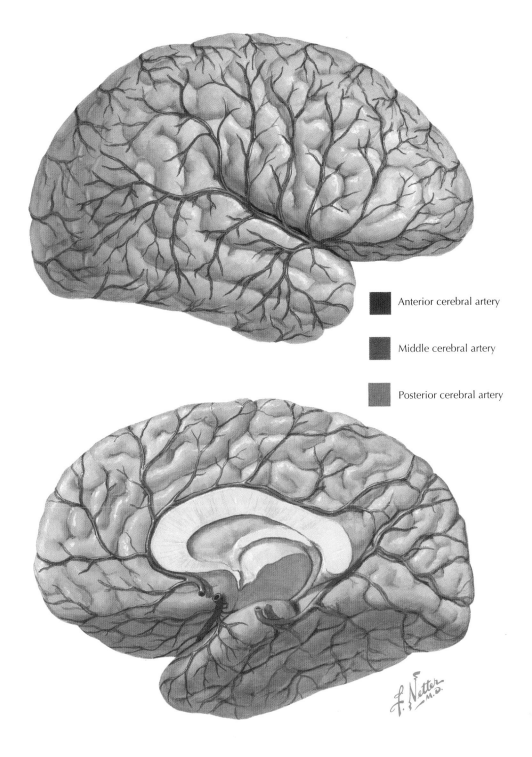

Anterior cerebral artery

Middle cerebral artery

Posterior cerebral artery

7.12 COLOR ILLUSTRATION OF TERRITORIES OF THE CEREBRAL ARTERIES

The specific midline and lateral territories of distribution of the ACA, MCA, and PCA illustrate the exclusive zones supplied by these major arteries and make particularly clear the watershed zones at the junctions of the major cerebral arteries.

A. Axial view

— Anterior cerebral artery

— Middle cerebral artery

— Internal carotid artery

— Posterior cerebral artery

— Basilar artery

— Vertebral artery

B. Lateral view

— Branches of middle cerebral artery
— Posterior cerebral artery
— Basilar artery
— Middle cerebral arteries
— Internal carotid arteries
— Vertebral arteries

— Midline portion, anterior cerebral artery

— Middle cerebral artery

— Anterior cerebral artery

— Internal carotid artery

— Basilar artery

— Vertebral artery

— Common carotid artery

— Subclavian artery

— Brachiocephalic trunk

— Aortic arch

C. Coronal full vessel view

7.13 MAGNETIC RESONANCE ANGIOGRAPHY: FRONTAL AND LATERAL VIEWS

A, Axial view. **B,** Lateral view. **C,** Coronal full vessel view. The technique of magnetic resonance angiography (MRA) exploits the properties of macroscopic blood flow to render images of cerebral blood vessels. Depending on the technique, the blood signal can be made to appear dark or bright; with conventional spin-echo pulse sequences, the blood vessels appear dark, and with gradient-echo pulse sequences, the blood vessels appear bright. There are two types of MRA that are defined mainly by the two fundamental flow effects in magnetic resonance: time-of-flight phenomena based on magnitude effects and phase contrast phenomena, based on phase-shift effect. The MRAs in these images were made by using the technique that exploits signal enhancement due to the effects of time of flight. Positive flow contrast is generated by inflow effects, whereas the background (stationary tissue) is saturated by the rapid, repeated application of the radiofrequency pulses; thus the blood signal is higher than that of stationary tissue.

Femorocerebral Angiography

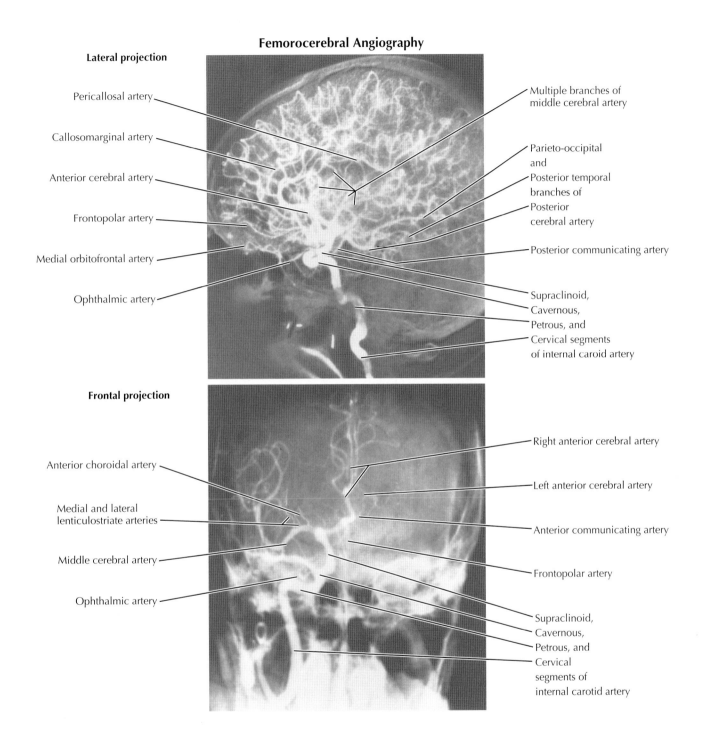

Lateral projection

Pericallosal artery

Callosomarginal artery

Anterior cerebral artery

Frontopolar artery

Medial orbitofrontal artery

Ophthalmic artery

Multiple branches of
middle cerebral artery

Parieto-occipital
and
Posterior temporal
branches of
Posterior
cerebral artery

Posterior communicating artery

Supraclinoid,
Cavernous,
Petrous, and
Cervical segments
of internal caroid artery

Frontal projection

Anterior choroidal artery

Medial and lateral
lenticulostriate arteries

Middle cerebral artery

Ophthalmic artery

Right anterior cerebral artery

Left anterior cerebral artery

Anterior communicating artery

Frontopolar artery

Supraclinoid,
Cavernous,
Petrous, and
Cervical
segments of
internal carotid artery

7.14 ANGIOGRAPHIC ANATOMY OF THE INTERNAL CAROTID CIRCULATION

The top plate is an angiogram that is a lateral view of the ICA circulation after injection of a radiopaque contrast agent into the ICA. The major branches of the ICA, particularly the ACA and MCA, are delineated. The bottom plate is an angiogram that is a frontal view of the ICA circulation after injection of a radiopaque contrast agent into the common carotid artery. The major branches of this arterial system are delineated. MRA is used commonly to investigate the status of the cerebral arteries, but angiography with contrast agents can provide excellent anatomical details for teaching purposes.

Arteries of Posterior Cranial Fossa

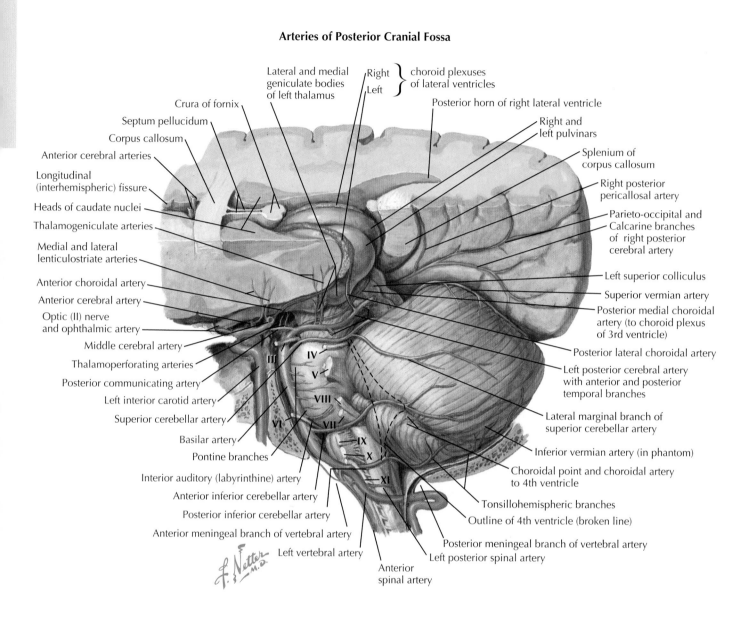

Crura of fornix
Septum pellucidum
Corpus callosum
Anterior cerebral arteries
Longitudinal (interhemispheric) fissure
Heads of caudate nuclei
Thalamogeniculate arteries
Medial and lateral lenticulostriate arteries
Anterior choroidal artery
Anterior cerebral artery
Optic (II) nerve and ophthalmic artery
Middle cerebral artery
Thalamoperforating arteries
Posterior communicating artery
Left interior carotid artery
Superior cerebellar artery
Basilar artery
Pontine branches
Interior auditory (labyrinthine) artery
Anterior inferior cerebellar artery
Posterior inferior cerebellar artery
Anterior meningeal branch of vertebral artery

Lateral and medial geniculate bodies of left thalamus

Right
Left } choroid plexuses of lateral ventricles

Posterior horn of right lateral ventricle
Right and left pulvinars
Splenium of corpus callosum
Right posterior pericallosal artery
Parieto-occipital and Calcarine branches of right posterior cerebral artery
Left superior colliculus
Superior vermian artery
Posterior medial choroidal artery (to choroid plexus of 3rd ventricle)
Posterior lateral choroidal artery
Left posterior cerebral artery with anterior and posterior temporal branches
Lateral marginal branch of superior cerebellar artery
Inferior vermian artery (in phantom)
Choroidal point and choroidal artery to 4th ventricle
Tonsillohemispheric branches
Outline of 4th ventricle (broken line)
Posterior meningeal branch of vertebral artery
Left posterior spinal artery
Anterior spinal artery
Left vertebral artery

III IV V VIII VI VII IX X XI

7.15 VERTEBROBASILAR ARTERIAL SYSTEM

The vertebral arteries unite at the midline to form the basilar artery. Medial penetrating branches extend into medial zones of the brain stem, supplying wedgelike territories. Infarcts in these branches can produce "alternating hemiplegias," contralateral motor deficits (corticospinal system damage above the decussation of the pyramids), and ipsilateral brain stem/ cranial nerve signs and symptoms. The vertebral and basilar arteries also give rise to larger short and long circumferential branches, such as the posterior inferior cerebellar artery, the anterior inferior cerebellar artery, and the superior cerebellar artery. Strokes in these arterial territories generally produce a constellation of ipsilateral brain stem sensory, motor, and autonomic symptoms and contralateral somatosensory symptoms. For example, an infarct in the posterior inferior cerebellar artery results in loss of pain and temperature

sensation on the contralateral body and the ipsilateral face. The end branch of the basilar artery is the PCA, which distributes to the visual cortex and inferior temporal lobe. Occlusion results in contralateral hemianopsia.

CLINICAL POINT

The vertebrobasilar system gives rise to several types of arterial branches. Those located most medially are the paramedian branches. An infarct in such a branch commonly involves ipsilateral damage to a cranial nerve and its function as well as contralateral hemiplegia because of involvement of the corticospinal tract before it decussates on its way to the spinal cord. These infarcts are known as alternating hemiplegias. The short and long circumferential arteries distribute into more lateral territories, and infarcts commonly result in a complex mixture of sensory, motor, and autonomic symptoms, as seen in the lateral medullary syndrome resulting from an infarct in the posterior inferior cerebellar artery.

Arteries of Posterior Cranial Fossa
Vertebral Angiograms: Arterial Phase

A. Lateral projection

Posterior lateral choroidal arteries
Superior cerebellar arteries
Posterior cerebral arteries
Thalamoperforating arteries

Posterior pericallosal artery
Parieto-occipital
Posterior temporal $\Big\}$ Branches of posterior cerebral artery
Calcarine

Posterior communicating arteries
Basilar artery
Anterior inferior cerebellar artery
Vertebral artery

Inferior vermian artery
Tonsillohemispheric branches
Posterior inferior cerebellar artery

B. Frontal projection

Posterior cerebral arteries
Superior cerebellar arteries

Anterior inferior cerebellar arteries
Basilar artery

Inferior vermian branches
or
Right and left posterior inferior cerebellar arteries
and
Left hemispheric branch of left posterior inferior cerebellar artery

Vertebral artery

7.16 ANGIOGRAPHIC ANATOMY OF THE VERTEBROBASILAR SYSTEM

These figures show angiograms of both lateral and frontal views of the vertebrobasilar (posterior) circulation after injection of a radiopaque contrast agent into the vertebral artery. The major arterial branches of this system are delineated.

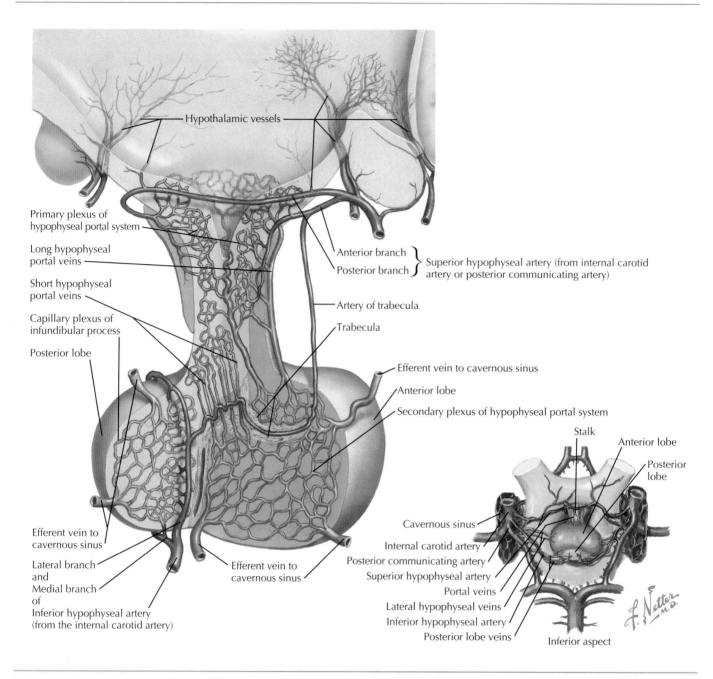

Hypothalamic vessels

Primary plexus of hypophyseal portal system

Long hypophyseal portal veins

Short hypophyseal portal veins

Capillary plexus of infundibular process

Posterior lobe

Anterior branch
Posterior branch
} Superior hypophyseal artery (from internal carotid artery or posterior communicating artery)

Artery of trabecula

Trabecula

Efferent vein to cavernous sinus

Anterior lobe

Secondary plexus of hypophyseal portal system

Stalk

Anterior lobe

Posterior lobe

Efferent vein to cavernous sinus

Lateral branch and Medial branch of Inferior hypophyseal artery (from the internal carotid artery)

Efferent vein to cavernous sinus

Cavernous sinus

Internal carotid artery

Posterior communicating artery

Superior hypophyseal artery

Portal veins

Lateral hypophyseal veins

Inferior hypophyseal artery

Posterior lobe veins

Inferior aspect

f. Netter
M.D.

7.17 VASCULAR SUPPLY TO THE HYPOTHALAMUS AND THE PITUITARY GLAND

The superior hypophyseal arteries (from the ICA or the posterior communicating artery) supply the hypothalamus and infundibular stalk and anastomose with branches of the inferior hypophyseal artery (from the ICA). A unique aspect of this arterial distribution is the hypophyseal portal system, whose primary plexus derives from small arterioles and capillaries that then send branches into the anterior pituitary gland. This plexus allows neurons producing hypothalamic releasing factors and inhibitory factors to secrete these factors into the hypophyseal portal system, which delivers a very high concentration directly into the secondary plexus in the anterior pituitary. Thus, anterior pituitary cells are bathed in releasing and inhibitory factors in very high concentrations. This private vascular communication channel allows the hypothalamus to exert fine control, both directly and through feedback, over the secretion of anterior pituitary hormones.

CLINICAL POINT

The primary hypophyseal portal system coalesces into long hypophyseal portal veins that give rise to a secondary hypophyseal plexus. This arrangement allows the secretion of releasing and inhibitory factors from nerve endings, whose cell bodies are located in the hypothalamus and other structures, into a private vascular system, to be delivered to the pituicytes in the anterior pituitary gland in extraordinarily high concentrations. The ultimate control of the releasing and inhibitory factors profoundly influences neuroendocrine secretion and its downstream effects in the entire body. For example, corticotrophin releasing hormone or factor induces the release of adrenocorticotropic hormone from the anterior pituitary, which is released into the systemic circulation and activates the adrenal cortex to release cortisol and other steroid hormones. This hypothalamo-pituitary-adrenal system helps to regulate glucose metabolism, insulin secretion, immune responses, adipose distribution, and a host of other vital functions. The corticotrophin releasing hormone neurons are under extensive regulatory control by neural inputs, hormonal feedback, and inflammatory mediators; these neurons help to orchestrate stress reactivity for the organism as a whole.

Anterior View

Posterior cerebral artery
Superior cerebellar artery
Basilar artery
Anterior inferior cerebellar artery
Posterior inferior cerebellar artery
Anterior spinal artery
Vertebral artery
Anterior radicular arteries
Ascending cervical artery
Deep cervical artery
Subclavian artery
Anterior radicular artery
Posterior intercostal artery
Artery of Adamkiewicz
(major anterior radicular artery)
Anterior radicular artery
Lumbar artery
Anastomotic loops to
posterior spinal arteries
Lateral sacral (or median sacral) artery

Cervical
vertebrae

Thoracic vertebrae

Lumbar vertebrae

Sacrum

Posterior View

Posterior inferior cerebellar artery
Posterior spinal arteries
Vertebral artery
Posterior radicular arteries
Deep cervical artery
Ascending cervical artery
Subclavian artery
Posterior radicular arteries
Posterior intercostal arteries
Posterior radicular arteries
Lumbar arteries
Anastomotic loops to anterior spinal artery
Lateral sacral (or median sacral) artery

7.18 ARTERIAL BLOOD SUPPLY TO THE SPINAL CORD: LONGITUDINAL VIEW

The major arterial blood supply to the spinal cord derives from the anterior spinal artery and the paired posterior spinal arteries, both branches of the vertebral artery. The actual blood flow through these arteries, derived from the posterior circulation, is inadequate to maintain the spinal cord beyond the cervical segments. Radicular arteries, deriving from the aorta, provide major anastomoses with the anterior and posterior spinal arteries and supplement the blood flow to the spinal cord. The largest of these anterior radicular arteries, often from the L2 region, is the artery of Adamkiewicz. Impaired blood flow through these critical radicular arteries, especially during surgical procedures that involve abrupt disruption of blood flow through the aorta, can result in spinal cord infarct.

Arteries of Cervical Cord Exposed from the Rear

Basilar artery
Posterior inferior cerebellar artery
Vertebral artery
Anterior spinal artery
Spinal ramus
Posterior spinal artery
Posterior radicular artery
Pre-laminar branch

Anterior spinal artery
Post-central branch
Anterior central artery
Spinal ramus
Neural branch
Anterior radicular artery
Posterior radicular artery
Internal spinal arteries
Posterior central artery
Pre-laminar branch
Posterior spinal artery

Arteries of Spinal Cord Diagrammatically Shown in Horizontal Section

7.19 ANTERIOR AND POSTERIOR SPINAL ARTERIES AND THEIR DISTRIBUTION

The anterior and posterior spinal arteries travel in the subarachnoid space and send branches into the spinal cord. The anterior spinal artery sends alternating branches into the anterior median fissure to supply the anterior two thirds of the spinal cord. Occlusion of one of these branches can result in ipsilateral flaccid paralysis in muscles supplied by the affected segments, ipsilateral spastic paralysis below the affected level (resulting from upper motor neuron axonal damage), and contralateral loss of pain and temperature sensation below the affected level (resulting from damage to the anterolateral spinothalamic/spinoreticular system). The posterior spinal artery branches supply the dorsal third of the spinal cord. Occlusion affects the ipsilateral perception of fine discriminative touch, vibratory sensation, and joint position sense below the level of the lesion (resulting from damage to fasciculi gracilis and cuneatus, the dorsal columns).

Posterior spinal arteries

Anterior spinal artery

Anterior radicular artery

Posterior radicular arteries

Branch to vertebral body and dura mater

Spinal branch

Dorsal ramus of posterior intercostal artery

Posterior intercostal arteries

Paravertebral anastomosis

Prevertebral anastomosis

Aorta

Section through Thoracic Spine

Right posterior spinal artery

Peripheral branches from pial plexus

Central branches to right side of spinal cord

Central branches to left side of spinal cord

Anterior radicular artery

Left posterior spinal artery

Zone supplied by penetrating branches from pial plexus

Pial arterial plexus

Zone supplied by central branches

Posterior radicular artery

Zone supplied by both central branches and branches from pial plexus

Anterior spinal artery

Posterior radicular artery

Anterior radicular artery

Schema of Arterial Distribution

Pial arterial plexus

7.20 ARTERIAL SUPPLY TO THE SPINAL CORD: CROSS-SECTIONAL VIEW

The major contribution to the arterial blood supply of the spinal cord below the cervical segments derives from the radicular arteries (*top*). This intercostal blood supply also distributes to adjacent bony and muscular structures. The penetrating vessels supplying the spinal cord derive from central branches of the anterior spinal artery and from a pial plexus of vessels that surround the exterior of the spinal cord.

CLINICAL POINT

Alternating branches arise from the anterior spinal artery into the anterior two thirds of the spinal cord. Following an infarct in the anterior spinal artery, acute radiating leg pain is experienced. Depending on the level, acute flaccid paraparesis or quadraparesis occurs, resolving to spastic paraparesis or quadraparesis with hyperreflexia as the result of the upper motor neuron lesion resulting from damage to the bilateral lateral funiculi. Only at the level of the infarct, where lower motor neurons are lost, does flaccid paralysis remain, along with hyporeflexia. Bilateral plantar extensor responses are seen. Bilateral loss of pain and temperature sensation is seen because of ischemia to the anterolateral territory of the spinothalamic/spinoreticular protopathic system. Descending fibers for control of the bladder and bowel travel in the lateral funiculus and are damaged by an anterior artery infarct. In a lesion of the anterior spinal artery above the T1 level, bilateral damage to descending central sympathetic fibers regulating T1 intermediolateral cell column outflow produces bilateral Horner's syndrome, with bilateral ptosis, myosis, and anhidrosis.

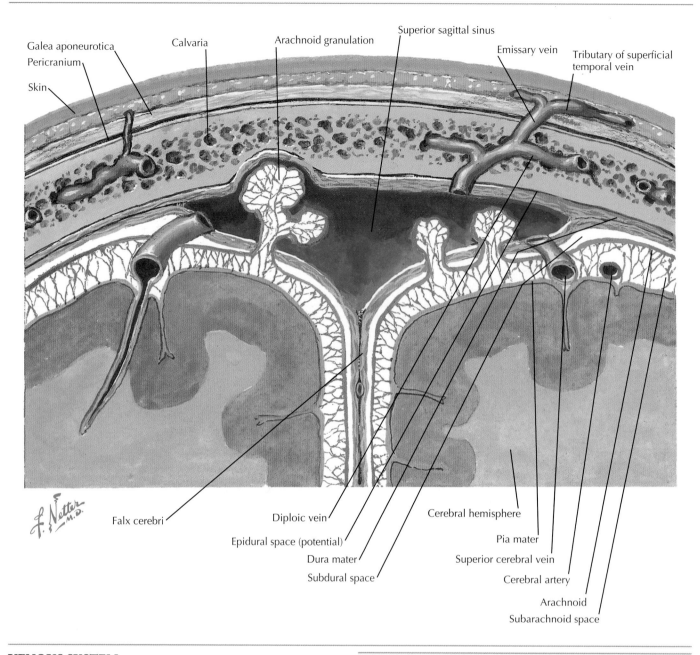

Galea aponeurotica
Pericranium
Skin
Calvaria
Arachnoid granulation
Superior sagittal sinus
Emissary vein
Tributary of superficial temporal vein

Falx cerebri
Diploic vein
Epidural space (potential)
Dura mater
Subdural space
Cerebral hemisphere
Pia mater
Superior cerebral vein
Cerebral artery
Arachnoid
Subarachnoid space

F. Netter M.D.

VENOUS SYSTEM

7.21 MENINGES AND SUPERFICIAL CEREBRAL VEINS

The superior sagittal sinus and other dural sinuses receive venous blood from a variety of veins, including superficial cerebral veins draining blood from the cortical surface, meningeal veins draining blood from the meninges, diploic veins draining blood from channels located between the inner and outer tables of the calvaria, and emissary veins, which link the venous sinuses and diploic veins with veins on the surface of the skull. These channels do not have valves and permit free communication between these venous systems and the venous sinuses. This is a significant factor in the possible spread of infections from foci outside the cranium to the venous sinuses.

CLINICAL POINT
Arachnoid granulations act as one-way valves that convey cerebrospinal fluid into the dural sinus, channeling it back into the venous circulation. The cerebral veins also extend across the subarachnoid space and enter into the superior sagittal sinus. With severe head trauma, these bridging veins can be torn, with resultant venous bleeding into the subdural space; this bleed dissects the dura from the arachnoid and becomes a space-occupying mass. It also brings about cerebral edema and swelling. Acute subdural hematomas can be life-threatening, especially in young individuals with head trauma. Chronic subdural hematomas often occur in the elderly with relatively minor trauma; the bridging veins tear because of some mild atrophy of the underlying hemisphere, making the course of the bridging veins more extended and more vulnerable to tearing. Slow accumulation of subdural blood eventually can result in increased intracranial pressure with headache, lethargy, confusion, seizures, and focal neurological abnormalities. Surgical drainage is often performed for large subdural hematomas, whereas small hematomas regress naturally in the elderly.

Scalp, Skull, Meningeal, and Cerebral Blood Vessels

Superior sagittal sinus
Diploic vein
Emissary vein
Arachnoid granulation
Cerebral vein penetrating subdural space to enter sinus (bridging veins)
Dura mater (two layers)
Frontal and parietal tributaries of superficial temporal vein
Frontal and parietal branches of superficial temporal artery
Arachnoid granulation indenting skull (foveola)
Venous lacuna
Inferior sagittal sinus
Thalamostriate and internal cerebral veins
Epidural space (potential)
Arachnoid
Subarachnoid space
Pia mater
Middle meningeal artery and vein
Deep middle and superficial temporal arteries and veins
Deep and superficial middle cerebral veins

Diploic and Emissary Veins of Skull

Frontal diploic vein
Anterior temporal diploic vein
Parietal emissary vein
Posterior temporal diploic vein
Occipital emissary vein
Occipital diploic vein
Mastoid emissary vein

7.22 VEINS: SUPERFICIAL CEREBRAL, MENINGEAL, DIPLOIC, AND EMISSARY

Venous blood drains from the skull, the meninges, and the cerebral cortex into the superior sagittal sinus and other dural sinuses. This is a point of vulnerability where potential infections and contamination from the more superficial venous drainage networks can be allowed into the central venous sinus channels.

Falx cerebri (cut)
Superior ophthalmic vein
Basilar plexus
Cavernous sinus
Tentorial artery
Superior and inferior petrosal sinuses
Tentorium cerebelli
Straight sinus
Falx cerebri (cut)
Confluence of sinuses
Superior sagittal sinus

Optic (II) nerve
Intercavernous (circular) sinus and pituitary gland
Internal carotid artery
Cavernous sinus
Sphenoparietal sinus
Superficial middle cerebral vein
Oculomotor (III) nerve
Trochlear (IV) nerve
Trigeminal (V) nerve
Middle meningeal vein
Abducens (VI) nerve
Superior petrosal sinus
Petrosal vein
Facial (VII) nerve and nervus intermedius
Vestibulocochlear (VIII) nerve
Glossopharyngeal (IX) nerve
Vagus (X) nerve
Jugular foramen
Sigmoid sinus
Accessory (XI) nerve
Hypoglossal (XII) nerve
Transverse sinus
Great cerebral vein (of Galen)
Opening of an inferior cerebral vein

Falx cerebri
Inferior sagittal sinus
Great cerebral vein (of Galen)
Sphenoparietal sinus
Intercavernous sinus
Superior petrosal sinus
Straight sinus
Inferior petrosal sinus
Sigmoid sinus
Jugular foramen
Transverse sinus
Confluence of sinuses
Occipital sinus

7.23 VENOUS SINUSES

The falx cerebri and tentorium cerebelli, protrusions of fused inner and outer dural membranes, confine the anterior, middle, and posterior fossae of the skull. Outer (superior sagittal) and inner (inferior sagittal) venous channels, found in split layers of the dura, drain blood from the superficial and deep regions of the central nervous system, respectively, into the jugular veins. The great cerebral vein of Galen and the straight sinus merge with the transverse sinus into the confluence of sinuses to drain the deep, more posterior regions of the central nervous system. Infection can be introduced into the cerebral circulation through these sinuses. Venous sinus thrombosis can cause stasis (a backup of the venous pressure), which results in inadequate perfusion of the regions where drainage should occur. The protrusions of dura, such as the tentorium cerebelli and falx cerebri, are tough, rigid membranes through which portions of the brain can herniate when intracranial pressure increases.

CLINICAL POINT

Venous sinus thrombosis commonly occurs with infection. Cavernous sinus thrombosis can occur as the result of infection in the paranasal sinuses or middle ear or following a furuncle in the region of the face. Anterior cavernous sinus thrombosis can result in severe pain and headache, ipsilateral visual loss, exophthalmos (protrusion of the eyeball), edema of the eyeball (chemosis), and palsies of the extraocular nerves (III, IV, VI) and V1 (ophthalmic division) that traverse the sinus. This lesion can expand to cause hemiparesis and can involve the interconnected cavernous sinus of the other side, the superior petrosal sinuses, and other venous structures.

The petrosal sinuses can undergo a process of thrombosis caused by the spread of infection in the middle ear. An inferior petrosal sinus thrombosis may cause damage to the VI (abducens) nerve; a superior petrosal sinus thrombosis can result in damage to the semilunar ganglion, producing facial pain. If the transverse sinus is thrombosed, cranial nerve deficits in nerves IX, X, and XI may occur.

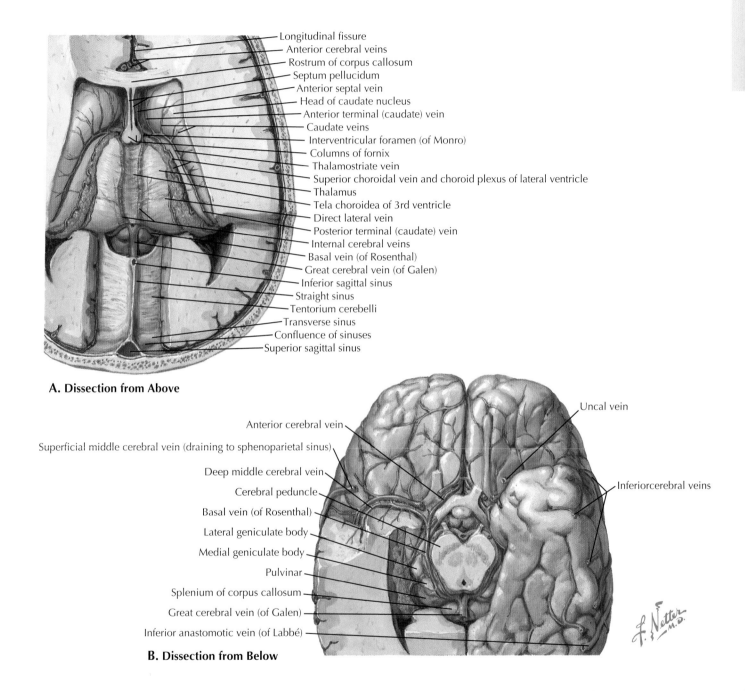

A. Dissection from Above

- Longitudinal fissure
- Anterior cerebral veins
- Rostrum of corpus callosum
- Septum pellucidum
- Anterior septal vein
- Head of caudate nucleus
- Anterior terminal (caudate) vein
- Caudate veins
- Interventricular foramen (of Monro)
- Columns of fornix
- Thalamostriate vein
- Superior choroidal vein and choroid plexus of lateral ventricle
- Thalamus
- Tela choroidea of 3rd ventricle
- Direct lateral vein
- Posterior terminal (caudate) vein
- Internal cerebral veins
- Basal vein (of Rosenthal)
- Great cerebral vein (of Galen)
- Inferior sagittal sinus
- Straight sinus
- Tentorium cerebelli
- Transverse sinus
- Confluence of sinuses
- Superior sagittal sinus

B. Dissection from Below

- Anterior cerebral vein
- Superficial middle cerebral vein (draining to sphenoparietal sinus)
- Deep middle cerebral vein
- Cerebral peduncle
- Basal vein (of Rosenthal)
- Lateral geniculate body
- Medial geniculate body
- Pulvinar
- Splenium of corpus callosum
- Great cerebral vein (of Galen)
- Inferior anastomotic vein (of Labbé)
- Uncal vein
- Inferiorcerebral veins

7.24 DEEP VENOUS DRAINAGE OF THE BRAIN

A, This superior view of the thalamus and basal ganglia reveals the venous drainage of deeper forebrain regions into the posterior venous sinuses. **B,** This basal view of the brain with the brain stem removed illustrates the drainage of forebrain and mesencephalic venous blood into the great cerebral vein of Galen, heading toward the straight sinus.

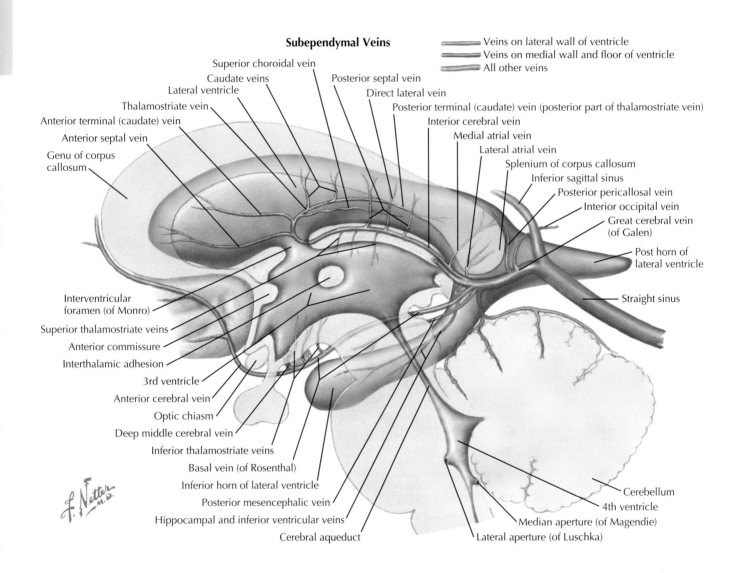

Subependymal Veins

Veins on lateral wall of ventricle
Veins on medial wall and floor of ventricle
All other veins

Superior choroidal vein
Caudate veins
Lateral ventricle
Thalamostriate vein
Anterior terminal (caudate) vein
Anterior septal vein
Genu of corpus callosum
Posterior septal vein
Direct lateral vein
Posterior terminal (caudate) vein (posterior part of thalamostriate vein)
Interior cerebral vein
Medial atrial vein
Lateral atrial vein
Splenium of corpus callosum
Inferior sagittal sinus
Posterior pericallosal vein
Interior occipital vein
Great cerebral vein (of Galen)
Post horn of lateral ventricle
Straight sinus

Interventricular foramen (of Monro)
Superior thalamostriate veins
Anterior commissure
Interthalamic adhesion
3rd ventricle
Anterior cerebral vein
Optic chiasm
Deep middle cerebral vein
Inferior thalamostriate veins
Basal vein (of Rosenthal)
Inferior horn of lateral ventricle
Posterior mesencephalic vein
Hippocampal and inferior ventricular veins
Cerebral aqueduct

Cerebellum
4th ventricle
Median aperture (of Magendie)
Lateral aperture (of Luschka)

7.25 DEEP VENOUS DRAINAGE OF THE BRAIN: RELATIONSHIP TO THE VENTRICLES

Subependymal regions of the central nervous system drain venous blood into the inferior sagittal sinus superiorly or into the great cerebral vein of Galen inferiorly, both of which drain into the straight sinus. Occlusion of a vein in this region causes a blockage of drainage and a backup of perfusion, with resultant ischemia of the tissue in the regions of drainage.

CLINICAL POINT

Venous thrombosis can occur following an infectious process, especially in the nearby sinuses, middle ear, or adjacent facial areas. Non-infectious causes of venous thrombosis include dehydration, cancer, polycythemia vera and other hyperviscosity syndromes, inflammatory conditions, and other disorders. The symptoms vary according to the affected focal territory and the spread of the underlying pathological process; they include severe headache, nausea and vomiting, weakness and sensory losses, sometimes aphasia, and sometimes coma.

Subependymal and Superficial Veins Opacified

A. Lateral projection

Caudate vein

Anterior terminal (caudate) vein

Posterior terminal (caudate) vein

Superior anastomotic vein (of Trolard)

Superior sagittal sinus

Inferior sagittal sinus

Internal cerebral vein

Great cerebral vein (of Galen)

Straight sinus

Anterior septal vein

Thalamostriate vein

Superior choroidal vein

Interior jugular vein

Transverse sinus

Inferior anastomotic vein (of Labbé)

Basal vein (of Rosenthal)

B. Frontal projection

Thalamostriate vein

Superior sagittal sinus

Straight sinus

Superficial cortical veins

Transverse sinus

Inferior jugular vein

Basal vein (of Rosenthal)

Internal cerebral vein

Great cerebral vein (of Galen)

7.26 CAROTID VENOGRAMS: VENOUS PHASE

These lateral and anterior venous-phase angiograms illustrate the superior sagittal sinus, the inferior sagittal sinus, and the great cerebral vein of Galen draining into the straight sinus, the transverse sinus, the basal vein of Rosenthal, and the internal jugular, through which the venous blood of the brain drains back to the heart.

A. Coronal view

- Superior sagittal sinus

- Transverse sinus
- Sigmoid sinus
- Internal jugular vein

- Cerebral veins
- Superior sagittal sinus
- Internal cerebral vein
- Great vein of Galen
- Basal vein of Rosenthal
- Straight sinus

- Confluence of sinus

- Transverse sinus

B. Lateral view

7.27 MAGNETIC RESONANCE VENOGRAPHY: CORONAL AND SAGITTAL VIEWS

Magnetic resonance venography uses the same principles of flow imaging used in MRA (see Fig. 7.13). The flow of venous blood in the brain is relatively slow and steady compared to the flow of arterial blood. Gradient echo sequences are sensitive to flow but are not sensitive to direction of flow. To distinguish arterial flow from venous flow, a presaturation slab must be applied downstream below the heart or upstream above the heart prior to placing imaging slices. In a typical magnetic resonance venography of the head, a saturation slab is placed at the level of the carotid bifurcation, and traveling saturation is placed inferiorly to the slice. Multiple two-dimensional thin slices are placed nearly perpendicular to the vessels. **A,** Coronal view. **B,** Sagittal view. These images illustrate the major cerebral veins and sinuses of the brain.

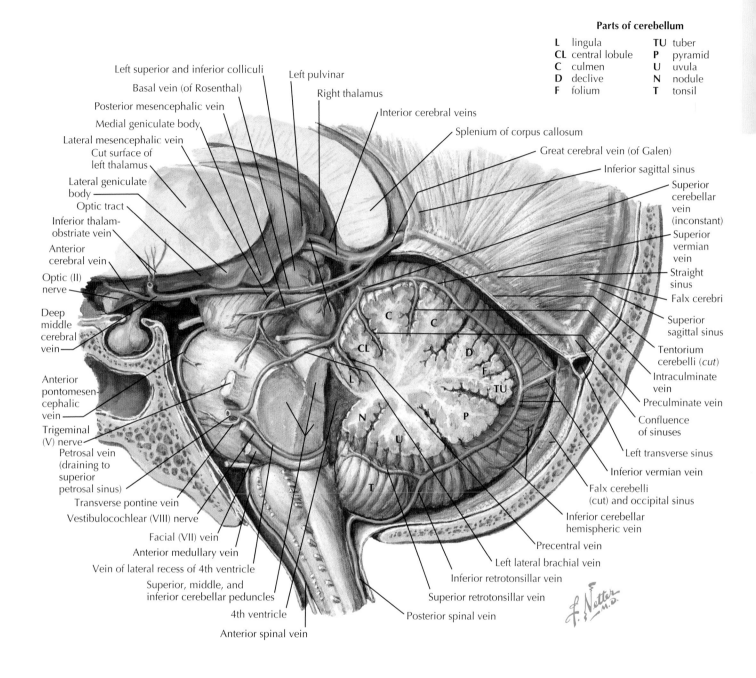

Parts of cerebellum

L	lingula	**TU**	tuber
CL	central lobule	**P**	pyramid
C	culmen	**U**	uvula
D	declive	**N**	nodule
F	folium	**T**	tonsil

Left superior and inferior colliculi

Basal vein (of Rosenthal)

Posterior mesencephalic vein

Medial geniculate body

Lateral mesencephalic vein

Cut surface of left thalamus

Lateral geniculate body

Optic tract

Inferior thalam-obstriate vein

Anterior cerebral vein

Optic (II) nerve

Deep middle cerebral vein

Anterior pontomesen-cephalic vein

Trigeminal (V) nerve

Petrosal vein (draining to superior petrosal sinus)

Transverse pontine vein

Vestibulocochlear (VIII) nerve

Facial (VII) vein

Anterior medullary vein

Vein of lateral recess of 4th ventricle

Superior, middle, and inferior cerebellar peduncles

4th ventricle

Anterior spinal vein

Left pulvinar

Right thalamus

Interior cerebral veins

Splenium of corpus callosum

Great cerebral vein (of Galen)

Inferior sagittal sinus

Superior cerebellar vein (inconstant)

Superior vermian vein

Straight sinus

Falx cerebri

Superior sagittal sinus

Tentorium cerebelli (cut)

Intraculminate vein

Preculminate vein

Confluence of sinuses

Left transverse sinus

Inferior vermian vein

Falx cerebelli (cut) and occipital sinus

Inferior cerebellar hemispheric vein

Precentral vein

Left lateral brachial vein

Inferior retrotonsillar vein

Superior retrotonsillar vein

Posterior spinal vein

7.28 VENOUS DRAINAGE OF THE BRAIN STEM AND THE CEREBELLUM

The venous drainage of the cerebellum and the brain stem is anatomically diverse. The veins of the posterior fossa drain the cerebellum and brain stem. The superior group drains the superior cerebellum and upper brain stem posteriorly into the great cerebral vein of Galen and the straight sinus or laterally into the transverse and superior petrosal sinuses. The anterior, or petrosal, group drains the anterior brain stem, the superior and inferior surfaces of the cerebellar hemispheres, and the lateral regions associated with the fourth ventricle into the superior petrosal sinus. The posterior, or tentorial, group drains the inferior portion of the cerebellar vermis and the medial portion of the superior and inferior cerebellar hemispheres into the transverse sinus or the straight sinus.

CLINICAL POINT

The confluence of sinuses occurs at the junction of the posterior fossa and the occipital lobe. The superior sagittal sinus drains into this confluence of sinuses as the blood flows ultimately toward the jugular vein. The most common sinus thrombosis is that of the superior sagittal sinus. Thrombosis in the posterior portion of this sinus results in headache, increased intracranial pressure with resultant papilledema (after 24 hours), and often a diminished state of consciousness or coma.

Veins of Spinal Cord and Vertebrae

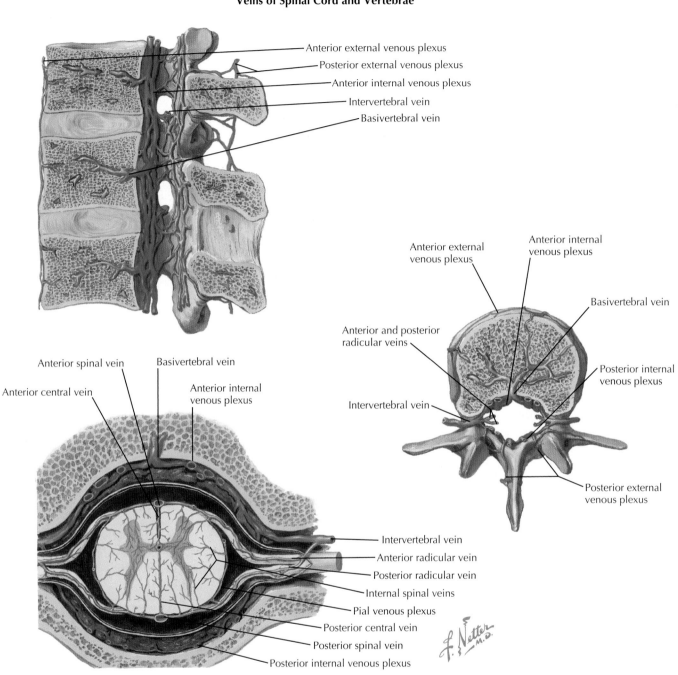

Anterior external venous plexus

Posterior external venous plexus

Anterior internal venous plexus

Intervertebral vein

Basivertebral vein

Anterior external venous plexus

Anterior internal venous plexus

Basivertebral vein

Anterior and posterior radicular veins

Posterior internal venous plexus

Intervertebral vein

Posterior external venous plexus

Anterior spinal vein

Basivertebral vein

Anterior central vein

Anterior internal venous plexus

Intervertebral vein

Anterior radicular vein

Posterior radicular vein

Internal spinal veins

Pial venous plexus

Posterior central vein

Posterior spinal vein

Posterior internal venous plexus

7.29 VENOUS DRAINAGE OF THE SPINAL CORD

An external and internal plexus of veins extends along the entire length of the vertebral column, forming a series of venous rings with extensive anastomoses around each vertebra. Blood from the spinal cord, the vertebrae, and the ligaments drains into these plexuses. Changes in intrathoracic pressure and cerebrospinal fluid pressure can be conveyed through these venous plexuses, affecting the venous volume. Ultimately, these venous plexuses drain through the intervertebral veins into vertebral, posterior intercostals, subcostal, and lumbar and lateral sacral veins.

CLINICAL POINT

A venous plexus is present in the epidural space surrounding the spinal cord, along with epidural fat. This epidural space is wide enough for the insertion of a catheter and infusion of local anesthesia. The local anesthesia is absorbed into this plexus and diffuses into the adjacent spinal cord, producing profound analgesia at and below the level of the infusion. This technique of epidural anesthesia often is used for analgesia in childbirth and also for a variety of surgeries in which epidural anesthesia is preferable to general anesthesia.

8

DEVELOPMENTAL NEUROSCIENCE

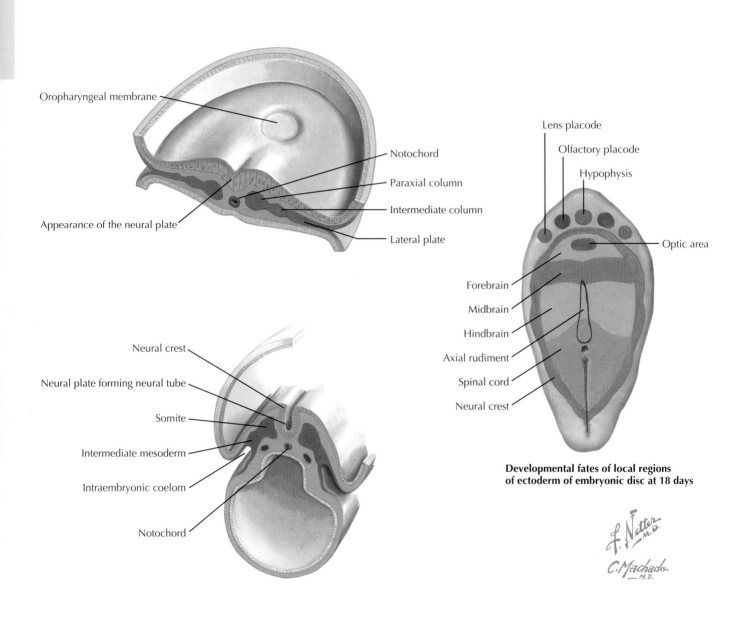

Oropharyngeal membrane

Notochord

Paraxial column

Intermediate column

Appearance of the neural plate

Lateral plate

Lens placode

Olfactory placode

Hypophysis

Optic area

Forebrain

Midbrain

Hindbrain

Axial rudiment

Spinal cord

Neural crest

Neural crest

Neural plate forming neural tube

Somite

Intermediate mesoderm

Intraembryonic coelom

Notochord

**Developmental fates of local regions
of ectoderm of embryonic disc at 18 days**

8.1 FORMATION OF THE NEURAL PLATE, NEURAL TUBE, AND NEURAL CREST

The neural plate, neural tube, and neural crest form at the 18-day stage of embryonic development. The underlying notochord induces the neural plate, and a midline neural groove forms. The elevated lateral margins become the neural folds, tissue destined to become the neural crest with future contributions to many components of the peripheral nervous system (PNS). At this very early stage of embryonic development, these neural precursors are vulnerable to toxic and other forms of insult.

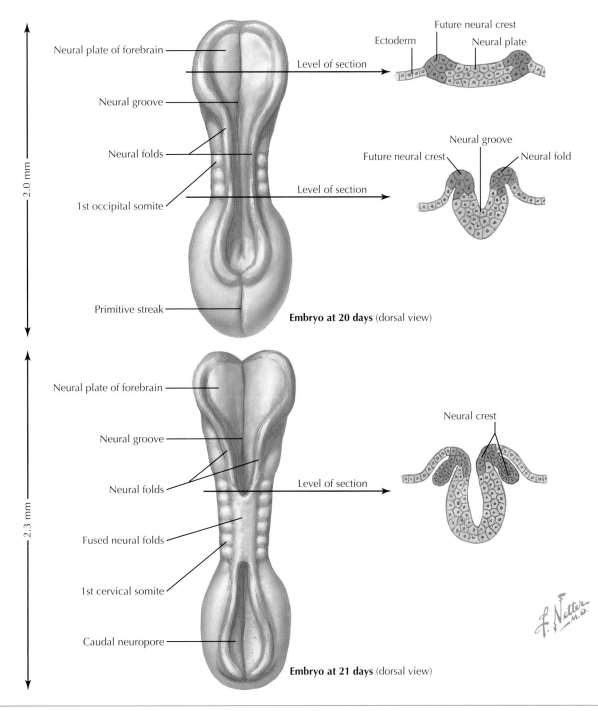

Neural plate of forebrain

Neural groove

Neural folds

1st occipital somite

Primitive streak

Ectoderm · Future neural crest · Neural plate

Level of section

Future neural crest · Neural groove · Neural fold

Level of section

Embryo at 20 days (dorsal view)

Neural plate of forebrain

Neural groove

Neural folds

Fused neural folds

1st cervical somite

Caudal neuropore

Neural crest

Level of section

Embryo at 21 days (dorsal view)

8.2 NEURULATION

In the 21- or 22-day-old-embryo, the neural plate, with its midline neorural groove, thickens and begins to fold and elevate along either side, allowing the two lateral edges to fuse at the dorsal midline to form the completed neural tube. The central canal, the site of the future development of the ventricular system, is in the center of the neural tube. This process of neurulation continues both caudally and rostrally. Disruption can occur because of failure of full neural tube formation caudally (spina bifida) or rostrally (anencephaly).

CLINICAL POINT

As the neural plate forms into a neural tube, the process of neurulation results in fused neural folds, starting centrally and moving both caudally and rostrally. Failure of the neural tube to close results in dysraphic defects, with altered development of associated muscles, bone, skin, and meninges. If the anterior neuropore fails to form, anencephaly results, with failure of the brain to develop, accompanied by facial defects. This condition is lethal. Failure of the posterior (caudal) neuropore to close results in spina bifida, with failure of the vertebral arches to fuse. A saccular protrusion from the lumbar region may contain meninges (meningocele) or meninges and spinal cord (meningomyelocele). Meningomyelocele is often accompanied by paraparesis, bowel and bladder dysfunction, sensory disruption at the level of the lesion, and accompanying hydrocephalus or Arnold-Chiari malformation, requiring a ventriculo-peritoneal or ventriculo-jugular shunt.

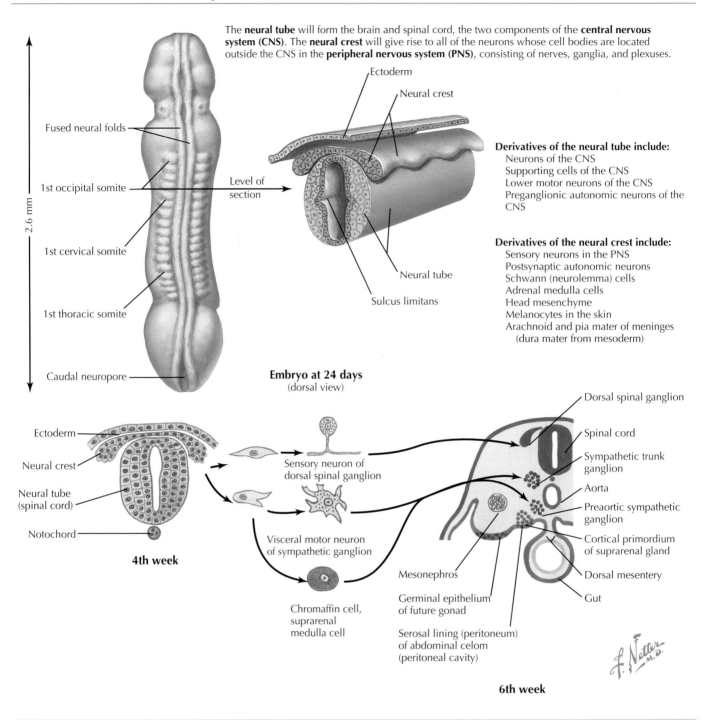

The **neural tube** will form the brain and spinal cord, the two components of the **central nervous system (CNS)**. The **neural crest** will give rise to all of the neurons whose cell bodies are located outside the CNS in the **peripheral nervous system (PNS)**, consisting of nerves, ganglia, and plexuses.

Ectoderm

Neural crest

Derivatives of the neural tube include:
Neurons of the CNS
Supporting cells of the CNS
Lower motor neurons of the CNS
Preganglionic autonomic neurons of the CNS

Derivatives of the neural crest include:
Sensory neurons in the PNS
Postsynaptic autonomic neurons
Schwann (neurolemma) cells
Adrenal medulla cells
Head mesenchyme
Melanocytes in the skin
Arachnoid and pia mater of meninges
(dura mater from mesoderm)

Fused neural folds

1st occipital somite

Level of section

1st cervical somite

Neural tube

1st thoracic somite

Sulcus limitans

2.6 mm

Caudal neuropore

Embryo at 24 days
(dorsal view)

Ectoderm

Neural crest

Neural tube (spinal cord)

Notochord

4th week

Sensory neuron of dorsal spinal ganglion

Visceral motor neuron of sympathetic ganglion

Chromaffin cell, suprarenal medulla cell

Mesonephros

Germinal epithelium of future gonad

Serosal lining (peritoneum) of abdominal celom (peritoneal cavity)

Dorsal spinal ganglion

Spinal cord

Sympathetic trunk ganglion

Aorta

Preaortic sympathetic ganglion

Cortical primordium of suprarenal gland

Dorsal mesentery

Gut

6th week

8.3 NEURAL TUBE DEVELOPMENT AND NEURAL CREST FORMATION

The dorsal and ventral halves of the neural tube are separated by the sulcus limitans, an external protrusion from the central canal that demarcates the alar plate above from the basal plate below. This important landmark persists at some sites in the adult ventricular system. The alar plate is the source of generation of many neurons with sensory function. The basal plate is the source of generation of many neurons with motor or autonomic function in the spinal cord and the brain stem. The neural crest cells at the edge of the neural folds unite and become a dorsal crest, the neural crest above the neural tube.

The neural tube and neural crest separate from the originating ectoderm.

CLINICAL POINT
The neural crest gives rise to a wide variety of neural elements of the PNS, including primary sensory neurons, postganglionic autonomic neurons, Schwann cells, adrenal medullary chromaffin cells, pia and arachnoid cells, melanocytes, and some mesenchyme of the head. A failure of the neural crest to develop and migrate properly is seen in Hirschsprung's disease (congenital megacolon), in which sensory signals from the colon are absent, and in familial dysautonomia, in which autonomic symptoms (cardiovascular dysfunction, gastrointestinal dysfunction) and sensory deficits (especially pain and temperature sensation) are present.

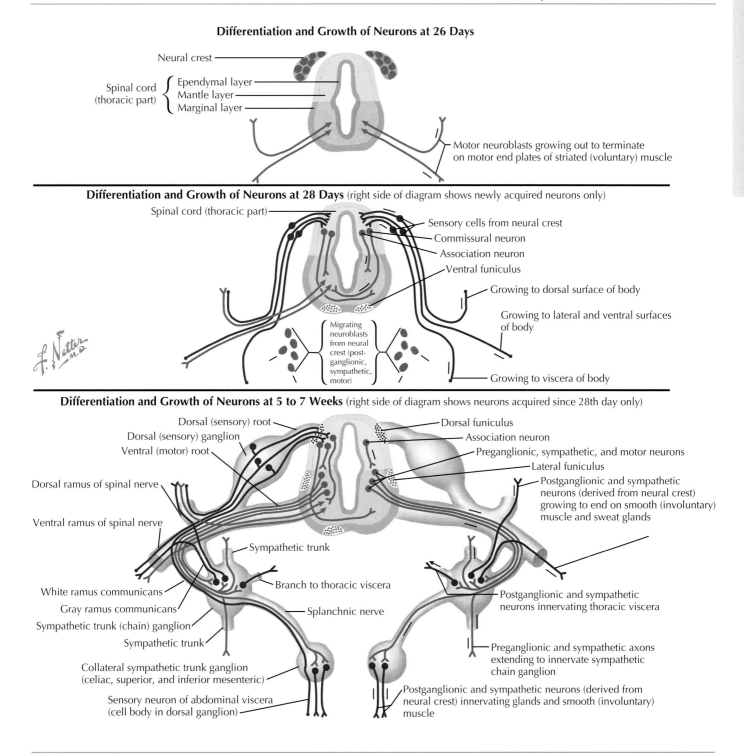

Differentiation and Growth of Neurons at 26 Days

Neural crest

Spinal cord (thoracic part) { Ependymal layer / Mantle layer / Marginal layer

Motor neuroblasts growing out to terminate on motor end plates of striated (voluntary) muscle

Differentiation and Growth of Neurons at 28 Days (right side of diagram shows newly acquired neurons only)

Spinal cord (thoracic part)

Sensory cells from neural crest
Commissural neuron
Association neuron
Ventral funiculus
Growing to dorsal surface of body
Growing to lateral and ventral surfaces of body

Migrating neuroblasts from neural crest (post-ganglionic, sympathetic, motor)

Growing to viscera of body

Differentiation and Growth of Neurons at 5 to 7 Weeks (right side of diagram shows neurons acquired since 28th day only)

Dorsal (sensory) root
Dorsal (sensory) ganglion
Ventral (motor) root
Dorsal ramus of spinal nerve
Ventral ramus of spinal nerve

Dorsal funiculus
Association neuron
Preganglionic, sympathetic, and motor neurons
Lateral funiculus
Postganglionic and sympathetic neurons (derived from neural crest) growing to end on smooth (involuntary) muscle and sweat glands

Sympathetic trunk
Branch to thoracic viscera
Splanchnic nerve

White ramus communicans
Gray ramus communicans
Sympathetic trunk (chain) ganglion
Sympathetic trunk
Collateral sympathetic trunk ganglion (celiac, superior, and inferior mesenteric)
Sensory neuron of abdominal viscera (cell body in dorsal ganglion)

Postganglionic and sympathetic neurons innervating thoracic viscera
Preganglionic and sympathetic axons extending to innervate sympathetic chain ganglion
Postganglionic and sympathetic neurons (derived from neural crest) innervating glands and smooth (involuntary) muscle

8.4 DEVELOPMENT OF PERIPHERAL AXONS

Peripheral axon development is a complex process of central and peripheral neurite extension, trophic and chemotactic factors, and axonal guidance and maintenance by innervated target tissues. Dorsal root ganglion cells are bipolar; a peripheral axonal process is associated with simple or complex sensory receptor cells, and a central axonal process extends into the central nervous system (CNS) to form connections with secondary sensory neurons. The lower motor neurons send motor axons to the developing skeletal muscles through the ventral roots or motor cranial nerves, forming neuromuscular junctions as sites of synaptic connectivity. Motor neurons that

fail to establish such contact with skeletal muscles die. Central preganglionic axons exit in the ventral roots and terminate on sympathetic ganglion cells in the sympathetic chain or collateral ganglia or on parasympathetic intramural ganglia near the organs innervated. Postganglionic axons form connections with target tissues, including smooth muscle, cardiac muscle, secretory glands, some metabolic cells (hepatocytes, fat cells), and cells of the immune system in parenchymal zones of many lymphoid organs. Sensory, motor, and autonomic symptoms can occur in peripheral neuropathies based on disruption of these connections.

Neural crest

Neural tube

Dorsal root ganglion

Dermatomyotome

Sympathetic chain ganglion (sympathetic for spinal nerves)

Collateral ganglion (sympathetic for visceral arteries)

Gut

Enteric plexus ganglia (parasympathetic input for muscle and glands)

Migration of neural crest cells forms peripheral ganglia of autonomic nervous system

Sensory neuroblast grows into dorsal horn and viscera

Splanchnic nerve

Gut

Motor neuroblasts form primitive axons, which migrate into ganglia and then innervate viscera

Autonomic Development

Autonomic nervous system mostly innervates splanchnopleure (viscera)

Dorsal root

Ventral root

Epaxial muscles

Dorsal ramus

Ventral ramus

Posterior division

Anterior division

Hypaxial muscles (extensors of limb)

Hypaxial muscles (flexors of limb)

Hypaxial muscles (flexors of arm and shoulder)

Motor neuroblasts form primitive axons and enter skeletal muscle of body wall

Posterior cutaneous nerve

Epaxial muscles

Dorsal ramus

Ventral ramus

Hypaxial muscles in thoracic and abdominal wall

Lateral cutaneous nerve

Anterior cutaneous nerve

Somatic Development

JOHN A. CRAIG—AD

Somatic nervous system innervates somatopleure (body wall)

8.5 SOMATIC VERSUS SPLANCHNIC NERVE DEVELOPMENT

Somatopleure and splanchnopleure constitute the embryonic basis for the subdivision of the PNS into spinal (somatic) nerves and splanchnic (autonomic) nerves. The somatopleure develops from ectoderm and the somatic portion of lateral plate mesoderm. Somite hypoblasts migrate into somatopleure to form the lateral and ventral aspects of the body wall, including the limbs. Splanchnopleure, derived from endoderm and lateral plate mesoderm, give rise to visceral organs. The ventral rami migrate into somatopleure, and splanchnic nerves grow into splanchnopleure. Thoracic and lumbar splanchnic nerves have sympathetic and visceral sensory axonal components. Pelvic splanchnic nerves (S2–S4) have parasympathetic and visceral sensory axonal components.

Changes in ventral dermatome pattern (cutaneous sensory nerve distribution) during limb development

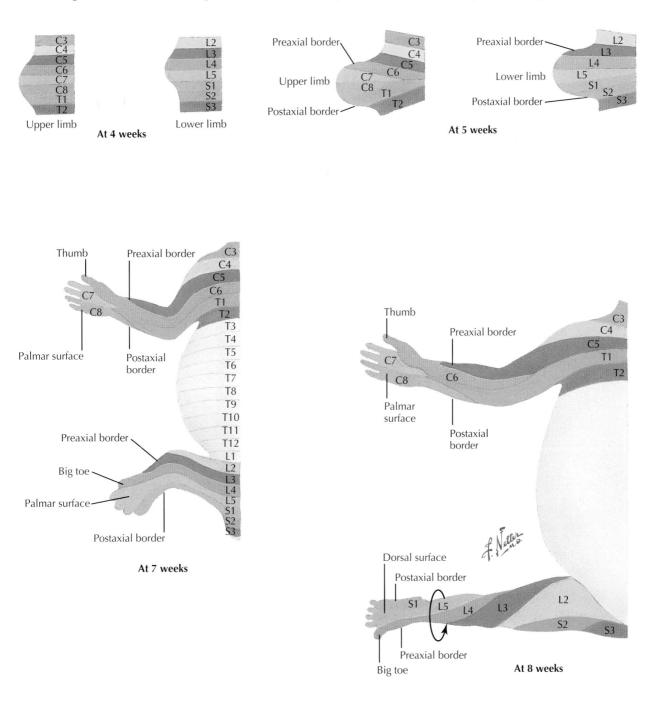

8.6 LIMB ROTATION AND DERMATOMES

Rotation of the lower limb results in a reversal of the preaxial and postaxial borders, producing a spiral arrangement of dermatomes. Spinal nerve segments on the anterior surface of the lower extremity extend medially and inferiorly; the great toe (hallux) is supplied by nerves from a more rostral dermatome (L4) than the little toe (S1). The lower extremity is an extension of the trunk, and the most caudal dermatomes (sacral and coccygeal) supply the perineum, not the foot. Cervical dermatomes maintain a relatively orderly distribution to the upper extremity with minimal rotation.

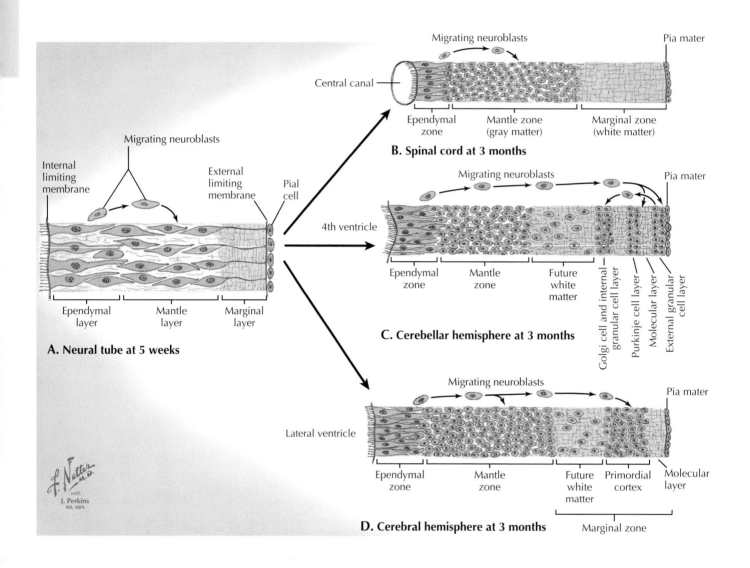

A. Neural tube at 5 weeks

B. Spinal cord at 3 months

C. Cerebellar hemisphere at 3 months

D. Cerebral hemisphere at 3 months

8.7 NEURAL PROLIFERATION AND DIFFERENTIATION: WALLS OF THE NEURAL TUBE

Early in development (5 weeks), neuroblasts in the ependymal layer lining the central canal move back and forth from the ependymal surface to the pial surface, replicating as they go. Neural migration follows distinctive patterns in different regions of the neural tube. In the spinal cord, neurons migrate into the inner mantle zone, leaving the outer marginal zone as a site for axonal pathways. In the cerebellar cortex, some neurons migrate to an outer location on the outer pial surface as an external granular layer, from which granular cells then migrate inward to synapse with other neurons present in deeper layers of the cerebellar cortex. In the cerebral cortex, neurons migrate to the outer zone, where the gray matter (neuronal cell bodies) remains on the surface, external to the white matter (nerve fibers). These developmental patterns reflect the anatomical organization of the mature structures, their blood supply, and their vulnerability to injury by tumors, vascular insults, trauma, and other disorders.

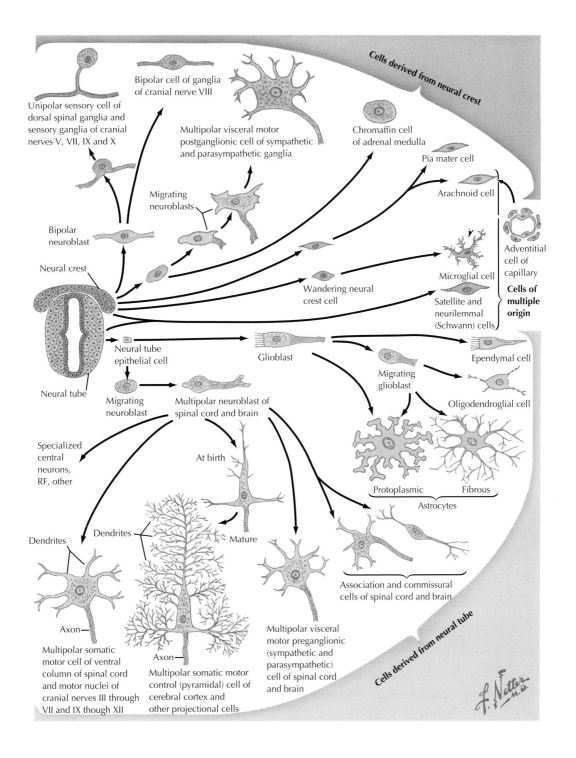

8.8 NEURAL TUBE AND NEURAL CREST DERIVATIVES

Neural tube ependymal cells give rise to neuroblasts, from which the neurons of the CNS are derived. They also give rise to the glioblasts, from which the mature ependymal cells, astrocytes, and oligodendroglia are derived. Microglia, the "scavenger cells" of the CNS, are derived mainly from mesodermal precursors. Cells of glial origin are the predominant cells that give rise to CNS tumors. The neural crest cells give rise to many peripheral neural structures, including primary sensory neurons, postganglionic autonomic neurons of both the sympathetic and parasympathetic systems, adrenal medullary chromaffin cells, and pial and arachnoid cells, Schwann cells (the supporting cells of the PNS), and some other specialized cell types. Neural crest cells can be damaged selectively in some disorders (e.g., familial dysautonomias) and also can give rise to specific tumor cell types such as pheochromocytomas.

Central nervous system at 28 days

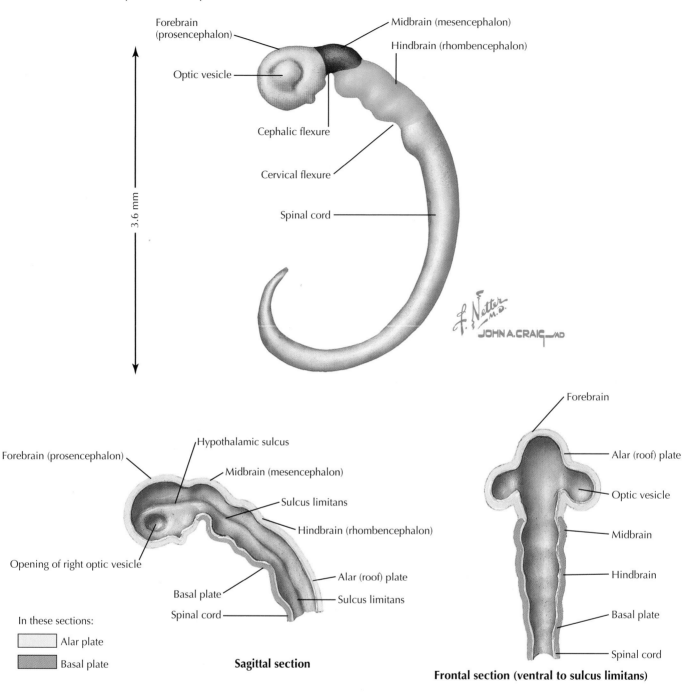

Forebrain (prosencephalon)

Optic vesicle

Midbrain (mesencephalon)

Hindbrain (rhombencephalon)

Cephalic flexure

Cervical flexure

Spinal cord

3.6 mm

Forebrain (prosencephalon)

Hypothalamic sulcus

Midbrain (mesencephalon)

Sulcus limitans

Hindbrain (rhombencephalon)

Opening of right optic vesicle

Basal plate

Spinal cord

Alar (roof) plate

Sulcus limitans

In these sections:

Alar plate

Basal plate

Sagittal section

Forebrain

Alar (roof) plate

Optic vesicle

Midbrain

Hindbrain

Basal plate

Spinal cord

Frontal section (ventral to sulcus limitans)

8.9 EARLY BRAIN DEVELOPMENT: THE 28-DAY-OLD EMBRYO

Some components of the neural tube expand differentially, resulting in bends or flexures that separate the neural tube into caudal to rostral components. The cervical flexure caudally and the cephalic flexure rostrally result from the differential expansion. Three regions of rapid cellular proliferation develop: the forebrain (prosencephalon) rostrally; the mesencephalon (midbrain) in the middle; and the hindbrain (rhombencephalon) caudally. The ventricular system bends and expands to accommodate the increasing neural growth. An outgrowth from the caudal part of the prosencephalon extends from the future diencephalon to become the optic cup, giving rise to the future retina and its central connections.

CLINICAL POINT

The optic vesicle develops from the prosencephalon, specifically the future diencephalon. As a consequence, the neuroretina is actually a central neural derivative and not a peripheral neural crest derivative. Therefore, the retina is supplied with CNS vasculature, and the ganglion cells of the retina (projecting into the optic nerve, chiasm, and tract) are actually CNS axons myelinated by oligodendroglia and surrounded by subarachnoid space and its cerebrospinal fluid. As a CNS tract, the optic nerve is subject to central demyelinating lesions as seen in multiple sclerosis. The retinal vasculature is the only CNS vasculature that is directly observable by ophthalmoscopy.

Cranial nerve VII (Facial) (sensory and motor)

Cranial nerve VI (abducens) (motor)

Cranial nerve V (trigeminal) (sensory and motor)

Cranial nerve IV (trochlear) (motor)

Midbrain (mesencephalon)

Cranial nerve III (oculomotor) (motor)

Forebrain (prosencephalon)
- Diencephalon
- Telencephalic vesicle

Optic cup

Infundibulum

1.0 mm

Coccygeal nerve (sensory and motor)

1st sacral nerve (sensory and motor)

1st lumbar nerve (sensory and motor)

Hindbrain (metencephalon)

Cranial nerve VIII (vestibulocochlear) (sensory)

Cranial nerve IX (glossopharyngeal) (sensory and motor)

Cranial nerve X (vagus) (sensory and motor)

Cranial nerve XI (accessory) (motor)

Cranial nerve XII (hypoglossal) (motor)

1st cervical nerve (sensory and motor)

1st thoracic nerve (sensory and motor)

Hindbrain (myelencephalon)

Central Nervous System: Cranial and Spinal Nerves at 36 Days

Sensory neurons and ganglia from neural crest

f. Netter M.D.
JOHN A. CRAIG—AD

In sagittal and frontal sections:
- Alar (roof) plate
- Basal plate

Sagittal section

Metencephalon (cerebellum, pons)

Alar plate

Basal plate

Sulcus limitans

Mesencephalon

Cerebral aqueduct

Diencephalon

3rd ventricle

Opening of right telencephalic vesicle

4th ventricle

Thin root of myelencephalon (medulla oblongata)

4th ventricle

Central canal

Spinal cord

Hypothalamic sulcus

Infundibulum

Opening of right optic stalk

Lamina terminalis

Frontal section (ventral to sulcus limitans)

Lamina terminalis

3rd ventricle

Telencephalic vesicle

Lateral ventricle

Alar plate

3rd ventricle

Optic stalk

Optic cup

Infundibular recess

Diencephalon

Mesencephalon

Cerebral aqueduct

Basal plate

Metencephalon (cerebellum, pons)

4th ventricle

Myelencephalon (medulla oblongata)

4th ventricle

Spinal cord

Central canal

Rhombencephalon

8.10 EARLY BRAIN DEVELOPMENT: THE 36-DAY-OLD EMBRYO

By day 36, the prosencephalon begins to expand rapidly as the future diencephalon (thalamus and hypothalamus) and telencephalon (basal ganglia, limbic forebrain, olfactory system, and cerebral cortex). This rapid growth is accompanied by the formation of the thin third ventricle for the diencephalon and the C-shaped lateral ventricles from the rostral end of the original central canal for the telencephalon. The rhombencephalon further develops into two distinct regions, the metencephalon (future pons and cerebellum) and the myelencephalon (future medulla). Distinct spinal nerves and cranial nerves begin to form as sensory and motor neurons differentiate and begin to connect with their appropriate targets in the periphery.

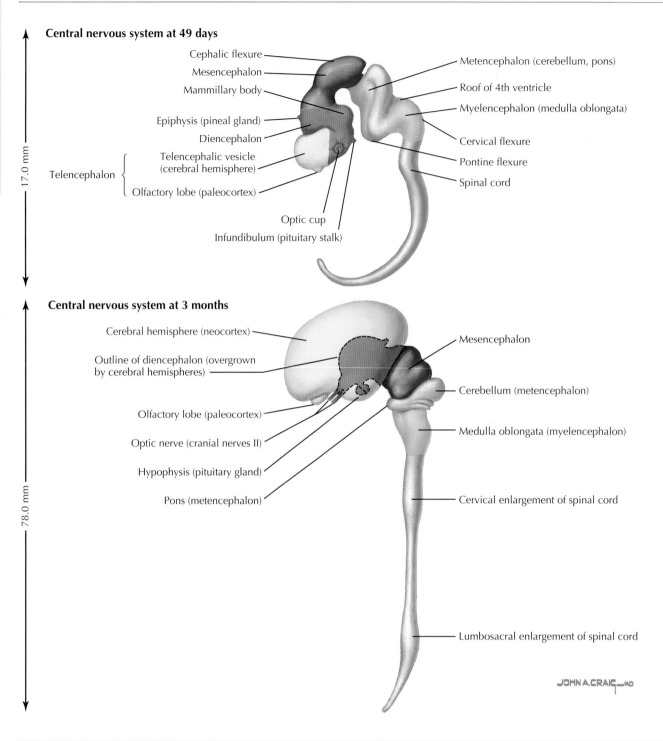

Central nervous system at 49 days

17.0 mm

Cephalic flexure
Mesencephalon
Mammillary body
Epiphysis (pineal gland)
Diencephalon
Telencephalic vesicle (cerebral hemisphere)
Telencephalon
Olfactory lobe (paleocortex)
Optic cup
Infundibulum (pituitary stalk)

Metencephalon (cerebellum, pons)
Roof of 4th ventricle
Myelencephalon (medulla oblongata)
Cervical flexure
Pontine flexure
Spinal cord

Central nervous system at 3 months

78.0 mm

Cerebral hemisphere (neocortex)
Outline of diencephalon (overgrown by cerebral hemispheres)
Olfactory lobe (paleocortex)
Optic nerve (cranial nerves II)
Hypophysis (pituitary gland)
Pons (metencephalon)

Mesencephalon
Cerebellum (metencephalon)
Medulla oblongata (myelencephalon)
Cervical enlargement of spinal cord
Lumbosacral enlargement of spinal cord

JOHN A. CRAIG—AD

8.11 EARLY BRAIN DEVELOPMENT: THE 49-DAY-OLD EMBRYO AND THE 3-MONTH-OLD EMBRYO

By 49 days of age, the diencephalons and telencephalon differentiate into distinct components: the thalamus dorsally and the hypothalamus ventrally from the diencephalons, and the olfactory lobe, basal ganglia, limbic forebrain structures, and cerebral cortex from the telencephalon. The metencephalon (pons) and myelencephalon (medulla) develop further and fold, separated by the pontine flexure dorsally. Between 49 days and 3 months, massive development of the telencephalon overrides and covers the diencephalon. The cerebellum forms from the rhombic lips of the metencephalon as neurons travel dorsally to overlie the

future pons and eventually most of the brain stem. The mesencephalon expands dorsally, forming the superior and inferior colliculi (quadrigeminal bodies). The continuing growth of the spinal cord as it connects with peripheral tissues in the developing limbs forms the cervical and lumbosacral enlargements.

CLINICAL POINT

The process by which the prosencephalon gives rise to the diencephalons and telencephalon is termed prosencephalization. A failure of this process to form the two hemispheres results in holoprosencephaly, with a single large forebrain ventricle, a poorly developed diencephalon, and aberrant development of telencephalic structures. This severe defect in forebrain formation is also accompanied by severe facial malformations.

Forebrain at 7 Weeks (transverse section)

Choroidal vein and artery
Telencephalic vesicle (cerebral hemisphere; neopallium)
Roof of median telocele (3rd ventricle)
Lateral telocele (lateral ventricle)
Opening between lateral and median teloceles (interventricular foramen)
Ependymal layer
Mantle layer
Marginal layer
Median telocele (3rd ventricle)

Telencephalon at 7½ Weeks (transverse section)

Choroidal vein and artery
Telencephalic vesicle (cerebral hemisphere; neopallium)
Roof of 3rd ventricle
Hippocampus (archipallium)
Lateral ventricle
Choroid plexus
Interventricular foramen
Ependymal layer
Mantle layer
Marginal layer
Anterior lobe of hypophysis (pituitary gland)
Corpus striatum (basal ganglion)
3rd ventricle
Infundibulum (pituitary stalk)

Forebrain at 2 Months (coronal section; anterior view)

Epiphysis (pineal gland)
Cerebral hemisphere (neopallium, cut edge)
Hippocampus (archipallium)
Choroid plexus
Choroid fissure
Thalamus
Corpus striatum (basal ganglion)
3rd ventricle
Optic (nerve) stalk
Diencephalon
Roof of 3rd ventricle
Lateral ventricle
Interventricular foramen
Lamina terminalis

Telencephalon at 2½ Months (right anterior view)

Right cerebral hemisphere (neopallium, cut edge)
Left cerebral hemisphere (neopallium)
Hippocampus (archipallium)
Choroid plexus protruding into right lateral ventricle along choroid fissure
Corpus striatum (basal ganglion)
Interventricular foramen
Opening of cavity of right olfactory lobe
Olfactory lobes (paleopallium)

Right Cerebral Hemisphere at 3 Months (medial aspect)

Corpus callosum
Commissure of fornix (hippocampal commissure)
Fornix
Anterior commissure
Lamina terminalis
Olfactory lobe (paleopallium)
3rd ventricle
Medial surface of right cerebral hemisphere (neopallium)
Choroidal vessels passing to choroid plexus, which protrudes into right lateral ventricle along choroid fissure
Hippocampus (archipallium)
Stria terminalis
Thalamus (cut surface)
Line of division between diencephalon and telencephalon

Cerebral Hemispheres at 3 Months (coronal section)

Falx cerebri
Ependymal layer
Mantle layer
Marginal layer
Neopallial cortex
Hippocampal cortex
Corpus striatum (basal ganglia) { Caudate nucleus / Lenticular nucleus }
Dura mater
Superior sagittal sinus
Inferior sagittal sinus
Lateral ventricle
Ependymal-pial covering of choroid plexus
Choroidal vein and artery
Internal capsule
Anterior commissure
Interventricular foramen
Choroid plexus of roof of 3rd ventricle
Optic recess of 3rd ventricle

F. Netter M.D.

8.12 FOREBRAIN DEVELOPMENT: 7 WEEKS THROUGH 3 MONTHS

Neurons of the developing telencephalon move rostrally, dorsally, and then around the diencephalon in a C shape toward the anterior pole of the temporal lobe. The hippocampal formation forms in a dorsal and anterior position and migrates in a C-shaped course into the anterior temporal lobe. The amygdala develops in a similar manner, giving rise to the stria terminalis pathway in a C shape. The lateral ventricles follow the same C-shaped developmental process anatomically. The caudate nucleus also extends around the telencephalon in a C-shaped pattern, with the large head of the nucleus remaining anterior and the much smaller body and tail following as a thinner C-shaped structure that ends ventrally in the temporal horn of the lateral ventricle. The corpus callosum and anterior commissure connect the two hemispheres. The internal capsule funnels centrally in the core of the forebrain on either side; the posterior limb continues caudally as the cerebral peduncle.

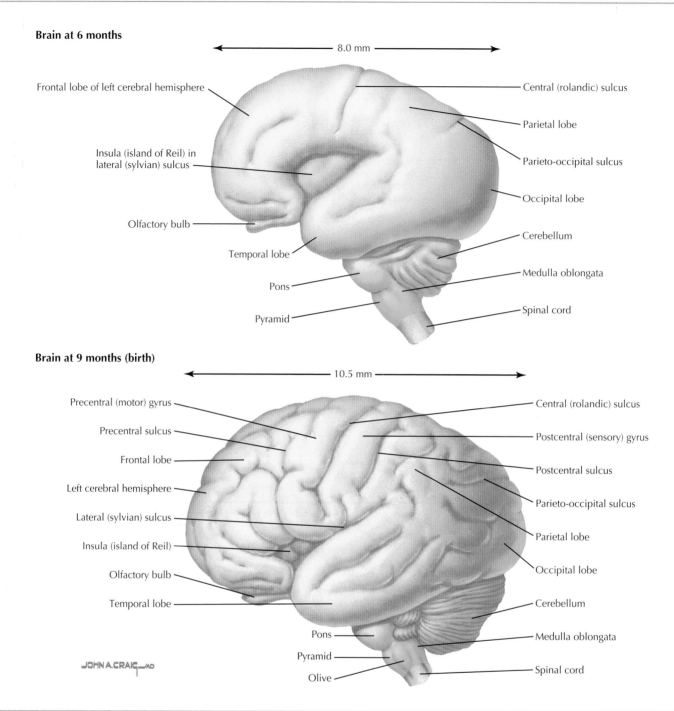

Brain at 6 months

8.0 mm

Frontal lobe of left cerebral hemisphere

Central (rolandic) sulcus

Parietal lobe

Insula (island of Reil) in lateral (sylvian) sulcus

Parieto-occipital sulcus

Occipital lobe

Olfactory bulb

Cerebellum

Temporal lobe

Medulla oblongata

Pons

Spinal cord

Pyramid

Brain at 9 months (birth)

10.5 mm

Precentral (motor) gyrus

Central (rolandic) sulcus

Precentral sulcus

Postcentral (sensory) gyrus

Frontal lobe

Postcentral sulcus

Left cerebral hemisphere

Parieto-occipital sulcus

Lateral (sylvian) sulcus

Parietal lobe

Insula (island of Reil)

Occipital lobe

Olfactory bulb

Temporal lobe

Cerebellum

Pons

Medulla oblongata

Pyramid

Spinal cord

Olive

JOHN A. CRAIG—AD

8.13 THE 6-MONTH AND 9-MONTH CENTRAL NERVOUS SYSTEMS

At 6 months, the brain stem has differentiated into the medulla, pons, and midbrain, with the developing cerebellum overlying them dorsally. Even though the diencephalon is rapidly developing, the overlying telencephalon shows massive growth rostrally, then caudally, downward, and forward into the temporal lobe. From 6 to 9 months of age, the cerebral cortex forms its characteristic convolutions with gyri and sulci, and the cerebellar cortex forms its distinctive folds, the folia. Within the forebrain, the major components of the basal ganglia, the limbic forebrain structures (i.e., the amygdala and hippocampal formation), the olfactory system, and the cerebral cortex develop rapidly. Most neurons are present at birth, except for some populations of granular cells in the cerebellum,

the dentate gyrus of the hippocampus, and the cerebral cortex, which form postnatally in response to environmental stimuli. The in utero and postnatal environments provide major influences on neural development and function.

CLINICAL POINT

The cerebral cortex develops through an orderly process of cell proliferation from the ventricular zone and then the subventricular zone, with proper cell migration and interconnectivity extending through prenatal life and well into postnatal life. A failure of proper cell proliferation and migration of cortical neurons can result in the failure of proper formation of gyri and sulci, giving a smooth cortical surface appearance called lissencephaly. In some situations, gyri can be unusually small (microgyria) or unusually large (pachygyria). These developmental defects may be accompanied by profound neural deficits and retardation.

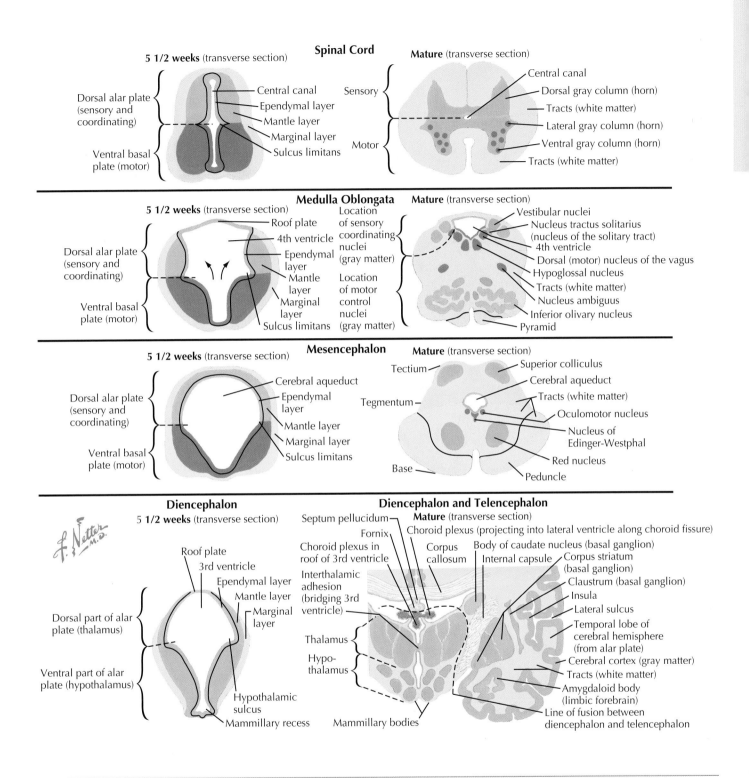

8.14 COMPARISON OF 5½-WEEK AND ADULT CENTRAL NERVOUS SYSTEM REGIONS

The relatively large ventricular system at 5½ weeks becomes comparatively smaller as the process of neuronal growth occurs. In adults, the central canal of the spinal cord becomes virtually obliterated and does not convey cerebrospinal fluid (CSF). The fourth ventricle opens up laterally; the sulcus limitans demarcates motor nuclei (medially) and sensory nuclei (laterally). The cerebral aqueduct remains very small. The third ventricle narrows down to a slit. The lateral ventricles expand massively into a C-shape. The basal plate forms motor and autonomic structures whose axons leave the CNS. The alar plate forms sensory derivatives in the spinal cord and brain stem, and structures that migrate ventrally (the inferior olivary complex, the pontine nuclei, and the red nucleus). The rhombic lips, an alar derivative of the metencephalon, give rise to the entire cerebellum. The diencephalon and telencephalon are also alar plate derivatives.

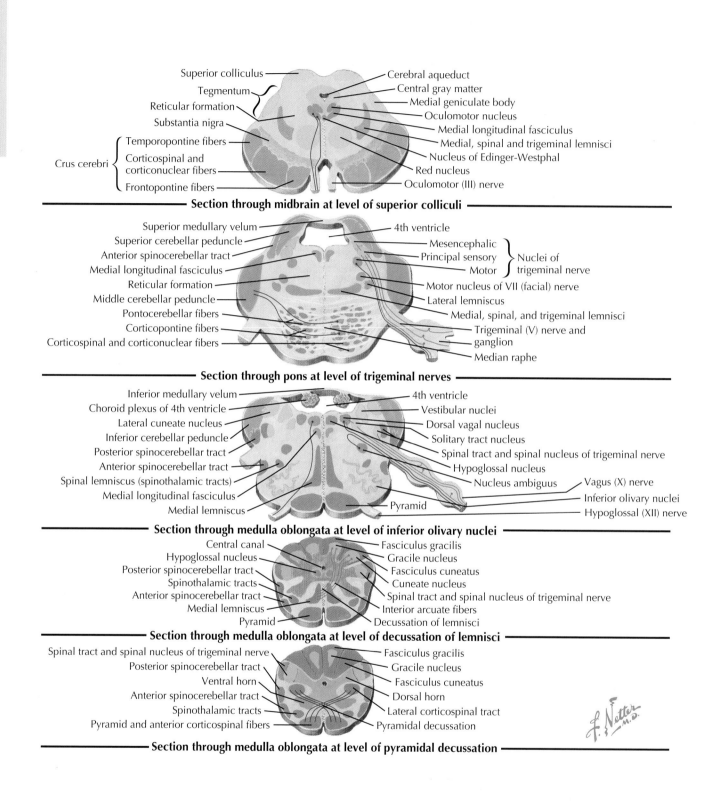

Superior colliculus — Cerebral aqueduct
Tegmentum — Central gray matter
Reticular formation — Medial geniculate body
Substantia nigra — Oculomotor nucleus
— Medial longitudinal fasciculus
Temporopontine fibers — Medial, spinal and trigeminal lemnisci
Crus cerebri { Corticospinal and corticonuclear fibers — Nucleus of Edinger-Westphal
Frontopontine fibers — Red nucleus
— Oculomotor (III) nerve

Section through midbrain at level of superior colliculi

Superior medullary velum — 4th ventricle
Superior cerebellar peduncle — Mesencephalic
Anterior spinocerebellar tract — Principal sensory } Nuclei of trigeminal nerve
Medial longitudinal fasciculus — Motor
Reticular formation — Motor nucleus of VII (facial) nerve
Middle cerebellar peduncle — Lateral lemniscus
Pontocerebellar fibers — Medial, spinal, and trigeminal lemnisci
Corticopontine fibers — Trigeminal (V) nerve and ganglion
Corticospinal and corticonuclear fibers — Median raphe

Section through pons at level of trigeminal nerves

Inferior medullary velum — 4th ventricle
Choroid plexus of 4th ventricle — Vestibular nuclei
Lateral cuneate nucleus — Dorsal vagal nucleus
Inferior cerebellar peduncle — Solitary tract nucleus
Posterior spinocerebellar tract — Spinal tract and spinal nucleus of trigeminal nerve
Anterior spinocerebellar tract — Hypoglossal nucleus
Spinal lemniscus (spinothalamic tracts) — Nucleus ambiguus — Vagus (X) nerve
Medial longitudinal fasciculus — Inferior olivary nuclei
Medial lemniscus — Pyramid — Hypoglossal (XII) nerve

Section through medulla oblongata at level of inferior olivary nuclei

Central canal — Fasciculus gracilis
Hypoglossal nucleus — Gracile nucleus
Posterior spinocerebellar tract — Fasciculus cuneatus
Spinothalamic tracts — Cuneate nucleus
Anterior spinocerebellar tract — Spinal tract and spinal nucleus of trigeminal nerve
Medial lemniscus — Interior arcuate fibers
Pyramid — Decussation of lemnisci

Section through medulla oblongata at level of decussation of lemnisci

Spinal tract and spinal nucleus of trigeminal nerve — Fasciculus gracilis
Posterior spinocerebellar tract — Gracile nucleus
Ventral horn — Fasciculus cuneatus
Anterior spinocerebellar tract — Dorsal horn
Spinothalamic tracts — Lateral corticospinal tract
Pyramid and anterior corticospinal fibers — Pyramidal decussation

Section through medulla oblongata at level of pyramidal decussation

8.15 ALAR AND BASAL PLATE DERIVATIVES IN THE BRAIN STEM

The general pattern of alar and basal plate derivatives seen in the spinal cord continues into the brain stem. The alar plate derivatives are the sensory nuclei (the rhombic lip from which the cerebellum is derived) and nuclei that migrate ventrally to form such structures as the inferior olivary nuclei, the pontine nuclei, the red nucleus, and others. The basal plate derivatives are the motor and preganglionic autonomic nuclei.

Adult derivatives of brain primordia

Adult neural structures derived from embryonic primordia

Sagittal view

Cerebral hemispheres (telencephalon)
Olfactory bulbs (CN I) (telencephalon)
Thalamus/3rd ventricle (diencephalon)
Optic chiasm (CN II) (diencephalon)
Pineal gland (diencephalon)
Neurohypophysis (diencephalon)
Tectum/aqueduct (mesencephalon)
Pons (metencephalon)
4th ventricle (metencephalon)
Cerebellum (metencephalon)
Medulla oblongata (myelencephalon)
Spinal cord

CN III
CN IV
CN VI
CN V
CN VII
CN VIII
CN IX
CN X
CN XI

Dorsal view

JOHN A. CRAIG—AD

Adult derivatives of the forebrain, midbrain, and hindbrain

Forebrain	Telencephalon	Cerebral hemispheres (neocortex) Olfactory cortex (paleocortex) Hippocampus (archicortex) Basal ganglia/corpus striatum Lateral and 3rd ventricles	Nerves: Olfactory (I)
	Diencephalon	Optic cup/nerves Thalamus Hypothalamus Mammillary bodies Part of 3rd ventricle	Optic (II)
Midbrain	Mesencephalon	Tectum (superior, inferior colliculi) Cerebral aqueduct Red nucleus Substantia nigra Crus cerebelli	Oculomotor (III) Trochlear (IV)
Hindbrain	Metencephalon	Pons Cerebellum	Trigeminal (V) Abducens (VI)
	Myelencephalon	Medulla oblongata	Facial (VII) Acoustic (VIII) Glossopharyngeal (IX) Vagus (X) Hypoglossal (XI)

8.16 ADULT DERIVATIVES OF THE FOREBRAIN, MIDBRAIN, AND HINDBRAIN

The telencephalon has four major components: the cerebral cortex, the limbic forebrain structures, the basal ganglia, and the olfactory system. The diencephalon consists of two major structures: the thalamus and hypothalamus and two smaller structures, the epithalamus and subthalamus. The thalamus has extensive interconnections with the cerebral cortex and serves as a gateway to the telencephalon. The hypothalamus receives extensive input from the limbic forebrain and a variety of visceral sensory sources, and regulates neuroendocrine and visceral autonomic functions. The midbrain consists of the colliculi, the tegmentum, and the cerebral peduncles. The colliculi convey visual (superior) and auditory (inferior) information to higher regions of the brain and to brain stem and reflex pathways. The tegmentum houses important motor, sensory, and autonomic structures and plays a crucial role in consciousness and sleep. The cerebral peduncles are caudal continuations of the posterior limb of the internal capsule, and play a particularly important role in motor functions. The cerebellum plays an important role in coordinating movement, posture, locomotion, and equilibrium. The medulla and pons integrate the sensory, motor, and autonomic functions of the body via extensive connections through the cranial nerves, which the spinal cord inputs.

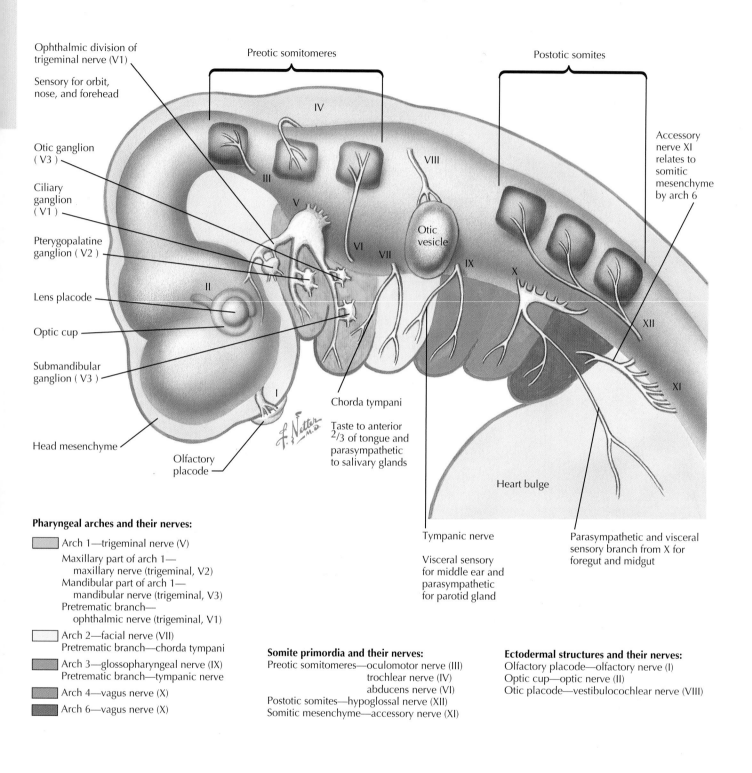

Ophthalmic division of trigeminal nerve (V1)

Sensory for orbit, nose, and forehead

Otic ganglion (V3)

Ciliary ganglion (V1)

Pterygopalatine ganglion (V2)

Lens placode

Optic cup

Submandibular ganglion (V3)

Head mesenchyme

Olfactory placode

Preotic somitomeres

Postotic somites

Accessory nerve XI relates to somitic mesenchyme by arch 6

Otic vesicle

Chorda tympani

Taste to anterior ²/₃ of tongue and parasympathetic to salivary glands

Heart bulge

Tympanic nerve

Visceral sensory for middle ear and parasympathetic for parotid gland

Parasympathetic and visceral sensory branch from X for foregut and midgut

Pharyngeal arches and their nerves:

Arch 1—trigeminal nerve (V)
Maxillary part of arch 1— maxillary nerve (trigeminal, V2)
Mandibular part of arch 1— mandibular nerve (trigeminal, V3)
Pretrematic branch— ophthalmic nerve (trigeminal, V1)

Arch 2—facial nerve (VII)
Pretrematic branch—chorda tympani

Arch 3—glossopharyngeal nerve (IX)
Pretrematic branch—tympanic nerve

Arch 4—vagus nerve (X)

Arch 6—vagus nerve (X)

Somite primordia and their nerves:
Preotic somitomeres—oculomotor nerve (III)
                    trochlear nerve (IV)
                    abducens nerve (VI)
Postotic somites—hypoglossal nerve (XII)
Somitic mesenchyme—accessory nerve (XI)

Ectodermal structures and their nerves:
Olfactory placode—olfactory nerve (I)
Optic cup—optic nerve (II)
Otic placode—vestibulocochlear nerve (VIII)

8.17 CRANIAL NERVE PRIMORDIA

The 12 pairs of cranial nerves exit the developing brain in sequence, except for cranial nerve XI, which exits most caudally. Cranial nerves I and II are CNS tracts, not peripheral nerves.

The cranial nerves relate to surface placodes, head somites, or the pharyngeal arches, and they innervate all of the structures and tissues that derive from them. The vagus nerve supplies arches 4 and 6.

Special sensory and somatomotor cranial nerve components

Nerve	Primordium innervated	Neuron components
Olfactory (I) Optic (II) Vestibulocochlear (VIII)	Olfactory placode Optic cup Otic placode	Special sensory (olfaction) Special sensory (vision) Special sensory (hearing and balance)

Oculomotor (III)
 	
Trochlear (IV)
Abducens (VI)
Hypoglossal (XII)
Accessory (XI)
	Preotic somitomere
	
	Preotic somitomere
	Preotic somitomere
	Postotic somites
	Somitic mesenchyme
	by arch 6
		Somatomotor to extraocular eye muscles
		Parasympathetics to ciliary ganglion (for pupil
		   constrictor and ciliary muscle)
		Somatomotor to superior oblique muscle
		Somatomotor to lateral rectus muscle
		Somatomotor to tongue muscles
		Somatomotor to sternocleidomastoid and trapezius
		   muscles

Pharyngeal arch cranial nerve components

Nerve	Arch	Neuron components
Trigeminal (V)	1	General sensory (face, orbit, nasal, and oral cavities) Branchiomotor (muscles of mastication, tensor tympani, tensor veli palatini)

Facial (VII)	2	Branchiomotor (muscles of facial expression, stylohyoid, posterior
		   digastric, stapedius)
		Special sensory (taste to anterior two thirds of tongue)
		Parasympathetic to pterygopalatine and submandibular ganglia (for
		   lacrimal glands, nasal mucosa, and salivary glands)

Glossopharyngeal (IX)	3	Visceral sensory to pharynx Branchiomotor to stylopharyngeus Parasympathetic to otic ganglion (for the parotid gland) Special sensory (taste to posterior tongue; carotid body and sinus)
Vagus (X)	4 and 6	Branchiomotor (pharynx and larynx) Visceral sensory (larynx, foregut below pharynx and midgut) General sensory to external acoustic meatus Parasympathetics (enteric ganglia of foregut and midgut) Special sensory (taste in laryngopharynx; carotid body and sinus)

Reprinted with permission from Cochard L. Netter's Atlas of Human Embryology. Philadelphia: Elsevier, 2002.

8.18 CRANIAL NERVE NEURON COMPONENTS

The pharyngeal arch nerves of the head and neck consist of several neuronal types. Most have branchiomotor neurons for skeletal muscles derived from arch mesenchyme, visceral sensory neurons for the inner endodermal linings of the arches (larynx and pharynx), and general sensory neurons for surface ectoderm or lining of the stomodeum. The somites give rise to extraocular muscles and intrinsic muscles of the tongue. The placodes and optic cup relate to the special sensory organs of the head. Cranial nerves III, VII, IX, and X have preganglionic parasympathetic components that innervate ganglia distant from their nerves of origin.

Somatic (GSE)	Parasympathetic (GVE)	Branchiomotor (SVE)
CN III	CN III	
CN IV		
CN VI		CN V
	CN VII	CN VII
	CN IX	CN IX
	CN X	CN X
CN XII		
CN XI		

CN III (GVE)
CN III (GSE)

Rhombomeres

Pharyngeal arches

Parasympathetic (GVE) column

Branchiomotor (SVE) column

Somatomotor (GSE) column

CN IV (GSE)
CN V (SVE)
CN VII (SVE)
CN VII (GVE)
CN VI (GSE)
CN IX (GVE)
CN IX (SVE)
CN XII (GSE)
CN X (SVE)
CN X (GVE)

Ventral horn
Lateral horn
Dorsal horn

Spinal cord

Note:
GSE = General somatic efferent
GVE = General visceral efferent
SVE = Special visceral efferent

JOHN A. CRAIG—AD
D. Mascaro

8.19 DEVELOPMENT OF MOTOR AND PREGANGLIONIC AUTONOMIC NUCLEI IN THE BRAIN STEM AND SPINAL CORD

Gray matter columns develop in the spinal cord for somatic lower motor neurons (ventral horn) and preganglionic autonomic neurons (lateral horn). These columns extend rostrally into the brain stem, maintaining the same general positional relationship to each other but organized into a series of separate but aligned nuclei. A third group of nuclei develop in the rhombencephalon as branchiomotor neurons supplying pharyngeal arch muscles. Both the somatic motor and the branchiomotor neurons are classified as lower motor neurons and have axons exiting the CNS to synapse on skeletal muscle fibers.

Optic vesicle

Surface ectoderm
Neuroectoderm (forebrain)
Mesenchyme
Optic cup
Lens placode

Optic stalk
Optic cup

Early eye develops as neuroectodermal outpouching (optic vesicle) of primitive forebrain and thickening of adjacent surface ectoderm (lens placode)

Lens vesicle
Hyaloid artery
Internal carotid artery

Lens placode invaginates to form the lens vesicle. The optic vesicle invaginates to form a double-layered optic cup that surrounds the lens vesicle and hyaloid vessels

Eyelid primordia

Mesenchymal condensation forms outer layers of globe (cornea and sclera)

Hyaloid artery

Inner layer of optic vesicle (visual retina)

Outer layer of optic vesicle (pigmented retina [epithelium])

Anterior chamber

Hyaloid vessels regress prior to birth

Fusion of visual retina and pigmented retinal epithelium

Orbicularis oculi (2nd pharyngeal arch)
Conjunctiva (surface ectoderm)
Corneal epithelium (surface ectoderm)
Cornea (mesenchyme)
Anterior chamber
Lens (surface ectoderm)
Iris (neuroectoderm)
Visual retina (neuroectoderm)
Pigmented retina (epithelium) (neuro-ectoderm)

Extraocular muscles (preotic somitomeres)
Sclera (mesenchyme)
Choroid (mesenchyme)

Optic nerve (neuroectoderm)

JOHN A. CRAIG—AD

Primordium	Derivative	Related nerve
Optic cup	Retina, optic nerve, ciliary and iris epithelium, and pupil constrictor and dilator muscles	Optic nerve (II)
Head mesenchyme	Cornea, sclera, meninges, choroid, ciliary muscle and connective tissue, and iris connective tissue	Ophthalmic nerve (VI)
Somites	Extraocular eye muscles	III, IV, and VI
Surface ectoderm	Eyelid epidermis, conjunctiva, lacrimal gland	Ophthalmic nerve (VI)
2nd pharyngeal arch	Orbicularis oculi muscle	Facial nerve (VII)
Lens placode	Lens	

8.20 DEVELOPMENT OF THE EYE AND ORBIT

The retina and optic nerve develop as a double-layered extension of the neural tube, the optic cup. This extension surrounds the lens vesicle of surface origin and has a ventral groove to accommodate blood vessels. The iris and ciliary body are formed in part from optic cup epithelium. The two layers of the optic cup never fully fuse and can be separated in the case of a retinal detachment. Connective tissues of mesodermal origin include the sclera, cornea, and vascular choroid layer. The extraocular muscles derive from somitomeres. The epidermis of the eyelids develops from surface ectoderm and is continuous with the conjunctiva and corneal epithelium.

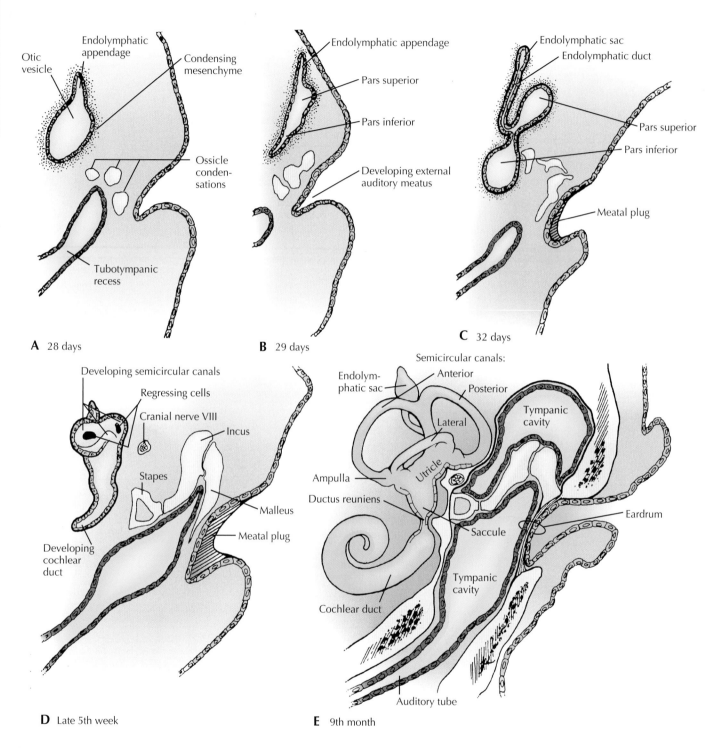

A 28 days

B 29 days

C 32 days

D Late 5th week

E 9th month

Reprinted with permission from Schoenwolf G, Bleyl S, Brauer P, et al. Larsen's Human Embryology, 4th ed. Philadelphia: Elsevier, 2008.

8.21 DEVELOPMENT OF THE EAR

The ear consists of the outer component (the auricle, external auditory meatus to the eardrum); the middle component (the ossicles [malleus, incus, stapes]); and the inner component (the bony and membranous labyrinths, the cochlea, and the semicircular canals). The outer ear derives from the first pharyngeal groove, the middle ear from the first pharyngeal pouch, and the inner ear from the otic placode.

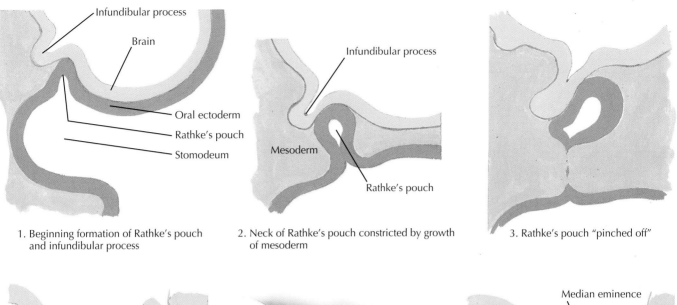

1. Beginning formation of Rathke's pouch and infundibular process

2. Neck of Rathke's pouch constricted by growth of mesoderm

3. Rathke's pouch "pinched off"

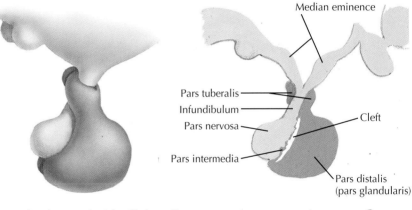

4. Pinched-off segment conforms to neural process, forming pars distalis, pars intermedia, and pars tuberalis

5. Pars tuberalis encircles infundibular stalk (lateral surface view)

6. Mature form

Pituitary hormones

From the anterior lobe (pars distalis)		From the posterior lobe (pars nervosa)
Follicle-stimulating hormone (FSH)	Thyroid-stimulating hormone (TSH)	Vasopressin
Luteinizing hormone (LH)	Adrenocorticotropic hormone (ACTH)	Oxytocin
Prolactin	Growth hormone (GH)	

8.22 DEVELOPMENT OF THE PITUITARY GLAND

The pituitary gland develops from outgrowth of two separate primordia. The anterior lobe (adenohypophysis) derives from the roof of the stomodeum and encircles the base of the posterior lobe (neurohypophysis). The posterior lobe derives from the brain and possesses axonal processes from the hypothalamus that secrete oxytocin and vasopressin into the general circulation. The anterior lobe contains pituicytes that respond to releasing and inhibitory factors from neurons of the brain that are delivered through the private vascular channel and the hypophyseal-portal system and secrete into this circulation hormones such as follicle-stimulating hormone, luteinizing hormone, prolactin, thyroid-stimulating hormone, adrenocorticotropic hormone, and growth hormone.

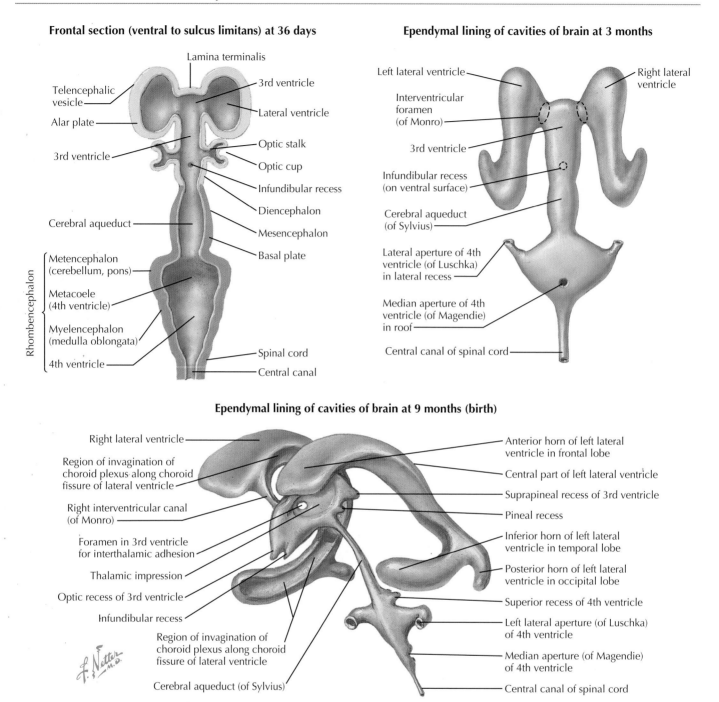

Frontal section (ventral to sulcus limitans) at 36 days

- Lamina terminalis
- Telencephalic vesicle
- 3rd ventricle
- Lateral ventricle
- Alar plate
- Optic stalk
- 3rd ventricle
- Optic cup
- Infundibular recess
- Diencephalon
- Cerebral aqueduct
- Mesencephalon
- Basal plate
- Rhombencephalon
  - Metencephalon (cerebellum, pons)
  - Metacoele (4th ventricle)
  - Myelencephalon (medulla oblongata)
  - 4th ventricle
- Spinal cord
- Central canal

Ependymal lining of cavities of brain at 3 months

- Left lateral ventricle
- Right lateral ventricle
- Interventricular foramen (of Monro)
- 3rd ventricle
- Infundibular recess (on ventral surface)
- Cerebral aqueduct (of Sylvius)
- Lateral aperture of 4th ventricle (of Luschka) in lateral recess
- Median aperture of 4th ventricle (of Magendie) in roof
- Central canal of spinal cord

Ependymal lining of cavities of brain at 9 months (birth)

- Right lateral ventricle
- Region of invagination of choroid plexus along choroid fissure of lateral ventricle
- Right interventricular canal (of Monro)
- Foramen in 3rd ventricle for interthalamic adhesion
- Thalamic impression
- Optic recess of 3rd ventricle
- Infundibular recess
- Region of invagination of choroid plexus along choroid fissure of lateral ventricle
- Cerebral aqueduct (of Sylvius)
- Anterior horn of left lateral ventricle in frontal lobe
- Central part of left lateral ventricle
- Suprapineal recess of 3rd ventricle
- Pineal recess
- Inferior horn of left lateral ventricle in temporal lobe
- Posterior horn of left lateral ventricle in occipital lobe
- Superior recess of 4th ventricle
- Left lateral aperture (of Luschka) of 4th ventricle
- Median aperture (of Magendie) of 4th ventricle
- Central canal of spinal cord

8.23 DEVELOPMENT OF THE VENTRICLES

The rapid growth of the brain stem and the forebrain alters the uniform appearance of the ventricles. The C-shaped lateral ventricles follow the growth of the telencephalon, with limited access into the third ventricle through the interventricular foramen of Monro. The narrow cerebral aqueduct remains very small in the upper mesencephalon and opens into the rhomboid-shaped and expanding fourth ventricle. The foramina of Magendie (medial) and Luschka (lateral) in the fourth ventricle allow flow from the ventricular system into the developing cisterns of the subarachnoid space. CSF reenters the venous system through the arachnoid granulations, one-way valves that allow drainage from the subarachnoid space into the dural (venous) sinuses, especially the superior sagittal sinus.

CLINICAL POINT

The C-shaped form of the ventricular system follows from the development of the primary brain vesicles, with the flexures and disproportionate neural development. The lateral ventricles are associated with the telencephalon, the third ventricle with the diencephalon, the cerebral aqueduct with the mesencephalon, and the fourth ventricle with the rhombencephalon (metencephalon [pons] and myelencephalon [medulla]). The foramina of Magendie and Luschka, which allow for the escape of CSF into the subarachnoid space, are already patent at the end of the first trimester. An obstruction of internal CSF flow results in internal hydrocephalus. A common site for such an obstruction is atresia of the cerebral aqueduct, with enlarged third and lateral ventricles. Another site of possible obstruction occurs with Dandy-Walker syndrome, a malformation of the fourth ventricle that includes atresia of the foramina of Magendie and Luschka, internal hydrocephalus of the entire ventricular system, hypoplasia of the cerebellum, and posterior fossa cyst formation.

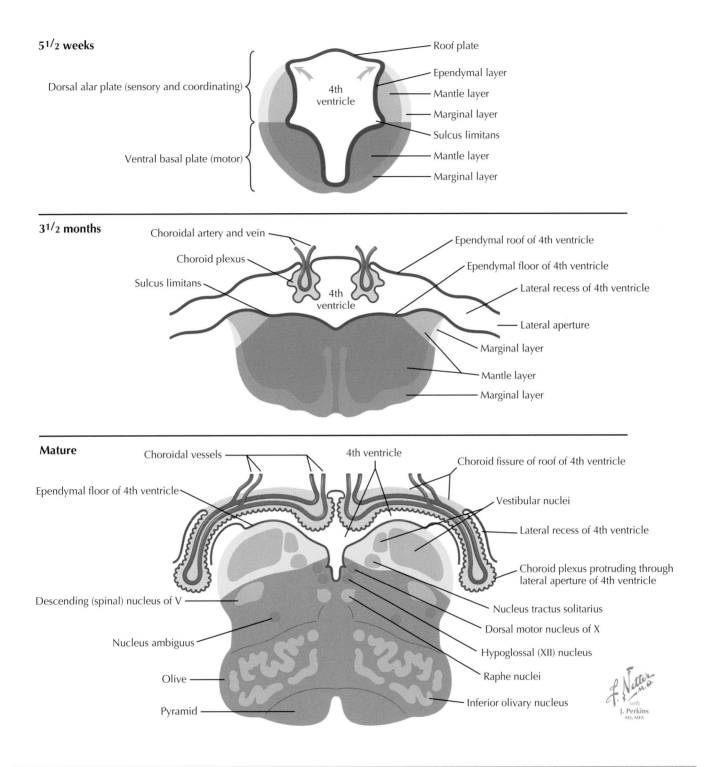

5¹/₂ weeks

Dorsal alar plate (sensory and coordinating)

4th ventricle

Ventral basal plate (motor)

Roof plate
Ependymal layer
Mantle layer
Marginal layer
Sulcus limitans
Mantle layer
Marginal layer

3¹/₂ months

Choroidal artery and vein
Choroid plexus
Sulcus limitans

4th ventricle

Ependymal roof of 4th ventricle
Ependymal floor of 4th ventricle
Lateral recess of 4th ventricle
Lateral aperture
Marginal layer
Mantle layer
Marginal layer

Mature

Choroidal vessels
4th ventricle
Choroid fissure of roof of 4th ventricle
Ependymal floor of 4th ventricle
Vestibular nuclei
Lateral recess of 4th ventricle
Choroid plexus protruding through lateral aperture of 4th ventricle
Descending (spinal) nucleus of V
Nucleus ambiguus
Olive
Pyramid
Nucleus tractus solitarius
Dorsal motor nucleus of X
Hypoglossal (XII) nucleus
Raphe nuclei
Inferior olivary nucleus

8.24 DEVELOPMENT OF THE FOURTH VENTRICLE

The expansion of the fourth ventricle from the original central canal of the rhombencephalon into its mature form is a complex process. The sulcus limitans is conspicuous early in development (5½ weeks), and the original lateral walls expand outward and lie down horizontally (3½ months) as the roof plate expands to both sides. As a result, the sulcus limitans becomes a landmark at the dorsal boundary of the medulla on the floor of the fourth ventricle, separating the motor structures medially from the sensory structures laterally. The lateral aperture of the fourth ventricle (the foramen of Luschka) opens into the subarachnoid space. In their mature form (bottom illustration), these paired lateral apertures are major channels between the internal and external circulation of the CSF and must remain open so as to prevent internal hydrocephalus.

Spinal bifida occulta

Dermal sinus

Dural sac

Cauda equina

Sinus with
squamous plug

Fat pad overlying spina bifida
occulta. Tuft of hair or only skin
dimple may be present, or there may
be no external manifestation. Dermal
sinus also present in this case (*arrow*)

Types of spina bifida aperta with protrusion of spinal contents

Meningocele

Meningomyelocele

Arnold-Chiari syndrome decompression

8.25 NEURAL TUBE DEFECTS

Spina bifida occurs when a vertebral arch fails to develop; the neural tube cannot move below the surface, and somite sclerotome cells cannot migrate over it to complete the vertebral arch. The spinal cord may be exposed on the surface (myeloschisis), which involves severe functional deficits or death and a high likelihood of infection. A protrusion may form, usually in the lumbar region, into which spinal cord and nerve roots may protrude (meningomyelocele) or in which CSF is present (meningocele). When these defects are repaired, the brain stem may herniate (Arnold-Chiari malformation), and extensive functional deficits may be present, such as loss of bladder and bowel function and loss of motor function and sensation in the lower extremities. In its most benign form, spina bifida occulta may be manifested by a small sinus or a tuft of hair at the site of defect.

Occipital encephalocele

Frontal encephalocele

Anencephaly

8.26 DEFECTS OF THE BRAIN AND SKULL

Defects of the rostral portion of the neural tube involve the brain and skull. If the occipital bone or other midline bones fail to ossify, meninges and possibly brain tissue may protrude into a sac (encephalocele). If the rostral (cranial) neuropore fails to close, the brain and much of the skull fail to develop (anencephaly) and the tissue that is present is exposed to the external environment. This condition is incompatible with life. The Arnold-Chiari malformation may occur with or without spina bifida such as in a meningomyelocele; in this malformation, the tonsils of the cerebellum herniate through the foramen magnum and can disrupt vital brain stem functions, resulting in death.

Section II: **REGIONAL NEUROSCIENCE**

9

PERIPHERAL NERVOUS SYSTEM

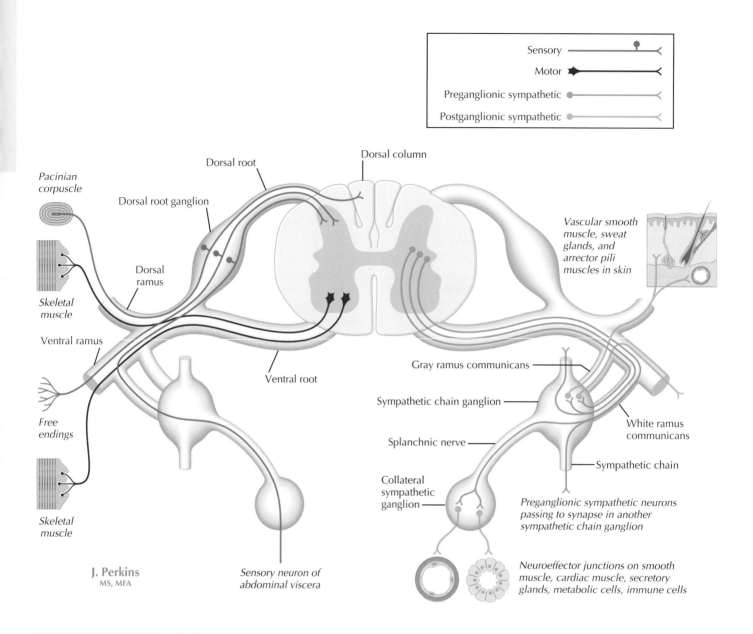

Sensory
Motor
Preganglionic sympathetic
Postganglionic sympathetic

Pacinian corpuscle

Dorsal root

Dorsal column

Dorsal root ganglion

Dorsal ramus

Skeletal muscle

Ventral ramus

Free endings

Skeletal muscle

Ventral root

J. Perkins
MS, MFA

Sensory neuron of abdominal viscera

Vascular smooth muscle, sweat glands, and arrector pili muscles in skin

Gray ramus communicans

Sympathetic chain ganglion

Splanchnic nerve

White ramus communicans

Sympathetic chain

Collateral sympathetic ganglion

Preganglionic sympathetic neurons passing to synapse in another sympathetic chain ganglion

Neuroeffector junctions on smooth muscle, cardiac muscle, secretory glands, metabolic cells, immune cells

INTRODUCTION AND BASIC ORGANIZATION

9.1 SCHEMATIC OF THE SPINAL CORD WITH SENSORY, MOTOR, AND AUTONOMIC COMPONENTS OF PERIPHERAL NERVES

Peripheral nerves consist of axons from primary sensory neurons, lower motor neurons (LMNs), and preganglionic and postganglionic autonomic neurons. The primary sensory axons have sensory receptors (transducing elements) at their peripheral (distal) ends, contiguous with the initial segment of the axon. The proximal portion of the axon enters the central nervous system (CNS) and terminates in secondary sensory nuclei associated with reflex, cerebellar, and lemniscal channels. LMNs in the anterior horn of the spinal cord send axons via the ventral (anterior) roots to travel in peripheral nerves to skeletal muscles, with which they form neuromuscular junctions. The autonomic preganglionic neurons send axons via the ventral roots to terminate in autonomic ganglia or in

the adrenal medulla. Postganglionic neurons send axons into splanchnic or peripheral nerves and form neuroeffector junctions with smooth muscle, cardiac muscle, secretory glands, metabolic cells, and cells of the immune system.

CLINICAL POINT

Peripheral nerves form through the union of dorsal and ventral roots and by subsequent branching, similar to the process that occurs through the brachial plexus. The resultant terminal peripheral nerves contain limited categories of axonal types, including LMN axons (both alpha and gamma); primary sensory axons (both myelinated and unmyelinated); and autonomic axons (mainly postganglionic sympathetic axons). Destructive lesions in peripheral nerves may cause flaccid paralysis of innervated skeletal muscles (with loss of tone and denervation atrophy); loss of some or all aspects of somatic sensation in the innervated territory; and some autonomic dysfunction resulting from loss of sympathetic innervation (e.g., vasodilation and lack of sweating). An irritative lesion of a peripheral nerve is usually manifested as pain radiating to the innervated territory.

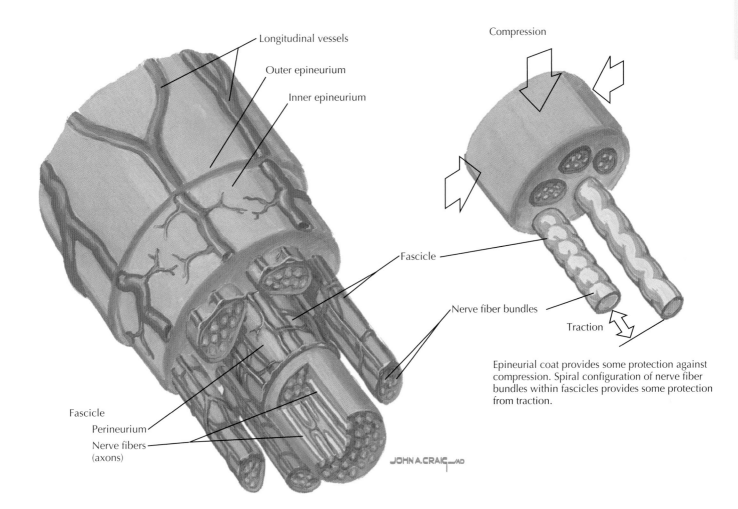

Longitudinal vessels

Outer epineurium

Inner epineurium

Fascicle

Nerve fiber bundles

Fascicle

Perineurium

Nerve fibers
(axons)

Compression

Traction

Epineurial coat provides some protection against compression. Spiral configuration of nerve fiber bundles within fascicles provides some protection from traction.

JOHN A. CRAIG_MD

9.2 ANATOMY OF A PERIPHERAL NERVE

A peripheral nerve is made up of unmyelinated and myelinated axons; the connective sheaths with which they are associated; and local blood vessels, the vasa nervorum. Unmyelinated axons are surrounded by the cytoplasm of Schwann cells, called Schwann cell sheaths. Each individual segment of a myelinated axon is enwrapped by a myelin sheath, provided by an individual Schwann cell. The bare space between each myelin sheath is called a node of Ranvier and is the site on the membrane where sodium channels are present and is also the site of initiation or reinitiation of the action potential. Endoneurium is loose, supportive, connective tissue that is found between individual axons within a fascicle. Fascicles of multiple axons are enwrapped by a sheath of supportive cells and collagenous connective tissue; this perineurium functions as a blood-nerve barrier and helps to protect the axons from local diffusion of potentially damaging substances. This perineurial barrier can be disrupted in neuropathic conditions such as diabetic neuropathy. The epineurium is the outermost layer of supportive connective tissue that enwraps the entire nerve.

Normal

Patent vessels

Normal epineurium

Severe acute compression

Vascular compression and ischemia

Severe chronic compression

Thickened epineurium

Axon

Patent microtubules

Compression of nerve with thinned myelin and closed microtubules

Myelin sheath

Thinned myelin in compressed area

Distortion of myelin or demyelination and axonal degeneration

Sunderland classification of nerve injury

Cell body

Axon

Epineurium
Perineurium
Endoneurium
Myelin sheath

Normal   First degree (neurapraxia)   Second degree (axonotmesis)   Third degree   Fourth degree   Fifth degree

JOHN A. CRAIG—AD

Classification of nerve injury by degree of involvement of various neural layers

9.3 PERIPHERAL NERVE INJURY AND DEGENERATION IN A COMPRESSION NEUROPATHY

If a peripheral nerve is compressed or damaged, a series of reactions takes place within the neurons whose axons have been damaged and in the supportive tissue. At the site of the injury, axonal damage and thinning of the myelination can occur. Distal to the site of the injury, the peripheral portion of the axon can degenerate (called Wallerian degeneration), resulting in the breaking up and dissolution of the peripheral axon. The Schwann cells myelinating the degenerating axons also break up and degenerate. However, the basement membrane remains intact, providing a scaffold through which future regenerating axons can be directed.

The central (proximal) portion of the neuron can undergo changes called central chromatolysis. The Nissl bodies break up into individual ribosomes, the cell body swells, and the neuron shifts its metabolism to structural and reparative synthetic products that attempt to save the neuron and permit it to try to recover from the injury. If successful, this process gradually reverses, and the neuron begins to sprout a peripheral axonal extension, seeking to reattach to the target from which it was disrupted. The Schwann cells proliferate and generate new myelin sheaths around the regrowing axon, but the intersegmental distances of the new myelin sheath are shorter than the original distances and the myelin sheath is thinner; thus, the regenerated axon shows a slower conduction velocity than the original intact axon.

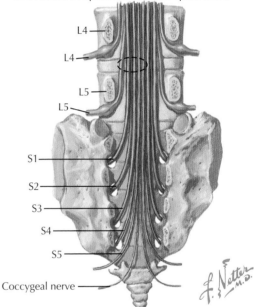

C1 { C1 spinal nerve exits above C1 vertebra

C8 { C8 spinal nerve exits below C7 vertebra (there are 8 cervical nerves but only 7 cervical vertebrae)

Base of skull

Cervical enlargement

Lumbar enlargement

Conus medullaris (termination of spinal cord)

Cauda equina

Internal terminal filum (pial part)

External terminal filum (pial part)

Sacrum

Termination of dural sac

Coccygeal nerve

Coccyx

- Cervical nerves
- Thoracic nerves
- Lumbar nerves
- Sacral and coccygeal nerves

Lumbar disc protrusion does not usually affect nerve exiting above disc. Lateral protrusion at disc level L4-5 affects L5 spinal nerve, not L4 spinal nerve. Protrusion at disc level L5-S1 affects S1 spinal nerve, not L5 spinal nerve

Coccygeal nerve

Medial protrusion at disc level L4-5 rarely affects L4 spinal nerve but may affect L5 spinal nerve and sometimes S1-4 spinal nerves.

9.4 RELATIONSHIP OF SPINAL NERVE ROOTS TO VERTEBRAE

The dorsal (posterior) and ventral (anterior) roots of the spinal cord segments extend from the spinal cord as peripheral axons, invested initially with meninges. As the axons enter the peripheral nervous system, they become associated with Schwann cells for myelination and support. The roots exit through the intervertebral foramina, compact openings between the vertebrae where herniated discs (nucleus pulposus) may impinge on the nerve roots and produce sensory or motor symptoms. Sensory and motor axons enter into the dorsal and ventral rami of peripheral nerves. Autonomic axons (myelinated) course from the ventral roots into the white (preganglionic) rami communicantes and synapse in autonomic ganglia. The ganglion cells give rise to postganglionic axons (unmyelinated) that course through the gray rami communicantes and join the peripheral nerves.

CLINICAL POINT

The longitudinal growth of the spinal column outstrips the longitudinal growth of the spinal cord; as a consequence, the spinal cord in adults ends adjacent to the L1 vertebral body. Nerve roots heading for intervertebral foramina below L1 extend caudally through the subarachnoid space in the lumbar cistern, forming the cauda equina. Damage to the cauda equina can occur as the result of tumors, such as ependymomas and lipomas, or of a prolapsed intervertebral disc. It is common for symptoms to occur gradually and be irregular because of the ample room in the lumbar cistern for nerve roots to move. Radicular pain often is experienced in a sciatic distribution, with progressive loss of sensation in radicular patterns. A more caudal location of the obstructing mass may lead to loss of sensation in regions of sacral innervation in the perineal (saddle) zone. Loss of bowel, bladder, and erectile function also may occur. More rostral lesions may result in flaccid paralysis of the legs.

A. Sensory channels - Reflex

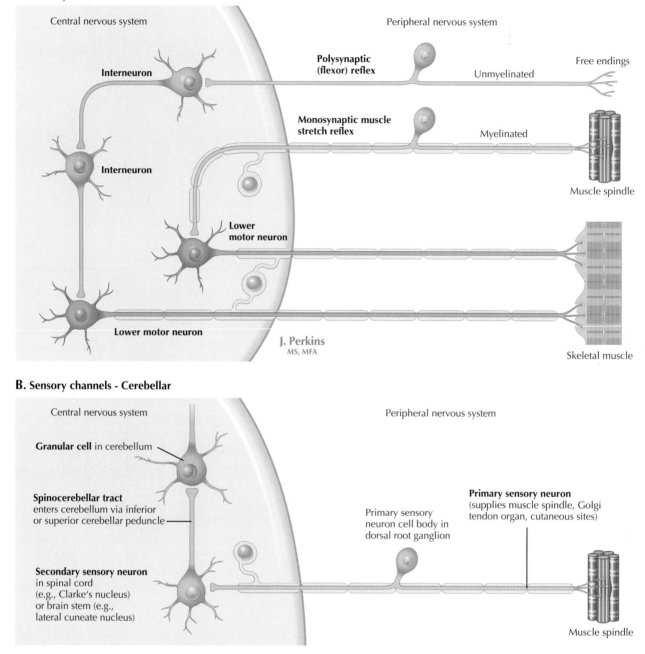

Central nervous system

Peripheral nervous system

Interneuron

Polysynaptic (flexor) reflex

Unmyelinated

Free endings

Monosynaptic muscle stretch reflex

Myelinated

Interneuron

Muscle spindle

Lower motor neuron

Lower motor neuron

J. Perkins
MS, MFA

Skeletal muscle

B. Sensory channels - Cerebellar

Central nervous system

Peripheral nervous system

Granular cell in cerebellum

Spinocerebellar tract
enters cerebellum via inferior
or superior cerebellar peduncle

Primary sensory neuron
(supplies muscle spindle, Golgi
tendon organ, cutaneous sites)

Primary sensory
neuron cell body in
dorsal root ganglion

Secondary sensory neuron
in spinal cord
(e.g., Clarke's nucleus)
or brain stem (e.g.,
lateral cuneate nucleus)

Muscle spindle

9.5 SENSORY CHANNELS: REFLEX AND CEREBELLAR

Primary sensory axons communicate with secondary sensory neurons in reflex, cerebellar, and lemniscal channels, carrying transduced information from the periphery into the CNS. **A,** The reflex channels interconnect primary sensory axons with anterior horn cells (LMNs) through one or more synapses to achieve unconscious reflex motor responses to sensory input. These responses can be elicited in an isolated spinal cord devoid of connections from the brain. The monosynaptic reflex channels connect primary sensory axons from muscle spindles, via the dorsal roots, directly with LMNs involved in muscle stretch reflex contraction; this is the only monosynaptic reflex seen in the human CNS. Polysynaptic reflex channels are directed particularly toward flexor (withdrawal) responses through one or more interneurons to produce coordinated patterns of muscle activity to remove a portion of the body from a potentially damaging or offending stimulus. This polysynaptic channel can spread ipsilaterally and contralaterally through many segments. **B,** Primary somatosensory axons carrying unconsciously processed information from muscles, joints, tendons, ligaments, and cutaneous sources enter the CNS via dorsal roots and synapse with secondary sensory neurons in the spinal cord or caudal brain stem. These secondary sensory neurons convey information, initially derived from the periphery, to the ipsilateral cerebellum via spinocerebellar pathways. The dorsal and ventral spinocerebellar pathways carry information from the lower body (T6 and below). The rostral spinocerebellar tract and the cuneocerebellar tract carry information from the upper body (above T6). Polysynaptic indirect spinocerebellar pathways (spino-olivo-cerebellar and spino-reticulo-cerebellar tracts) also are present.

Sensory Channels - Lemniscal

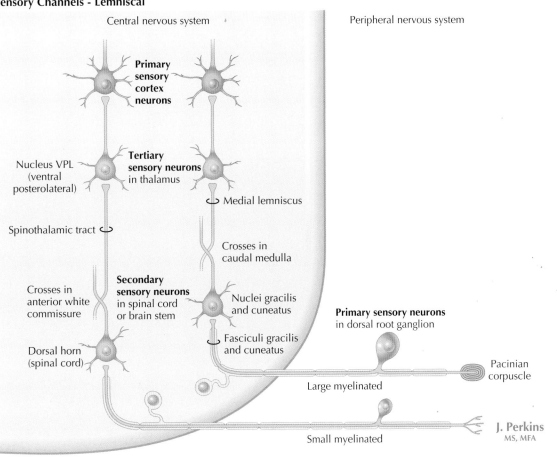

Central nervous system

Peripheral nervous system

Primary sensory cortex neurons

Nucleus VPL (ventral posterolateral)

Tertiary sensory neurons in thalamus

Medial lemniscus

Spinothalamic tract

Crosses in caudal medulla

Crosses in anterior white commissure

Secondary sensory neurons in spinal cord or brain stem

Nuclei gracilis and cuneatus

Primary sensory neurons in dorsal root ganglion

Dorsal horn (spinal cord)

Fasciculi gracilis and cuneatus

Pacinian corpuscle

Large myelinated

J. Perkins
MS, MFA

Small myelinated

9.6 SENSORY CHANNELS: LEMNISCAL

Primary sensory axons carrying sensory information destined for conscious perception arise from receptors in superficial and deep tissue. These axons enter the CNS via the dorsal roots and terminate on secondary sensory nuclei in the spinal cord or brain stem. Secondary sensory axons from these nuclei cross the midline (decussate), ascend as lemniscal pathways, and terminate in the contralateral thalamus. These specific thalamic nuclei then project to specific regions of the primary sensory cortex, where fine-grained analysis of incoming, consciously perceived sensory information takes place. Somatosensory information is directed into two sets of channels, protopathic and epicritic. The epicritic information (fine, discriminative sensation; vibratory sensation; joint position sense) is transduced by primary sensory neurons (dorsal root ganglion cells) that send myelinated axons to neurons in the medulla; the nucleus gracilis (lower body, T6 and below); and the nucleus cuneatus (upper body, above T6). Nuclei gracilis and cuneatus give rise to the medial lemniscus, a crossed secondary sensory pathway that terminates in the ventral posterolateral nucleus of the thalamus. This thalamic nucleus has reciprocal projections with cortical neurons in the postcentral gyrus (Brodmann's areas 3, 1, and 2). This entire epicritic somatosensory system is highly topographically organized, with each region of the body represented in each nucleus and axonal pathway. The protopathic information (pain, temperature sensation, light moving touch) is transduced by primary sensory neurons (dorsal root ganglion cells) that project mainly via small myelinated and unmyelinated axons to neurons in the dorsal horn of the spinal cord. These spinal cord neurons give rise to the spinothalamic tract (spinal lemniscus), a secondary sensory pathway that terminates in separate neuronal sites in the ventral posterolateral nucleus of the thalamus. This portion of the ventral posterolateral nucleus communicates mainly with the primary sensory cortex (SI) and a secondary area of somatosensory cortex (SII) posterior to the lateral postcentral gyrus. Some unmyelinated nociceptive protopathic axons that terminate in the dorsal horn of the spinal cord interconnect with a cascade of spinal cord interneurons that project mainly into the reticular formation of the brain stem (the spinoreticular pathway). This more diffuse pain system is processed through nonspecific thalamic nuclei with projections to somatosensory cortices and more widespread regions of cortex. This system can result in the perception of excruciating, long-lasting pain that may exceed the duration and intensity of direct peripheral stimuli.

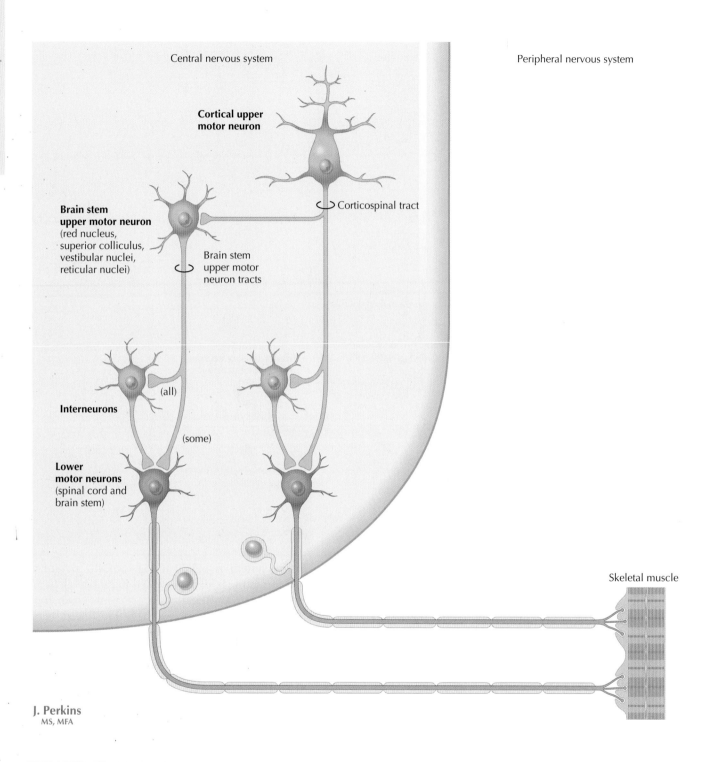

Central nervous system

Peripheral nervous system

**Cortical upper
motor neuron**

Corticospinal tract

**Brain stem
upper motor neuron**
(red nucleus,
superior colliculus,
vestibular nuclei,
reticular nuclei)

Brain stem
upper motor
neuron tracts

(all)

Interneurons

(some)

**Lower
motor neurons**
(spinal cord and
brain stem)

Skeletal muscle

J. Perkins
MS, MFA

9.7 MOTOR CHANNELS: BASIC ORGANIZATION OF LOWER AND UPPER MOTOR NEURONS

LMNs are found in the anterior horn of the spinal cord and in motor cranial nerve nuclei in the brain stem. Their axons exit via the ventral roots or cranial nerves to supply skeletal muscles. LMN synapses with muscle fibers form neuromuscular junctions and release the neurotransmitter acetylcholine, which acts on nicotinic receptors on the skeletal muscle fibers. A motor unit consists of an LMN, its axon, and the muscle fibers the axon innervates. LMNs are regulated and coordinated by groups of upper motor neurons (UMNs) found in the brain. Brain stem UMNs regulate basic tone and posture. Cortical UMNs (from corticospinal and corticobulbar tracts) regulate consciously directed, or volitional, movements. Cortical UMNs also have extensive connections with brain stem UMNs and may help to coordinate their activities. The cerebellum and basal ganglia aid in the coordination of movement and in pattern selection, respectively, via connections with UMNs; the cerebellum and basal ganglia do not connect with LMNs directly.

Central nervous system

Peripheral nervous system

Limbic forebrain structures
(e.g., amygdaloid nucleus,
some cortical areas)

Hypothalamus

Hypothalamus

Brain stem
nuclei and
"centers"

Hypophyseal portal system

Anterior pituitary hormones

Preganglionic sympathetic neuron
Intermediolateral
cell column in lateral
horn of spinal cord
(T1–L2)

Sensory neuron in
dorsal root ganglion

Reflex connections

Target tissue

Sympathetic ganglion cell

J. Perkins
MS, MFA

9.8 AUTONOMIC CHANNELS

Preganglionic neurons for the sympathetic nervous system (SNS) are found in the lateral horn (intermediolateral cell column) of the thoracolumbar (T1–L2) spinal cord (thoracolumbar system). Preganglionic neurons for the parasympathetic nervous system (PsNS) are found in nuclei of cranial nerves (CNs) III, VII, IX, and X and in the intermediate gray matter of the spinal cord between S2 and S4 (the craniosacral system). Preganglionic axons exit the CNS via cranial nerves or ventral roots and terminate in chain ganglia or collateral ganglia (the SNS) or in intramural ganglia in or near the organ innervated (the PsNS). Postganglionic autonomic axons innervate smooth muscle, cardiac muscle, secretory glands, metabolic cells, and cells of the immune system. The SNS is a fight-or-flight system that responds to emergency demands. The PsNS is a homeostatic, reparative system active in more quiescent activities and in digestive and eliminative functions. Preganglionic responses are coordinated by autonomic UMN equivalents from the brain stem (autonomic centers), the hypothalamus, and the limbic forebrain structures. Inputs that affect visceral functions or elicit emotional responsiveness are conveyed through these central autonomic regulatory systems, which help to coordinate appropriate autonomic responses. These central autonomic regulatory systems coordinate autonomic responses that affect both visceral functions and neuroendocrine outflow from the pituitary gland.

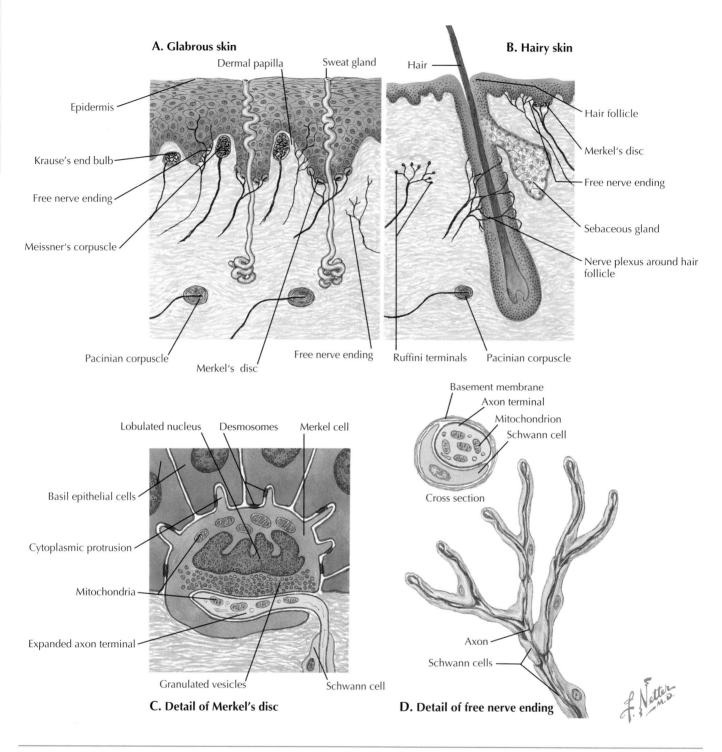

A. Glabrous skin

Dermal papilla
Sweat gland
Epidermis
Krause's end bulb
Free nerve ending
Meissner's corpuscle
Pacinian corpuscle
Merkel's disc
Free nerve ending

B. Hairy skin

Hair
Hair follicle
Merkel's disc
Free nerve ending
Sebaceous gland
Nerve plexus around hair follicle
Ruffini terminals
Pacinian corpuscle

Lobulated nucleus
Desmosomes
Merkel cell
Basil epithelial cells
Cytoplasmic protrusion
Mitochondria
Expanded axon terminal
Granulated vesicles
Schwann cell

C. Detail of Merkel's disc

Basement membrane
Axon terminal
Mitochondrion
Schwann cell
Cross section
Axon
Schwann cells

D. Detail of free nerve ending

9.9 CUTANEOUS RECEPTORS

Cutaneous receptors are found at the distal ends of the primary sensory axon; they act as dendrites, in which threshold stimuli lead to the firing of an action potential at the initial segment of the primary sensory axon. Although specific types of sensory receptors are thought to code for consciously perceived perceptions, there is not an exact correlation. Glabrous skin and hairy skin contain a wide variety of sensory receptors for detecting mechanical, thermal, or nociceptive (consciously perceived as painful) stimuli applied on the body surface. These receptors include bare nerve endings (nociception, thermal sensation) and encapsulated endings. The latter include pacinian corpuscles (rapidly adapting mechanoreceptors for detecting vibration or brief touch); Merkel's discs (slowly adapting mechanoreceptors for detecting maintained deformation or sustained touch on the skin); Meissner's corpuscles (rapidly adapting mechanoreceptors for detecting moving touch); Ruffini endings (slowly adapting mechanoreceptors for detecting steady pressure applied to hairy skin); hair follicle receptors (rapidly adapting); and Krause end bulbs (possibly thermoreceptors). The initial segment of the primary sensory axon is immediately adjacent to the sensory receptor.

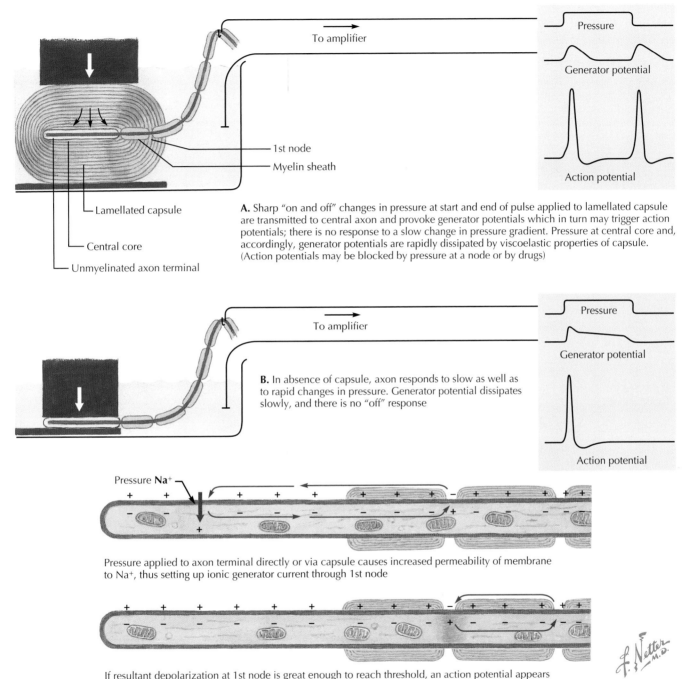

A. Sharp "on and off" changes in pressure at start and end of pulse applied to lamellated capsule are transmitted to central axon and provoke generator potentials which in turn may trigger action potentials; there is no response to a slow change in pressure gradient. Pressure at central core and, accordingly, generator potentials are rapidly dissipated by viscoelastic properties of capsule. (Action potentials may be blocked by pressure at a node or by drugs)

B. In absence of capsule, axon responds to slow as well as to rapid changes in pressure. Generator potential dissipates slowly, and there is no "off" response

Pressure applied to axon terminal directly or via capsule causes increased permeability of membrane to Na$^+$, thus setting up ionic generator current through 1st node

If resultant depolarization at 1st node is great enough to reach threshold, an action potential appears which is propagated along nerve fiber

9.10 PACINIAN CORPUSCLES

Pacinian corpuscles are mechanoreceptors that transform mechanical force or displacement into action potentials in large-diameter primary sensory axons. The mechanical stimulus is modified by the viscoelastic properties of the contributing lamellae of the pacinian corpuscle and the associated accessory cells. An action potential results when a generator potential of sufficient magnitude to bring the initial segment of the axon to threshold is elicited. The onset and cessation of mechanical deformation enhance ionic permeability in the axon, optimizing the physiological response of the pacinian corpuscle to vibratory stimuli.

A. Carotid body and carotid sinus

Glossopharyngeal (IX) nerve

Carotid sinus nerve

Veins from carotid body

External carotid artery

Carotid body

Artery to carotid body

Superior thyroid artery

Common carotid artery

Vagus (X) nerve

Superior cervical sympathetic trunk ganglion

Retromandibular and facial veins

Lingual vein

Internal jugular vein

Internal carotid artery

Carotid sinus

B. Carotid body

Synaptic ending

Nerve fibers

Type II (sheath) cells

Nerve fibers

Fibroblast

Capillaries

Basement membrane

Endothelial cells

Type I (glomus) cells

C. Carotid sinus

Intima

Media

Adventitia

Free nerve endings

Thin elastic media

Encapsulated endings

9.11 INTEROCEPTORS

Interoceptors, including internal nociceptors, chemoreceptors, and stretch receptors, inform the CNS about the internal state of the body. The carotid body, a specialized chemoreceptor for detecting carbon dioxide (in a hypoxic state) or to a lesser extent low blood pH resulting in increased respiration, is associated with afferent axons of CN IX that project to the caudal nucleus solitarius in the medulla. The carotid sinus, a thin-walled region of the carotid artery, contains encapsulated and bare nerve endings that act as stretch receptors. These stretch receptors respond to increased arterial pressure as baroreceptors, send primary afferents to the caudal nucleus solitarius via CN IX, and elicit reflex bradycardia and decrease in blood pressure.

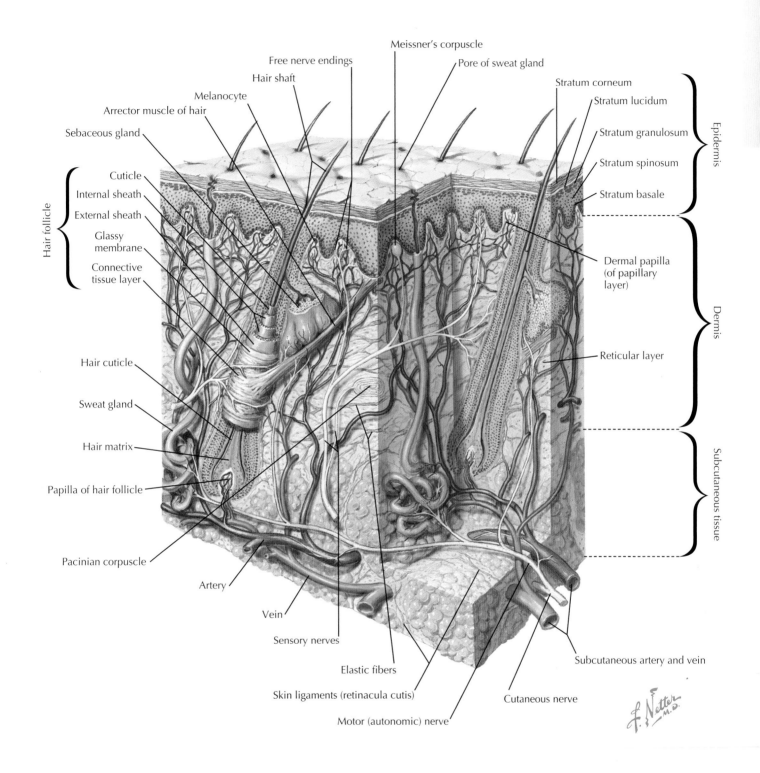

Free nerve endings

Hair shaft

Melanocyte

Arrector muscle of hair

Sebaceous gland

Meissner's corpuscle

Pore of sweat gland

Stratum corneum

Stratum lucidum

Stratum granulosum

Stratum spinosum

Stratum basale

Epidermis

Cuticle

Internal sheath

External sheath

Glassy membrane

Connective tissue layer

Hair follicle

Dermal papilla (of papillary layer)

Reticular layer

Dermis

Hair cuticle

Sweat gland

Hair matrix

Papilla of hair follicle

Subcutaneous tissue

Pacinian corpuscle

Artery

Vein

Sensory nerves

Elastic fibers

Skin ligaments (retinacula cutis)

Motor (autonomic) nerve

Subcutaneous artery and vein

Cutaneous nerve

9.12 **SKIN AND ITS NERVES**

The skin is supplied with a variety of receptor types (see Fig. 9.9) that transduce slowly and rapidly adapting mechanical stimuli and deformation into electrical impulses in primary afferent fibers. The bare nerve endings are associated mainly with nociceptors, peripheral arborizations of unmyelinated axons. Some nociceptors and thermoreceptors are associated with small myelinated axons. These axons collectively contribute somatosensory information to the spinothalamic/spinoreticular lemniscal system for protopathic sensation. The more complex encapsulated receptors contribute somatosensory information to the dorsal column/medial lemniscal system for epicritic sensation and are associated with larger myelinated axons.

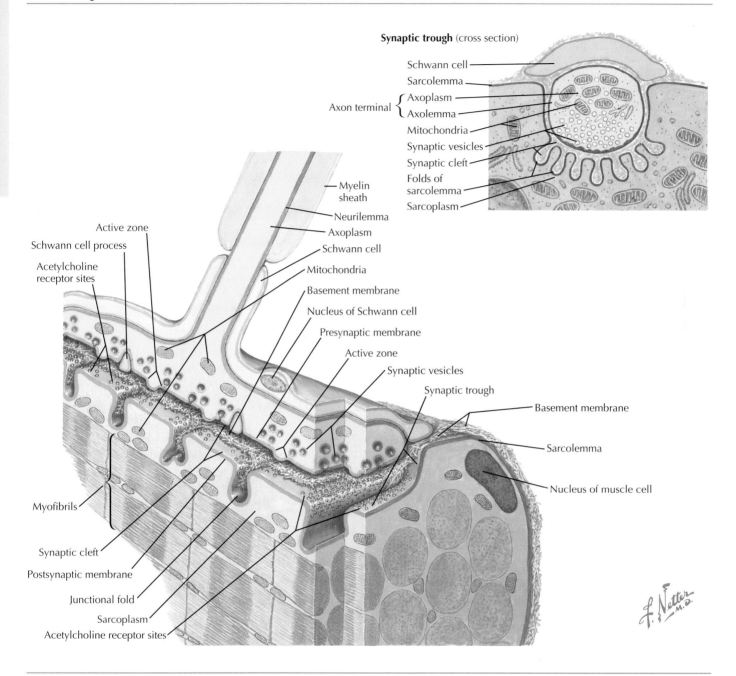

Synaptic trough (cross section)

Schwann cell
Sarcolemma
Axon terminal { Axoplasm
Axolemma
Mitochondria
Synaptic vesicles
Synaptic cleft
Folds of sarcolemma
Sarcoplasm

Active zone
Schwann cell process
Acetylcholine receptor sites

Myelin sheath
Neurilemma
Axoplasm
Schwann cell
Mitochondria
Basement membrane
Nucleus of Schwann cell
Presynaptic membrane
Active zone
Synaptic vesicles
Synaptic trough
Basement membrane
Sarcolemma
Nucleus of muscle cell

Myofibrils
Synaptic cleft
Postsynaptic membrane
Junctional fold
Sarcoplasm
Acetylcholine receptor sites

9.13 THE NEUROMUSCULAR JUNCTION AND NEUROTRANSMISSION

Axons of LMNs that synapse on skeletal muscle form expanded terminals called neuromuscular junctions (motor end plates). The motor axon loses its myelin sheath and expands into an extended terminal that resides in a trough in the muscle fiber and is covered by a layer of Schwann cell cytoplasm. The postsynaptic membrane is thrown into secondary folds. When an action potential invades the motor terminal, several hundred vesicles simultaneously release their acetylcholine (ACh) into the synaptic cleft. The ACh binds to nicotinic receptors on the muscle sarcolemma, initiating a motor end-plate potential, which is normally of sufficient magnitude to result in the firing of a muscle action potential, leading to contraction of the muscle fiber. A single muscle fiber has only one neuromuscular junction, but a motor axon may innervate multiple muscle fibers.

CLINICAL POINT

An action potential that invades the motor end plate results in a calcium-mediated simultaneous release of multiple quanta (vesicles) of ACh. This released ACh acts on nicotinic cholinergic receptors on the postjunctional membrane, normally resulting in a muscle contraction (excitation-contraction coupling). In myasthenia gravis, antibodies against the cholinergic nicotinic receptors greatly reduce the number of active receptors available for stimulation by released ACh. The size and number of ACh quanta appear to be normal. As a consequence, there is easy fatiguability of involved muscles with repeated attempts at contraction. Ocular, facial, and bulbar muscles are the most likely to be affected by this disease, with resultant ptosis, drooping face, diplopia with strabismus, and dysarthria, dysphonia, and dysphagia. Limb muscles (mainly proximal) are involved only in advanced myasthenia gravis. The muscles do not show wasting and atrophy because they are not denervated; muscle stretch reflexes are elicitable.

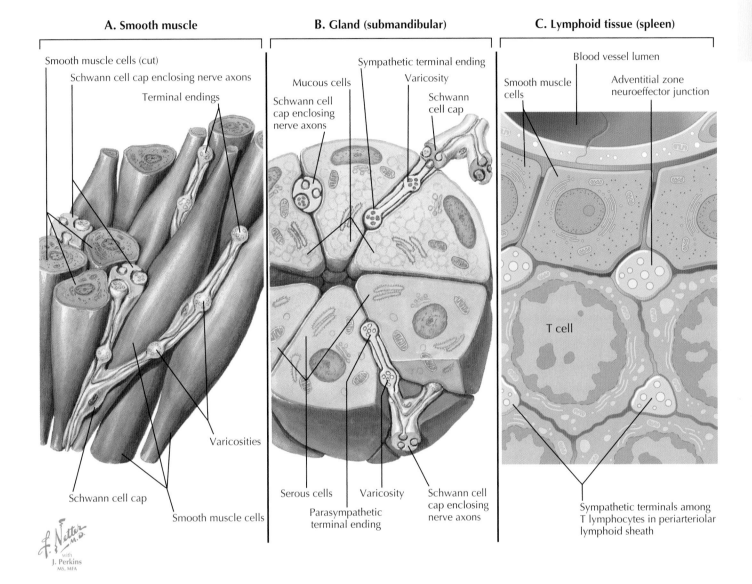

A. Smooth muscle

Smooth muscle cells (cut)

Schwann cell cap enclosing nerve axons

Terminal endings

Varicosities

Schwann cell cap

Smooth muscle cells

B. Gland (submandibular)

Sympathetic terminal ending

Varicosity

Schwann cell cap

Mucous cells

Schwann cell cap enclosing nerve axons

Serous cells

Varicosity

Parasympathetic terminal ending

Schwann cell cap enclosing nerve axons

C. Lymphoid tissue (spleen)

Blood vessel lumen

Adventitial zone neuroeffector junction

Smooth muscle cells

T cell

Sympathetic terminals among T lymphocytes in periarteriolar lymphoid sheath

9.14 NEUROEFFECTOR JUNCTIONS

Autonomic postganglionic axons form neuroeffector junctions with cardiac muscle, smooth muscle **(A)**, secretory glands **(B)**, metabolic cells such as hepatocytes and fat cells, and cells of the immune system **(C)**. These nerve endings use mainly norepinephrine for the SNS and acetylcholine for the PsNS. These endings do not form classic CNS or motor endplate synapses; instead, they terminate as neuroeffector junctions, releasing neurotransmitter into interstitial spaces. This permits a widespread diffusion of the neurotransmitter as a paracrine secretion, initiating postsynaptic responses on cells with appropriate receptors (including many types of cells of the immune system). Some close appositions also are found, such as SNS endings on lymphocytes. Not all smooth muscle cells are innervated by neuroeffector junctions; they are coupled by gap junctions and can contract together when the innervated smooth muscle cell contracts.

Levels of Principal Dermatomes

C5	Clavicles
C5, 6, 7	Lateral parts of upper limbs
C8; T1	Medial sides of upper limbs
C6	Thumb
C6, 7, 8	Hand
C8	Ring and little fingers
T4	Level of nipples

T10	Level of umbilicus
T12	Inguinal or groin regions
L1, 2, 3, 4	Anterior and inner surfaces of lower limbs
L4, 5; S1	Foot
L4	Medial side of great toe
L5; S1, 2	Outer and posterior sides of lower limbs
S1	Lateral margin of foot and little toe
S2, 3, 4	Perineum

SOMATIC NERVOUS SYSTEM

9.15 DERMATOMAL DISTRIBUTION

A dermatome is the cutaneous area supplied by a single spinal nerve root; the cell bodies are located in dorsal root ganglia. The spinal nerve roots are distributed to structures according to their associations with spinal cord segments. The nerve roots supplying neighboring dermatomes overlap. Thus, sectioning or dysfunction of a single dorsal root produces hypoesthesia (diminished sensation), not anesthesia (total loss of sensation) in the region supplied predominantly by that dermatome, as shown in the figure. Dermatomal anesthesia requires damage to at least three dorsal roots: the central dorsal root and the roots above and below it. In contrast, an irritative lesion such as a herniated intervertebral disc may produce sharp, radiating pain within the distribution of the affected dermatome. As the limb buds for the lower extremities develop, they draw out the nerve roots that correspond with their mesodermal cores and ectodermal coverings. The developing lower limbs rotate medially around a longitudinal axis, with a resultant oblique orientation of the dermatomes. The L1 and L2 dermatomes can be found in sites adjacent to S2 and S3 dermatomes because of the intervening segments migrating into more distal parts of the lower limbs. Knowledge of dermatomes is important for localizing peripheral nerve root lesions and distinguishing them from peripheral nerve lesions.

From ophthalmic division of trigeminal nerve (V₁)

Supraorbital nerve

Supratrochlear nerve

Palpebral branch of lacrimal nerve

Infratrochlear nerve

External nasal branch of anterior ethmoidal nerve

From maxillary division of trigeminal nerve (V₂)

Infraorbital nerve

Zygomaticofacial nerve

Zygomaticotemporal nerve

From mandibular division of trigeminal nerve (V₃)

Mental nerve

Buccal nerve

Auriculotemporal nerve

Auricular branch of vagus nerve (X)

Medial branches of dorsal rami of cervical spinal nerves

Greater occipital nerve (C2)

3rd occipital nerve (C3)

From 4th, 5th, 6th, and 7th nerves in succession below

Branches from cervical plexus

Lesser occipital nerve (C2, 3)

Great auricular nerve (C2, 3)

Transverse cervical nerve (C2, 3)

Supraclavicular nerves (C3, 4)

Ophthalmic nerve (V₁)

Maxillary nerve (V₂)

Trigeminal nerve (V)

Mandibular nerve (V₃)

Dorsal rami of cervical spinal nerves

Note: Auricular branch of vagus nerve to external acoustic meatus and small area on posteromedial surface of auricle

Branches from cervical plexus

9.16 CUTANEOUS NERVES OF THE HEAD AND NECK

Cutaneous nerves of the head and neck derive from dorsal rami of cervical spinal nerves, from branches from the cervical plexus, and from all three divisions of the trigeminal nerve (CN V).

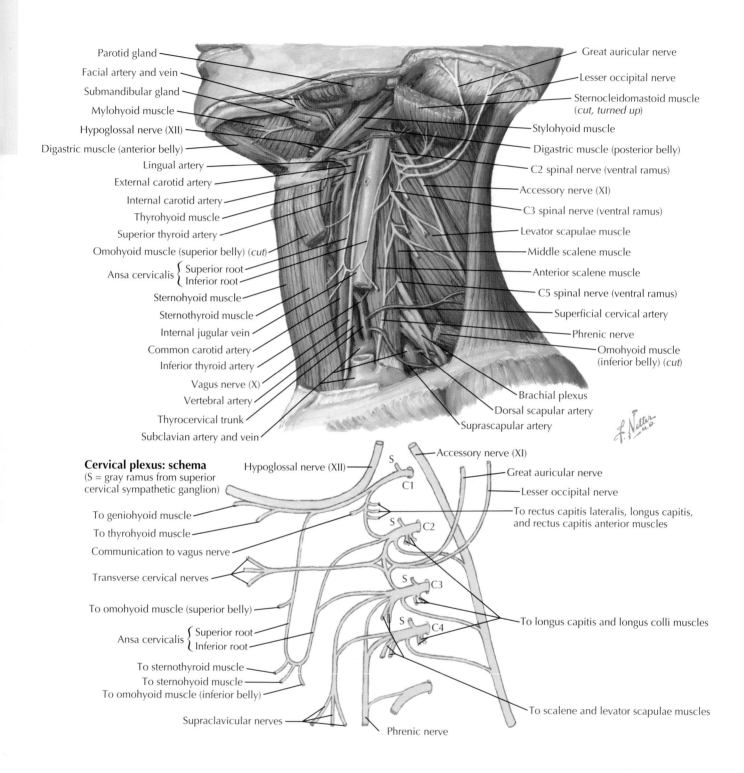

Parotid gland
Facial artery and vein
Submandibular gland
Mylohyoid muscle
Hypoglossal nerve (XII)
Digastric muscle (anterior belly)
Lingual artery
External carotid artery
Internal carotid artery
Thyrohyoid muscle
Superior thyroid artery
Omohyoid muscle (superior belly) (cut)
Ansa cervicalis { Superior root
Inferior root
Sternohyoid muscle
Sternothyroid muscle
Internal jugular vein
Common carotid artery
Inferior thyroid artery
Vagus nerve (X)
Vertebral artery
Thyrocervical trunk
Subclavian artery and vein

Great auricular nerve
Lesser occipital nerve
Sternocleidomastoid muscle (cut, turned up)
Stylohyoid muscle
Digastric muscle (posterior belly)
C2 spinal nerve (ventral ramus)
Accessory nerve (XI)
C3 spinal nerve (ventral ramus)
Levator scapulae muscle
Middle scalene muscle
Anterior scalene muscle
C5 spinal nerve (ventral ramus)
Superficial cervical artery
Phrenic nerve
Omohyoid muscle (inferior belly) (cut)
Brachial plexus
Dorsal scapular artery
Suprascapular artery

Cervical plexus: schema
(S = gray ramus from superior
cervical sympathetic ganglion)

Hypoglossal nerve (XII)
S
C1

Accessory nerve (XI)
Great auricular nerve
Lesser occipital nerve
To rectus capitis lateralis, longus capitis, and rectus capitis anterior muscles

To geniohyoid muscle
To thyrohyoid muscle
Communication to vagus nerve
Transverse cervical nerves
To omohyoid muscle (superior belly)
Ansa cervicalis { Superior root
Inferior root
To sternothyroid muscle
To sternohyoid muscle
To omohyoid muscle (inferior belly)
Supraclavicular nerves

S
C2
S
C3
S
C4

To longus capitis and longus colli muscles

To scalene and levator scapulae muscles

Phrenic nerve

9.17 CERVICAL PLEXUS IN SITU

This diagram of the cervical plexus in situ and the schema below demonstrate the distribution of branches from the C1–C4
nerve roots into the associated peripheral nerves and branches
to the innervated muscles.

Greater occipital nerve
(from dorsal ramus of C2)

Accessory (XI) nerve

Hypoglossal (XII) nerve

Geniohyoid muscle

Thyrohyoid muscle

Superior root (descendens
hypoglossi) of ansa cervicalis

Inferior root (descendens
cervicalis) of ansa cervicalis

Transverse cervical nerve

Omohyoid muscle

Sternothyroid muscle

Sternohyoid muscle

Ansa cervicalis (ansa hypoglossi)

Phrenic nerve

Sternocleidomastoid
muscle (lower end)

C1
C2
C3
C4
C5

Lesser occipital nerve

Sternocleidomastoid muscle
(upper end)

Great auricular nerve

Nerves to anterior and lateral rectus
capitis muscles, and longus capitis
and longus colli muscles

Nerves to longus capitis, longus
colli and levator scapulae muscles

Trapezius muscle

Nerves to longus colli, scalenus anterior
and scalenus medius muscles

Communication to
brachial plexus

Supraclavicular nerves (medial,
intermediate and lateral)

——— Motor fibers

——— Sensory fibers

· · · · · Proprioceptive fibers

9.18 CERVICAL PLEXUS

The cervical plexus lies deep to the sternocleidomastoid muscle. Its branches convey motor fibers to many cervical muscles and to the diaphragm. Its sensory fibers convey exteroceptive information from parts of the scalp, neck, and chest as well as proprioceptive information from muscles, tendons, and joints. Sympathetic sudomotor and vasomotor fibers travel with this plexus to blood vessels and glands. The superficial branches perforate the cervical fascia to supply cutaneous structures; the deep branches supply mainly muscles and joints.

CLINICAL POINT

The cervical plexus is formed from the anterior primary rami of C1–C4, deep to the sternocleidomastoid muscle and in front of the scalenus medius and levator scapulae muscles. Sensory branches include the greater and lesser occipital nerves, great auricular nerve, cutaneous cervical nerves, and supraclavicular nerves. The motor branches include the ansa hypoglossi, branches to scalenus medius and levator scapulae muscles, the phrenic nerve, and branches to the spinal accessory nerve. Lesions of the cervical plexus are uncommon, usually resulting from trauma, mass lesions, or as sequelae to surgery such as carotid endarterectomy. Involvement of motor branches results in disruption of muscular function, such as shoulder elevation and head rotation and flexion with spinal accessory nerve damage. Involvement of sensory branches results in loss of cutaneous sensation or in pain and paresthesias in regions of the head or neck supplied by these branches.

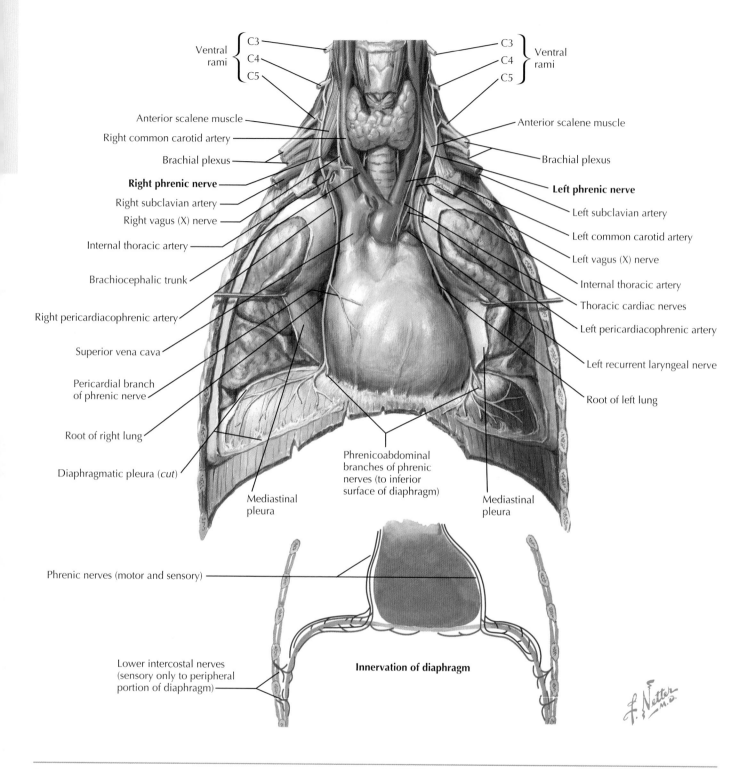

Innervation of diaphragm

9.19 PHRENIC NERVE

The left and right phrenic nerves are the motor nerves that supply both sides of the diaphragm from the C3, C4, and C5 ventral roots. The phrenic nerve also contains many sensory nerve fibers that supply the fibrous pericardium, the mediastinal pleura, and central areas of the diaphragmatic pleura. Sympathetic postganglionic nerve fibers also travel with this nerve. Coordinated contraction of the diaphragm relies on central control of firing of LMNs through dendrite bundles in the spinal cord.

CLINICAL POINT

The phrenic nerves derive from the C3–C5 ventral roots and provide the motor supply to the diaphragm. Lesions of the phrenic nerve usually occur in the mediastinum, not the cervical plexus. Pathological processes, such as enlarged mediastinal nodes, aortic aneurysms, mediastinal tumors, sequelae of surgery, and demyelination from Guillain-Barré syndrome, can damage these nerves. Unilateral damage to the phrenic nerve results in paralysis of the diaphragm on the ipsilateral side, which can usually be tolerated at rest but not following exertion. Bilateral phrenic nerve damage results in diaphragmatic paralysis with extreme dyspnea and hypoventilation.

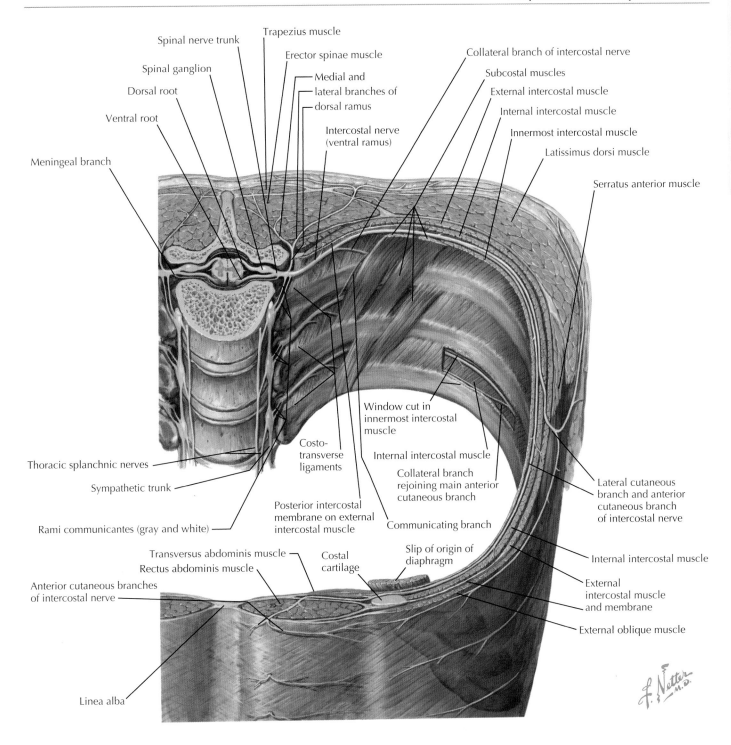

Spinal nerve trunk

Spinal ganglion

Dorsal root

Ventral root

Meningeal branch

Trapezius muscle

Erector spinae muscle

Medial and lateral branches of dorsal ramus

Intercostal nerve (ventral ramus)

Collateral branch of intercostal nerve

Subcostal muscles

External intercostal muscle

Internal intercostal muscle

Innermost intercostal muscle

Latissimus dorsi muscle

Serratus anterior muscle

Thoracic splanchnic nerves

Sympathetic trunk

Rami communicantes (gray and white)

Costo-transverse ligaments

Posterior intercostal membrane on external intercostal muscle

Window cut in innermost intercostal muscle

Internal intercostal muscle

Collateral branch rejoining main anterior cutaneous branch

Communicating branch

Lateral cutaneous branch and anterior cutaneous branch of intercostal nerve

Transversus abdominis muscle

Rectus abdominis muscle

Anterior cutaneous branches of intercostal nerve

Costal cartilage

Slip of origin of diaphragm

Internal intercostal muscle

External intercostal muscle and membrane

External oblique muscle

Linea alba

9.20 THORACIC NERVES

The 12 pairs of thoracic nerves are derived from dorsal and ventral roots of their corresponding segments. These nerves do not form plexuses; they distribute cutaneous branches to the thoracic dermatomes and send other sensory fibers to deeper muscular structures, vessels, periosteum, parietal pleura, the peritoneum, and breast tissue. The thoracic nerves also send motor fibers to muscles of the thoracic and abdominal wall and carry preganglionic and postganglionic sympathetic nerve fibers into and out of the sympathetic chain. Muscles of the thoracic and abdominal wall, supplied by these nerves, act as accessory respiratory muscles and may assist in breathing in times of dyspnea or phrenic nerve impairment.

3 Trunks

5 Roots
(ventral rami)

3 Ventral divisions
3 Dorsal divisions

Contribution from C4

Dorsal scapular
nerve; C5

Dorsal ramus

Suprascapular
nerve; C5, 6

To phrenic
nerve; C5

C5

3 Cords

To subclavius
muscle; C5, 6

C6

Superior

Lateral pectoral
nerve; C5, 6, 7

C7

Middle

C8

Terminal
branches
(2 from
each cord)

Lateral

Inferior

T1

Musculocutaneous
nerve; C(4), 5, 6, 7

Axillary nerve; C5, 6

Posterior

Long
thoracic
nerve;
C5, 6, 7

Contribution
from T2

To longus colli and
scalene muscles;
C5, 6, 7, 8

Subscapular
nerves; C5, 6

Radial nerve; C5,
6, 7, 8; T1

1st rib

Medial

1st intercostal nerve

Median nerve; C(5),
6, 7, 8; T1

Medial pectoral nerve; C8; T1

Some contributions
inconstant

Medial cutaneous nerve of forearm; C8; T1

Medial cutaneous nerve of arm; T1

Thoracodorsal nerve; C6, 7, 8

Ulnar nerve; C(7), 8; T1

Supraclavicular Branches		Infraclavicular Branches		Infraclavicular Branches	
From plexus roots		*From lateral cord*		Ulnar	C(7), 8; T1
To longus colli and scalene muscles	C5, 6, 7, 8	Lateral pectoral	C5, 6, 7	Medial root of median	C8; T1
Dorsal scapular	C5	Musculocutaneous	C(4), 5, 6, 7	*From posterior cord*	
Branch to phrenic	C5	Lateral root of median	C(5), 6, 7	Upper subscapular	C5, 6, (7)
Long thoracic	C5, 6, 7	*From medial cord*		Lower subscapular	C5, 6
From superior trunk		Medial pectoral	C8; T1	Axillary (circumflex humeral)	C5, 6
Suprascapular	C5, 6	Medial cutaneous nerve of arm	T1	Thoracodorsal	C5, 6
To subclavius muscle	C5, 6	Medial cutaneous nerve of forearm	C8; T1	Radial	C5, 6, 7, 8

9.21 BRACHIAL PLEXUS

The brachial plexus is formed by the union of the ventral roots of C5 through C8 plus T1, with a smaller contribution from C4. Sensory and sympathetic fibers also distribute in the brachial plexus. The roots give rise to three trunks, three ventral and three dorsal divisions, three cords as well as numerous terminal branches, the peripheral nerves. This plexus is vulnerable to birth injury (superior plexus paralysis), which causes paralysis of the deltoid, biceps, brachial, and brachioradialis muscles, with sparing of the hands, and causes sensory loss over the deltoid area and radial aspect of the forearm and hand. Pressure by a cervical rib can cause inferior plexus injury (C8, T1 injury), which results in paralysis of small hand muscles and flexors of the hand, with ulnar sensory loss and possible Horner's syndrome.

birth, including displacement of the head to the opposite side and depression of the shoulder on the same side (Erb-Duchenne palsy); by radiation damage, from congenital causes, and by tumors. Such lesions may result in paresis of shoulder abduction and external rotation and in paresis of elbow flexion caused by damage to the motor nerve supply to the deltoid, supraspinatus, infraspinatus, biceps, supinator, and brachioradialis muscles. The arm hangs down and is rotated medially; the forearm is pronated. The biceps and brachioradialis muscle stretch reflexes are absent. Sensory loss is experienced over the deltoid region and along the radial side of the forearm.

Lesions of the lower brachial plexus, particularly those affecting C8 and T1 contributions, can result from traction on an abducted arm, a breech delivery (Dejerine-Klumpke paralysis), an apical lung tumor, a cervical rib, radiation damage, or a tumor. These lesions result in paralysis of finger flexion and paralysis of all the small muscles of the hand; a claw hand results. Sensory loss is present along the ulnar surface of the forearm and hand. Ipsilateral Horner's syndrome is sometimes seen due to damage to T1 preganglionic outflow to the superior cervical ganglion, with resultant ptosis, miosis, and hemianhydrosis.

CLINICAL POINT
Lesions in the upper brachial plexus, particularly those affecting C5 and C6 contributions, can be caused by traction from a difficult

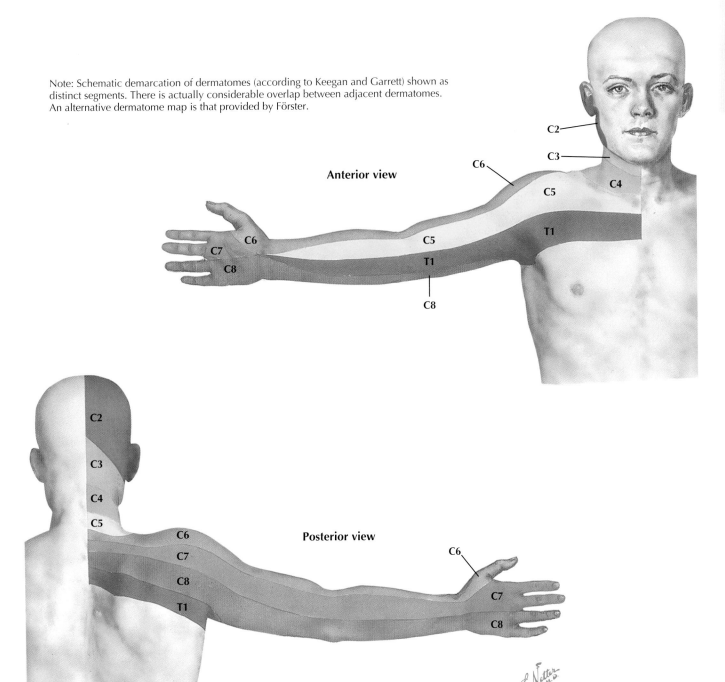

Note: Schematic demarcation of dermatomes (according to Keegan and Garrett) shown as distinct segments. There is actually considerable overlap between adjacent dermatomes. An alternative dermatome map is that provided by Förster.

Anterior view

Posterior view

9.22 DERMATOMES OF THE UPPER LIMB

Because of the distribution of nerve fibers in the brachial plexus and the interchange of sensory and motor fibers through the trunks, divisions, and cords, the orderly segmental distribution of cervical dermatomes is obscured to some degree.

However, the arrangement of dermatomes in the upper limb is explicable embryologically as limb buds extend. The more proximal dermatomes are elongated strips located along the outer sides of the limbs, whereas the more distal dermatomes are found medially.

Anterior (palmar) view

Posterior (dorsal) view

Supraclavicular nerves
(from cervical plexus – C3, 4)

Axillary nerve
Superior lateral cutaneous
nerve of arm (C5, 6)

Radial nerve
Inferior lateral cutaneous
nerve of arm (C5, 6)

Lateral cutaneous nerve of forearm
(C5, 6 [7]) (terminal part of
musculocutaneous nerve)

Radial nerve
Superficial branch (C6, 7, 8)

Median nerve
Palmar branch
and Palmar
digital branches
(C6, 7, 8)

Intercosto-
brachial
nerve (T2)
and medial
cutaneous
nerve of arm
(C8, T1, 2)

Medial
cutaneous
nerve of
forearm
(C8, T1)

Ulnar nerve (C8, T1)

Palmar branch

Palmar digital
branches

Dorsal branch
and dorsal digital
branches

Proper palmar
digital branches

Supraclavicular nerves
(from cervical plexus – C3, 4)

Axillary nerve
Superior lateral cutaneous nerve
of arm (C5, 6)

Radial nerve
Posterior cutaneous
nerve of arm (C5, 6, 7, 8)
Inferior lateral cutaneous nerve of arm
Posterior cutaneous nerve of forearm
(C[5], 6, 7, 8)

Lateral cutaneous nerve of forearm
(C5, 6, [7]) (terminal part of musculocutaneous nerve)

Radial nerve
Superficial branch and dorsal
digital branches (C6, 7, 8)

Median nerve
Proper palmar digital branches

Note: Division is variable between ulnar and radial innervation on dorsum of hand and often aligns with middle of 3rd digit instead of 4th digit as shown.

9.23 CUTANEOUS INNERVATION OF THE UPPER LIMB

The cutaneous innervation of the limb derives from the musculocutaneous, axillary, radial, median, and ulnar nerves. These nerves are the terminal branches of the brachial plexus. Unlike the distributions of the dorsal nerve roots, the cutaneous sensory distributions of these peripheral nerves to the upper limb do not overlap. Thus, a peripheral nerve injury or compression results in a zone of anesthesia corresponding to its distribution. Irritative lesions result in pain and paresthesias that occur in the same corresponding distribution.

Dorsal scapular nerve

Suprascapular nerve

Supraspinatus muscle

Levator scapulae muscle (supplied also by branches from C5 and C6)

Rhomboideus minor muscle

Rhomboideus major muscle

Infraspinatus muscle

Teres major muscle

Lower subscapular nerve

Posterior cutaneous nerve of arm (branch of radial nerve in axilla)

Triceps brachii muscle
- Long head
- Lateral head
- Medial head

Triceps tendon

Medial epicondyle

Olecranon

Anconeus muscle

Extensor digitorum muscle

Extensor carpi ulnaris muscle

Dorsal Scapular Nerve (C5),
Suprascapular Nerve (C5, C6),
Axillary Nerve (C5, C6) and
Radial Nerve (C5, C6, C7, C8; T1)
Above Elbow (viewed from behind)

Deltoid muscle

Teres minor muscle

Axillary nerve

Upper lateral cutaneous nerve of arm

Radial nerve

Lower lateral cutaneous nerve of arm

Posterior cutaneous nerve of forearm

Lateral intermuscular septum

Brachialis muscle (lateral part)

Brachioradialis muscle

Extensor carpi radialis longus muscle

Extensor carpi radialis brevis muscle

9.24 THE SCAPULAR, AXILLARY, AND RADIAL NERVES ABOVE THE ELBOW

The dorsal scapular nerve (C5) supplies the levator scapulae and rhomboid muscles; it aids in elevation and adduction of the scapula toward the spinal column. A nerve lesion leads to lateral displacement of the vertebral border of the scapula and to rhomboid atrophy (difficult to detect). The suprascapular nerve (C5–C6) supplies the supraspinatus and infraspinatus muscles; it aids in lifting and in outward rotation of the arm. A lesion results in weakness in the first 15 degrees of abduction and in external rotation of the arm. The axillary nerve (C5–C6) supplies the deltoid and teres minor muscles; it aids in abduction of the arm to the horizontal and in outward rotation of the arm. A lesion may be caused by dislocation of the shoulder joint or a fracture of the surgical neck of the humerus and results in deltoid atrophy, in weakness in abduction from 15 degrees to 90 degrees, and in loss of cutaneous sensation over the lower half of the deltoid. The radial nerve (C5–C8) in the upper arm supplies the triceps, anconeus, brachioradialis, extensor carpi radialis, extensor digitorum, and supinator muscles and aids in the extension and flexion of the elbow. A lesion may be caused by a fracture of the midshaft of the humerus that affects the nerve within the spiral groove and leads to paralysis of extension and flexion of the elbow and of supination of the forearm. The wrist and fingers cannot be extended, and wristdrop occurs.

Radial nerve

Superficial branch

Deep terminal branch

Lateral epicondyle

Anconeus muscle

Brachioradialis muscle

Extensor carpi radialis longus muscle

Supinator muscle

Extensor carpi radialis brevis muscle

Extensor carpi ulnaris muscle

Extensor digitorum muscle and extensor digiti minimi muscle

Extensor indicis muscle

Extensor pollicis longus muscle

Abductor pollicis longus muscle

Extensor pollicis brevis muscle

Posterior interosseous nerve (deep branch of radial nerve)

Superficial branch of radial nerve

Dorsal digital nerves

Radial Nerve in Forearm (C5, C6, C7, C8; T1) (viewed from behind and slightly laterally)

Extensor supinator group of muscles

From axillary nerve

Upper lateral cutaneous nerve of arm

Lower lateral cutaneous nerve of arm

Posterior cutaneous nerve of arm

From radial nerve

Posterior cutaneous nerve of forearm

Superficial branch of radial nerve

Cutaneous innervation from radial and axillary nerves

9.25 RADIAL NERVE IN THE FOREARM

In the forearm, the radial nerve (C6–C8) supplies motor fibers to the (1) extensor carpi radialis; (2) extensor digitorum; (3) extensor digiti V; (4) extensor carpi ulnaris; (5) supinator; (6) abductor pollicis longus; (7) extensor pollicis brevis and longus; and (8) extensor indicis proprius muscles. It supplies the posterior upper arm, an elongated zone of the posterior forearm, and the posterior hand, thumb, and lateral 2½ fingers. A lesion results in paralysis of extension and flexion of the elbow, paralysis of supination of the forearm, paralysis of extension of the wrist and fingers, and paralysis of abduction of the thumb as well as loss of sensation over the radial aspect of the posterior forearm and the dorsum of the hand.

Musculocutaneous Nerve (C5, C6, C7)
(only muscles innervated by
musculocutaneous nerve are depicted)

Musculocuotaneous nerve

Coracobrachialis muscle

Biceps brachii muscle (*turned back*)

Brachialis muscle

Articular branch

Lateral cutaneous nerve of forearm

Anterior branch

Posterior branch

Medial
Posterior
Lateral cords of brachial plexus

Medial cutaneous nerves of
forearm and arm

Ulnar nerve

Median nerve

Radial nerve

Axillary nerve

**Cutaneous
innervation**

f. Netter
M.D.

9.26 MUSCULOCUTANEOUS NERVE

The musculocutaneous nerve (C5–C6) supplies the biceps brachii, coracobrachialis, and brachialis muscles; it aids in flexion of the upper and lower arm, supination of the lower arm, and elevation and adduction of the arm. The nerve supplies sensory innervation to the lateral forearm. A lesion may be caused by a fracture of the humerus and results in the wasting of the muscles supplied, weakness of flexion of the supinated arm, and loss of sensation on the lateral forearm.

Median Nerve (C6, C7, C8; T1)
(only muscles innervated
by median nerve are depicted)

Musculocutaneous nerve

Median nerve

Pronator teres muscle (humeral head)

Articular branch

Flexor carpi radialis muscle

Palmaris longus muscle

Pronator teres muscle (ulnar head)

Flexor digitorum superficialis muscle (*turned up*)

Flexor digitorum profundus muscle (lateral portion supplied via anterior interosseous nerve; medial portion by ulnar nerve)

Anterior interosseous nerve

Flexor pollicis longus muscle

Pronator quadratus muscle

Palmar branch

Abductor pollicis brevis

Opponens pollicis

Flexor pollicis brevis (superficial head; deep head supplied by ulnar nerve)

Thenar muscles

1st and 2nd lumbrical muscles

Branches to dorsum of middle and distal phalanges

Medial

Posterior

Lateral cords of brachial plexus

Medial cutaneous nerve of arm

Medial cutaneous nerve of forearm

Axillary nerve

Radial nerve

Ulnar nerve

Flexor retinaculum

Anastomotic branch to ulnar nerve

Common
Proper } Palmar digital nerves

Cutaneous innervation

9.27 MEDIAN NERVE

The median nerve (C5–T1) supplies motor fibers to the (1) flexor carpi radialis; (2) pronator teres; (3) palmaris longus; (4) flexor digitorum superficialis and profundus; (5) flexor pollicis longus; (6) abductor pollicis brevis; (7) flexor pollicis brevis; (8) opponens pollicis brevis; and (9) lumbrical muscles of the index and middle fingers. It supplies sensory innervation to the palm and adjacent thumb, the index and middle fingers, and the lateral half of the fourth finger. A lesion (caused by carpal tunnel syndrome) results in weakness in flexion of the fingers, the abduction and opposition of the thumb, and loss of sensation or painful sensation in the radial distribution in the hand (thumb, index finger, half of middle finger) that often radiates back to the wrist. A higher lesion also produces weakness in pronation of the forearm.

Transverse carpal ligament

Median nerve

Palmar cutaneous branch of median nerve

Thenar muscles
Abductor pollicis brevis

Carpal tunnel

Opponens pollicis

Flexor pollicis brevis (superficial head)

1st and 2nd lumbrical muscles

Digital nerves

Distribution of branches of median nerve in hand

Ulnar nerve in Guyon's canal

Transverse carpal ligament (roof of carpal tunnel)

Median nerve in carpal tunnel

Flexor tendons in carpal tunnel

Activities or medical conditions that increase contents and pressure within tunnel may result in nerve compression.

Long-term compression can result in thenar muscle weakness and atrophy.

Thenar atrophy

Sensory distribution of median nerve

9.28 CARPAL TUNNEL SYNDROME

The median nerve travels through the carpal tunnel in the wrist. The carpal tunnel is a tightly confined space restricted by the presence of the transverse carpal ligament. Repetitive movements of the wrist (e.g., repeated computer activity), chronic extension of the wrist (e.g., bicycling), and even sleeping with the wrist bent can compress the median nerve in the carpal tunnel. The mechanism of damage to the nerve may be direct compression on the nerve and also may involve an accompanying reduction in blood flow to the nerves through the vasa

nervorum. This produces a painful neuropathy characterized by tingling and paresthesias or pain (sometimes severe) on the median side of the palm and in the thumb, the index finger, and the adjacent half of the middle finger, often radiating back to the wrist. The pain is severe enough to awaken the patient. There also may be weakness in the innervated muscles with atrophy in the thenar eminence. Nerve conduction velocity studies show slowing of motor and sensory axons. An electromyogram may show denervation of innervated muscles such as the abductor pollicis brevis.

Ulnar Nerve (C8; T1)
(only muscles innervated
by ulnar nerve are depicted)

Ulnar nerve (no branches above elbow)

Articular branch (behind medial condyle)

Flexor digitorum profundus muscle
(medial portion only; lateral portion
supplied by anterior interosseous
branch of median nerve)

Cutaneous innervation

Flexor carpi ulnaris muscle (*drawn aside*)

Dorsal branch

Palmar branch

Superficial branch

Deep branch

Flexor pollicis brevis muscle
(deep head only; superficial
head and other thenar muscles
supplied by median nerve)

Adductor pollicis muscle

Palmaris brevis
Abductor digiti minimi
Flexor digiti minimi brevis
Opponens digiti minimi

} Hypothenar muscles

Common palmar digital nerve

Anastomotic branch to median nerve

Palmar and dorsal interossei muscles

3rd and 4th lumbrical muscles (*turned down*)

Proper palmar digital nerves (dorsal digital nerves are from dorsal branch)

Branches to dorsum of middle and distal phalanges

f. Netter m.d.

9.29 ULNAR NERVE

The ulnar nerve (C8–T1) supplies motor fibers to the (1) flexor carpi ulnaris; (2) flexor digitorum profundus; (3) adductor pollicis; (4) abductor digiti V; (5) opponens digiti V; (6) flexor digiti brevis V; (7) interosseus dorsal and palmar; and (8) lumbrical muscles of the fourth and little fingers. It supplies sensory innervation to the dorsal and palmar medial surface of the hand for the little finger and the medial half of the fourth

finger. A lesion results in wasting of hand muscles; weakness of wrist flexion and ulnar deviation of the hand; weakness of abduction and adduction of fingers, known as claw hand (hyperextension of the fingers at metacarpophalangeal joints and flexion at the interphalangeal joints); and loss of sensation in the ulnar distribution in the hand (dorsal and palmar surfaces of the medial hand, the little finger, and the medial half of the fourth finger).

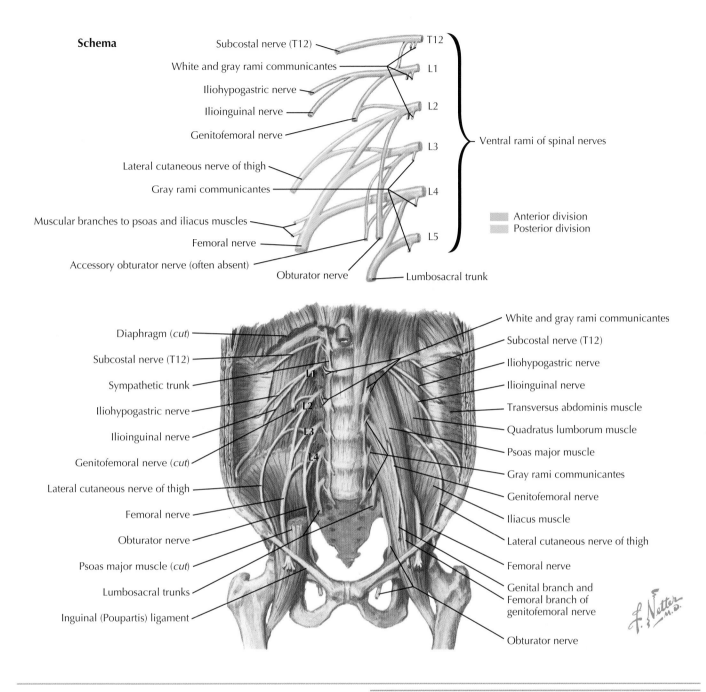

Schema

Subcostal nerve (T12)

White and gray rami communicantes

Iliohypogastric nerve

Ilioinguinal nerve

Genitofemoral nerve

Lateral cutaneous nerve of thigh

Gray rami communicantes

Muscular branches to psoas and iliacus muscles

Femoral nerve

Accessory obturator nerve (often absent)

Obturator nerve

T12

L1

L2

L3

L4

L5

Ventral rami of spinal nerves

Anterior division
Posterior division

Lumbosacral trunk

Diaphragm (cut)

Subcostal nerve (T12)

Sympathetic trunk

Iliohypogastric nerve

Ilioinguinal nerve

Genitofemoral nerve (cut)

Lateral cutaneous nerve of thigh

Femoral nerve

Obturator nerve

Psoas major muscle (cut)

Lumbosacral trunks

Inguinal (Poupartis) ligament

White and gray rami communicantes

Subcostal nerve (T12)

Iliohypogastric nerve

Ilioinguinal nerve

Transversus abdominis muscle

Quadratus lumborum muscle

Psoas major muscle

Gray rami communicantes

Genitofemoral nerve

Iliacus muscle

Lateral cutaneous nerve of thigh

Femoral nerve

Genital branch and
Femoral branch of
genitofemoral nerve

Obturator nerve

9.30 LUMBAR PLEXUS

The lumbar plexus is formed from the anterior primary rami of the L1 through L4 roots within the posterior substance of the psoas muscle. The L1 (and some of L2) root forms the iliohypogastric and ilioinguinal nerves and the genitofemoral nerves. These nerves contribute innervation to the transverse and the oblique abdominal muscles. The remaining roots form the femoral, obturator, and lateral femoral cutaneous nerves. Lesions in the lumbar plexus are unusual because of the protection of the plexus within the psoas muscle. Such lesions result in weakness of hip flexion, weakness of adduction of the thigh and extension of the leg, and decreased sensation on the anterior thigh and leg.

CLINICAL POINT

A lumbar plexopathy results in characteristic weakness and sensory losses in nerve roots L2–L4 and involves the distribution of both the obturator and femoral nerves. The most characteristic motor losses are weakness of hip flexion and adduction and weakness of extension of the leg. The motor loss can sometimes occur as the principal finding in a plexopathy but must be distinguished from radiculopathy. Sensory loss over the anterior (and medial) aspect of the thigh may or may not be seen. The patellar reflex usually is diminished. Some lumbar plexopathies present with a patchy motor loss in one or both legs; sometimes the cause is very clear, as in postradiation lumbar plexopathy following treatment of a retroperitoneal tumor or nodes or in a plexopathy that accompanies pregnancy. And sometimes the cause is not clear, and may include an ischemic diabetic plexopathy, a tumor with infiltration, vasculitis, or trauma. Lumbar plexopathies are usually distinguished from radiculopathies because the latter are painful and are accompanied by a nerve root distribution.

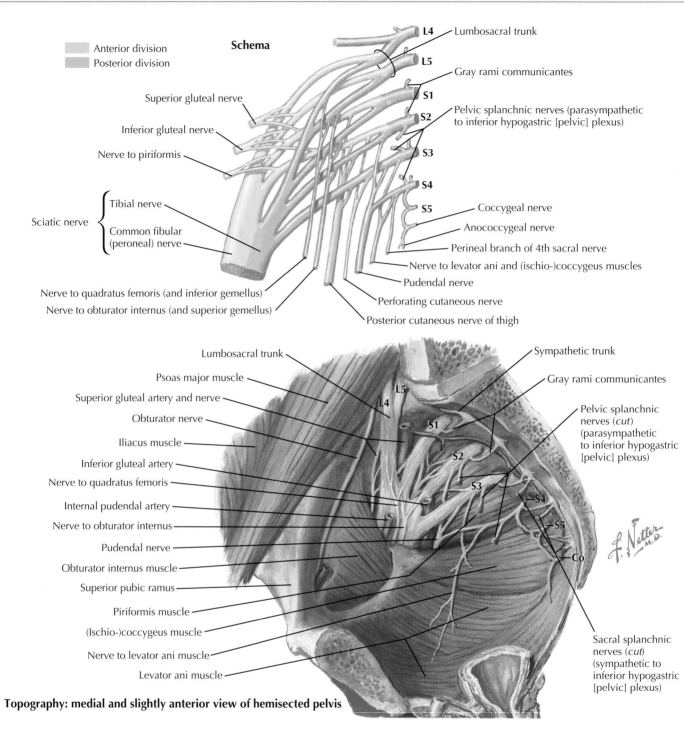

Schema

Anterior division
Posterior division

Lumbosacral trunk — L4
L5
Gray rami communicantes
S1
S2 — Pelvic splanchnic nerves (parasympathetic to inferior hypogastric [pelvic] plexus)
S3
S4
S5 — Coccygeal nerve
Anococcygeal nerve
Perineal branch of 4th sacral nerve
Nerve to levator ani and (ischio-)coccygeus muscles
Pudendal nerve
Perforating cutaneous nerve
Posterior cutaneous nerve of thigh

Superior gluteal nerve
Inferior gluteal nerve
Nerve to piriformis

Sciatic nerve { Tibial nerve
Common fibular (peroneal) nerve

Nerve to quadratus femoris (and inferior gemellus)
Nerve to obturator internus (and superior gemellus)

Lumbosacral trunk
Psoas major muscle
Superior gluteal artery and nerve
Obturator nerve
Iliacus muscle
Inferior gluteal artery
Nerve to quadratus femoris
Internal pudendal artery
Nerve to obturator internus
Pudendal nerve
Obturator internus muscle
Superior pubic ramus
Piriformis muscle
(Ischio-)coccygeus muscle
Nerve to levator ani muscle
Levator ani muscle

Sympathetic trunk
Gray rami communicantes
Pelvic splanchnic nerves (cut) (parasympathetic to inferior hypogastric [pelvic] plexus)

L5
L4
S1
S2
S3
S4
S5
Co

Sacral splanchnic nerves (cut) (sympathetic to inferior hypogastric [pelvic] plexus)

Topography: medial and slightly anterior view of hemisected pelvis

9.31 SACRAL AND COCCYGEAL PLEXUSES

The sacral and coccygeal plexuses are formed from the roots of the L4–S4 segments, located anterior to the piriformis muscle. The major branches include the superior (L4–S1) and inferior (L5–S2) gluteal nerves, the posterior femoral cutaneous nerve (S1–S3), the sciatic nerve (L4–S3) and its tibial and common peroneal divisions, and the pudendal nerve (S2–S4). The pudendal nerve supplies the perineal and sphincter muscles, which aid in closing the sphincters of the bladder and the rectum. Lesions of the sacral plexus result in weakness of the posterior thigh and muscles of the leg and feet, with decreased sensation in the posterior thigh and a perianal/saddle location.

CLINICAL POINT
Sacral plexopathies usually present as weakness and loss of sensation in the distribution of the gluteal, tibial, and peroneal nerves. The leg weakness can be significant; it includes weakness of hip extension and abduction, weakness of flexion of the leg, and weakness of ankle movements (plantarflexors and dorsiflexors). Weakness may occur in the gluteal muscles if the plexopathy involves more proximal regions of the plexus. Sensory loss can occur in the posterior region of the thigh, the anterolateral and posterior leg, and the plantar surface and dorsolateral portion of the foot. Saddle sensory loss may or may not be present. Some autonomic involvement also may occur, with vascular changes and trophic alterations characteristic of autonomic damage.

Lateral femoral cutaneous nerve

Femoral nerve

Obturator nerve

Iliacus muscle

Psoas major muscle (lower part)

Articular twig

Sartorius muscle (*divided*)

Pectineus muscle

Quadriceps femoris

Rectus femoris muscle (*divided*)

Vastus intermedius muscle

Vastus medialis muscle

Vastus lateralis muscle

Articularis genus muscle

T12
L1
L2
L3
L4

Lumbar plexus

Lumbosacral trunk

Femoral Nerve (L2, L3, L4) and Lateral Femoral Cutaneous Nerve (L2, L3)

Lateral femoral cutaneous nerve

Anterior cutaneous branches of femoral nerve

Sartorius muscle (*divided*)

Saphenous nerve

Infrapatellar branch of saphenous nerve

Medial crural cutaneous branches of saphenous nerve

Cutaneous innervation

Note: Only muscles innervated by the femoral nerve are shown.

9.32 FEMORAL AND LATERAL FEMORAL CUTANEOUS NERVES

The femoral nerve (mainly L2–L4) innervates the iliopsoas, sartorius, and quadriceps femoris muscles. It contributes to flexion and outward rotation of the hip, flexion and inward rotation of the lower leg, and extension of the lower leg around the knee joint. It supplies sensory fibers to the anterior thigh and to the anterior and medial surface of the leg and foot. A lesion results in weakness of extension of the leg and flexion of the hip and leg, with quadriceps atrophy and in loss of sensation in territories of sensory distribution. The lateral femoral cutaneous nerve supplies sensation to the skin and fascia of the anterior and lateral surfaces of the thigh to the level of the knee. Compression of the nerve at the inguinal ligament or near the surface (caused by a tight-fitting garment) may result in loss of sensation or paresthesias and pain on the anterior and lateral surfaces of the ipsilateral thigh.

Obturator Nerve (L2, L3, L4)

Iliohypogastric nerve

Ilioinguinal nerve

Genitofemoral nerve

Lateral femoral
cutaneous nerve

Femoral nerve

Obturator nerve

Posterior branch

Articular branch

Anterior branch

Posterior branch

Cutaneous branch

Articular branch
to knee joint

Hiatus of adductor canal

L1
L2   Lumbar plexus
L3
L4

Lumbosacral trunk

Obturator externus muscle

Adductor brevis muscle

Adductor longus muscle (*divided*)

Adductor magnus muscle
(partly supplied by sciatic nerve)

Gracilis muscle

Cutaneous
innervation

Note: Only muscles innervated
by the obturator nerve are shown.

9.33 OBTURATOR NERVE

The obturator nerve (L2–L4) supplies the pectineus; adductor (longus, brevis, and magnus) gracilis; and external obturator muscles. This nerve controls adduction and rotation of the thigh. A small cutaneous zone on the internal thigh is supplied by sensory fibers. A lesion of the obturator nerve results in weakness of adduction of the thigh and a tendency to abduct the thigh in walking. There also is weakness of external rotation of the thigh. A small zone of anesthetic skin on the medial thigh is present.

Sciatic Nerve (L4, L5; S1, S2, S3) and Posterior Femoral Cutaneous Nerve (S1, S2, S3)

Posterior femoral cutaneous nerve

Inferior cluneal nerve

Perineal branches

Tibial segment of sciatic nerve

Long head *(divided)* of biceps femoris muscle

Adductor magnus muscle (also supplied by obturator nerve)

Semitendinosus muscle

Semimembranosus muscle

Tibial nerve

Articular branch

Plantaris muscle

Medial sural cutaneous nerve

Gastrocnemius muscle

Sural nerve

Soleus muscle

Tibial nerve

Medial calcaneal branches

Medial and lateral plantar nerves

Greater sciatic foramen

Sciatic nerve

Common peroneal segment of sciatic nerve

Short head of biceps femoris muscle

Long head *(divided)* of biceps femoris muscle

Common peroneal nerve

Articular branch

Lateral sural cutaneous nerve

Peroneal communicating branch

Lateral calcaneal branches

Lateral dorsal cutaneous nerve

Cutaneous innervation

Posterior femoral cutaneous nerve

From sciatic nerve
- Common peroneal nerve (via lateral sural cutaneous nerve)
- Superficial peroneal nerve
- Sural nerve
- Tibial nerve (via medial calcaneal branches)

Sciatic and Posterior Femoral Cutaneous Nerves

9.34 SCIATIC AND POSTERIOR FEMORAL CUTANEOUS NERVES

The sciatic nerve is formed from the roots of the L4–S3 segments. The superior and inferior gluteal nerve branch proximally, just before the sciatic nerve's formation. The superior gluteal nerve (L4–S1) supplies the gluteus medius and minimus, tensor fascia lata, and piriformis muscles. It contributes to abduction and inward rotation and some outward rotation of the thigh and to flexion of the upper leg at the hip. The inferior gluteal nerve (L4–S1) supplies the gluteus maximus, obturator internus, gemelli, and quadratus muscles. It contributes to extension of the thigh at the hip and to outward rotation of the thigh. A lesion results in difficulty climbing stairs and

rising from a sitting position. The sciatic nerve proper supplies the biceps femoris, semitendinosus, and semimembranosus muscles (hamstrings) and regulates flexion of the lower leg. Because it branches into the tibial and common peroneal nerves, major lesions of the sciatic nerve result in weakness of leg flexion, weakness of all muscles below the knee, and loss of sensation in the posterior thigh, posterior and lateral aspects of the leg, and sole of the foot. Such lesions may result from a fracture of the pelvis or femur, nerve compression, a herniated disc, or diabetes. The posterior femoral cutaneous nerve (S1–S3) supplies sensory innervation to the posterior thigh, lateral part of the perineum, and lower portion of the buttock.

Tibial Nerve (L4, L5; S1, S2, S3)

Tibial nerve
Medial sural cutaneous nerve *(cut)*
Articular branches
Plantaris muscle
Gastrocnemius muscle
Nerve to popliteus muscle
Popliteus muscle
Crural interosseous nerve
Soleus muscle
Flexor digitorum longus muscle
Tibialis posterior muscle
Flexor hallucis longus muscle
Sural nerve *(cut)*
Lateral calcaneal branch
Medial calcaneal branch
Flexor retinaculum *(cut)*

Common peroneal nerve
From tibial nerve
Articular branch
Lateral sural cutaneous nerve *(cut)*

Medial calcaneal branches (S1, 2)
Medial plantar nerve (L4, 5)
Lateral plantar nerve (S1, 2)
Sural nerve (S1, 2)
Saphenous nerve (L3, 4)

Cutaneous innervation of sole

Flexor retinaculum *(cut)*
Tibial nerve
Medial plantar nerve to:
Flexor digitorum brevis muscle
Abductor hallucis muscle;
Flexor hallucis brevis muscle
1st lumbrical muscle,
Articular branch,
Cutaneous branches,
Proper plantar digital nerves

Medial and lateral calcaneal branches
Lateral plantar nerve to:
Quadratus plantae muscle,
Abductor digiti minimi muscle
Deep branch to:
1st, 2nd, 3rd plantar interossei muscles;
2nd, 3rd, 4th lumbrical muscles;
Adductor hallucis muscle,
articular branches
Superficial branch to:
Flexor digiti minimi brevis muscle,
4th interossei muscles,
Proper plantar digital nerves,
cutaneous branches

9.35 **TIBIAL NERVE**

The tibial nerve (L4–S2) supplies innervation to (1) the gastrocnemius and soleus muscles (the main plantar flexors of the foot); (2) the tibialis posterior (plantar flexion and inversion); (3) the flexor digitorum longus (plantar flexor and toe flexor); (4) the flexor hallucis longus (plantar flexor and great toe flexor); and (5) the muscles of the foot, including the abductor digiti minimi pedis, flexor digiti minimi, adductor hallucis, interosseous, and third and fourth lumbrical muscles. Sensory branches supply the skin over the lateral calf, foot, heel, and small toe (sural nerve) and the medial aspect of the heel and the sole of the foot. A lesion can occur because of compression in the tarsal tunnel, a tumor, or diabetes; it results in weakness of plantar flexion and inversion of the foot, weakness of toe flexion, and loss of sensation in the lateral calf and the plantar region of the foot.

CLINICAL POINT

The tibial nerve in the popliteal fossa can be used for evaluation of conduction velocity and of specific reflexes. This nerve may be directly stimulated by electrical current. Surface recording electrodes are placed over a distal innervated muscle, and the nerve is stimulated in one or more places, resulting in an indirect evaluation of motor conduction velocity and the muscle response to tibial nerve stimulation. Sensory conduction velocity evaluation is a bit more straightforward; the stimulating electrode is placed at a distal site, and compound action potentials are recorded over at least two proximal sites. A more complex evaluation of reflexes involves evaluation of the muscle stretch (monosynaptic) reflex. With recording electrodes placed over the distal muscle (triceps surae), the tibial nerve is gradually stimulated first by weak and then by stronger electrical current in the popliteal fossa. The first axons that are stimulated are the Ia afferents, which conduct action potentials into the spinal cord and excite the homonymous LMN, whose axon then sends action potentials down to the innervated muscle. This is a long-latency response, called the H wave or H reflex because it involves both the sensory and the motor arms of the muscle stretch reflex. As current strength is increased, the LMN axon is finally stimulated directly, and the muscle response (direct muscle activation) occurs and with a far shorter latency. This H reflex evaluation is useful in assessment of axonal neuropathies and demyelinating neuropathies.

Common peroneal nerve *(in phantom)*

Tendon of biceps femoris muscle

Common peroneal nerve

Head of fibula

Peroneus longus muscle

Superficial peroneal nerve

Branches of lateral sural cutaneous nerve

Peroneus longus muscle

Peroneus brevis muscle

Medial dorsal cutaneous nerve

Intermediate dorsal cutaneous nerve

Superior extensor retinaculum

Inferior extensor retinaculum *(cut)*

Lateral dorsal cutaneous nerve (branch of sural nerve)

Proper dorsal digital nerves

Common Peroneal Nerve (L4, L5; S1, S2)

Lateral sural cutaneous nerve *(in phantom)*

Articular branches

Anterior tibial recurrent branch

Extensor digitorum longus muscle

Deep peroneal nerve

Tibialis anterior muscle

Extensor digitorum longus muscle

Extensor hallucis longus muscle

Lateral branch of deep peroneal nerve to: Extensor hallucis brevis muscle and Extensor digitorum brevis muscle

Medial branch of deep peroneal nerve

Proper dorsal digital nerves

Cutaneous innervation

Lateral sural cutaneous nerve

Superficial peroneal nerve

Deep peroneal nerve

Sural nerve

Common Peroneal Nerve

9.36 COMMON PERONEAL NERVE

The common peroneal nerve (L4–S1) branches into the deep peroneal nerve, supplying (1) the tibialis anterior (foot dorsiflexion and inversion); (2) the extensor hallucis longus (foot dorsiflexion and great toe extension); (3) the extensor digitorum longus (extension of the toes and foot dorsiflexion); and (4) the extensor digitorum brevis muscles (extension of toes) and the superficial peroneal nerve, which supplies the peroneus longus and brevis muscles (plantar flexion and foot eversion). Sensory branches supply the lateral aspect of the leg below the knee and the skin on the dorsal surface of the foot. This nerve may be damaged by compression, a fracture at the head of the fibula, or diabetes, resulting in weakness of dorsiflexion and eversion of the foot, weakness of toe extension (dorsiflexion), and loss of sensation in the lateral aspect of the lower leg and the dorsum of the foot.

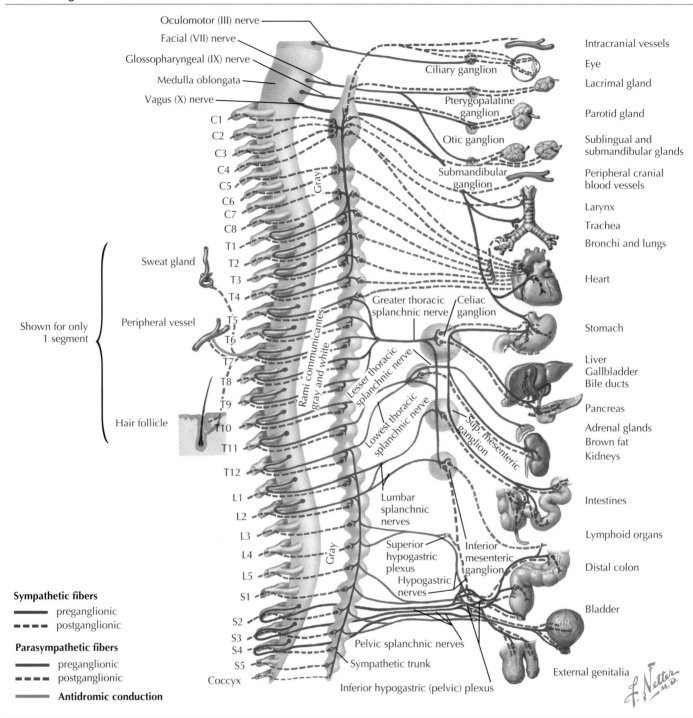

Oculomotor (III) nerve
Facial (VII) nerve
Glossopharyngeal (IX) nerve
Medulla oblongata
Vagus (X) nerve

Intracranial vessels
Eye
Lacrimal gland
Parotid gland
Sublingual and submandibular glands
Peripheral cranial blood vessels
Larynx
Trachea
Bronchi and lungs
Heart
Stomach
Liver
Gallbladder
Bile ducts
Pancreas
Adrenal glands
Brown fat
Kidneys
Intestines
Lymphoid organs
Distal colon
Bladder
External genitalia

Ciliary ganglion
Pterygopalatine ganglion
Otic ganglion
Submandibular ganglion
Greater thoracic splanchnic nerve
Celiac ganglion
Lesser thoracic splanchnic nerve
Lowest thoracic splanchnic nerve
Sup. mesenteric ganglion
Lumbar splanchnic nerves
Superior hypogastric plexus
Inferior mesenteric ganglion
Hypogastric nerves
Pelvic splanchnic nerves
Sympathetic trunk
Inferior hypogastric (pelvic) plexus

Gray
Rami communicantes gray and white
Gray

Sweat gland
Peripheral vessel
Hair follicle
Shown for only 1 segment

C1 C2 C3 C4 C5 C6 C7 C8 T1 T2 T3 T4 T5 T6 T7 T8 T9 T10 T11 T12 L1 L2 L3 L4 L5 S1 S2 S3 S4 S5 Coccyx

Sympathetic fibers
—— preganglionic
- - - - postganglionic

Parasympathetic fibers
—— preganglionic
- - - - postganglionic
—— Antidromic conduction

AUTONOMIC NERVOUS SYSTEM

9.37 GENERAL SCHEMA

The autonomic nervous system is a two-neuron chain. The preganglionic neuron arises from the brain stem or spinal cord and synapses on postganglionic neurons in the sympathetic chain or collateral ganglia (sympathetic) or on intramural ganglia (parasympathetic) near the organ innervated. The sympathetic division, derived from neurons in the T1–L2 lateral horn, prepares the body for fight-or-flight mobilization for emergency responses. The parasympathetic division, derived from neurons in the brain stem (CNs III, VII, IX, and X) and the sacral spinal cord (S2–S4 intermediate gray) regulates reparative, homeostatic, and digestive functions. These autonomic systems achieve their actions through innervation of smooth

muscle, cardiac muscle, secretory (exocrine) glands, metabolic cells (hepatocytes, fat cells), and cells of the immune system. Normally, both autonomic divisions work together to regulate visceral activities such as respiration, cardiovascular function, digestion, and some endocrine functions.

CLINICAL POINT

Pure autonomic failure is a gradual deterioration of sympathetic postganglionic neurons; it occurs in middle-aged individuals and is observed more commonly in men than in women. This syndrome includes neurogenic orthostatic hypotension (syncope or dizziness when standing), inability to sweat, urinary tract dysfunction, erectile dysfunction, and retrograde ejaculation. Pure autonomic failure can be present without evidence of involvement of the CNS. Catecholamine challenge results in robust reactivity in target organs caused by denervation hypersensitivity.

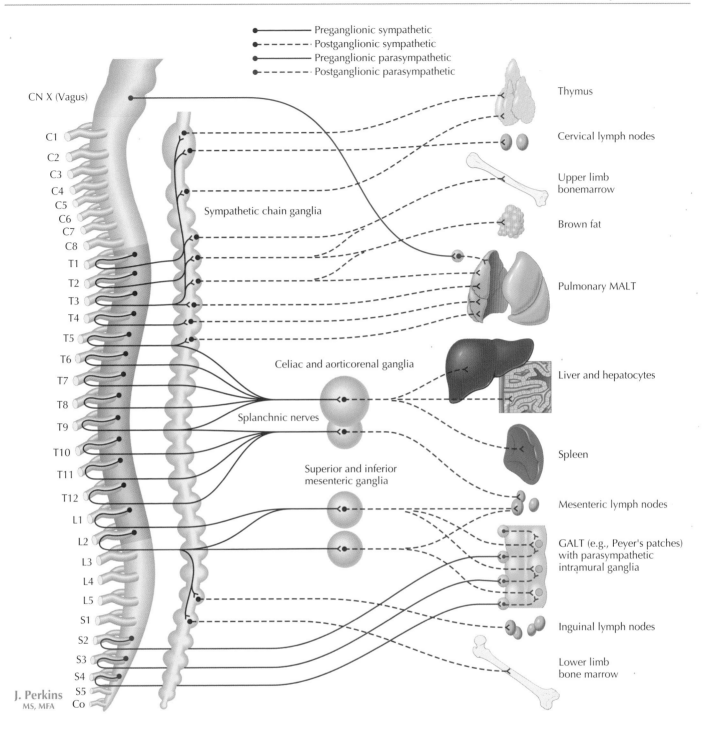

Preganglionic sympathetic
Postganglionic sympathetic
Preganglionic parasympathetic
Postganglionic parasympathetic

CN X (Vagus)

C1
C2
C3
C4
C5
C6
C7
C8
T1
T2
T3
T4
T5
T6
T7
T8
T9
T10
T11
T12
L1
L2
L3
L4
L5
S1
S2
S3
S4
S5
Co

J. Perkins
MS, MFA

Sympathetic chain ganglia

Celiac and aorticorenal ganglia

Splanchnic nerves

Superior and inferior
mesenteric ganglia

Thymus

Cervical lymph nodes

Upper limb
bonemarrow

Brown fat

Pulmonary MALT

Liver and hepatocytes

Spleen

Mesenteric lymph nodes

GALT (e.g., Peyer's patches)
with parasympathetic
intramural ganglia

Inguinal lymph nodes

Lower limb
bone marrow

9.38 AUTONOMIC INNERVATION OF THE IMMUNE SYSTEM AND METABOLIC ORGANS

The autonomic nervous system innervates the vasculature, smooth muscle tissue, and parenchyma of organs of the immune system mainly through the sympathetic division. In the bone marrow and thymus, sympathetic fibers modulate cell proliferation, differentiation, and mobilization. In the spleen and lymph nodes, sympathetic fibers modulate innate immune reactivity, and the magnitude and timing of acquired immune responses, particularly the choice of cell-mediated (Th1 cytokines) as opposed to humoral (Th2 cytokines) immunity. Autonomic nerve fibers regulate immune responses and inflammatory responses in the mucosa-associated lymphoid tissue (MALT) in the lungs, the gut-associated lymphoid tissue (GALT), and the skin. Extensive neuropeptidergic innervation, derived from both the autonomic nervous system and the primary sensory neurons, also is present in the parenchyma of lymphoid organs. Many subsets of lymphoid cells express cognate receptors for catecholamines (alpha and beta receptor subsets) and neuropeptides; the expression of these neurotransmitter receptors is highly regulated by both lymphoid and neural molecular signals. Postganglionic sympathetic nerve fibers also directly innervate hepatocytes and fat cells. (Th = T helper cells)

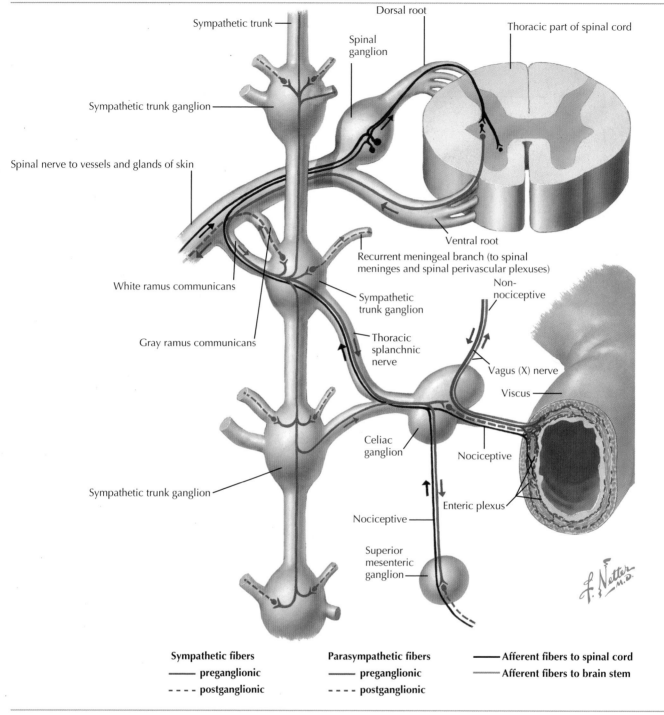

Sympathetic trunk

Dorsal root

Spinal ganglion

Thoracic part of spinal cord

Sympathetic trunk ganglion

Spinal nerve to vessels and glands of skin

Ventral root

Recurrent meningeal branch (to spinal meninges and spinal perivascular plexuses)

White ramus communicans

Sympathetic trunk ganglion

Non-nociceptive

Gray ramus communicans

Thoracic splanchnic nerve

Vagus (X) nerve

Viscus

Celiac ganglion

Nociceptive

Sympathetic trunk ganglion

Enteric plexus

Nociceptive

Superior mesenteric ganglion

Sympathetic fibers	Parasympathetic fibers	——— Afferent fibers to spinal cord
——— preganglionic	——— preganglionic	——— Afferent fibers to brain stem
- - - postganglionic	- - - postganglionic	

9.39 REFLEX PATHWAYS

Autonomic reflex pathways consist of a sensory (afferent) component, interneurons in the CNS, and autonomic efferent components that innervate the peripheral tissue responding to the afferent stimulus. The afferents can be either autonomic (e.g., from the vagus nerve) and processed by brain stem nuclei such as the nucleus solitarius; or they can be somatic (e.g., nociception) and processed by spinal cord neurons. The preganglionic sympathetic or parasympathetic neurons are activated through interneurons to produce a reflex autonomic response (e.g., contraction of vascular smooth muscle to alter blood pressure and increase heart rate and contractility). The efferent connectivity can be relayed via splanchnic or somatic nerves because of the complexity of autonomic efferent pathways.

CLINICAL POINT

Autonomic reflex pathways are vital for maintenance of homeostasis. Sensory signals associated with standing result in vascular constriction induced by sympathetic neurons to maintain blood pressure, prevent pooling of blood in the lower extremities, and maintain appropriate perfusion of the brain and other vital organs. Nociceptive stimulation may result in reflex elevation of heart rate, blood pressure, and other characteristics of sympathetic activation. Stimulation of the perioral region, particularly in an infant during feeding, activates a parasympathetic state to enhance digestion and diminish sympathetic activation, thereby promoting growth and development. Problems can arise when autonomic reflexes are disrupted, or when hyperactivation of reflex pathways elevates either parasympathetic or sympathetic activity. In such circumstances, there is often a counterpart activation of the other system, as when paradoxical parasympathetic activation leads to compensatory sympathetic activation. This can increase the likelihood of problems such as arrhythmia or even cardiac arrest.

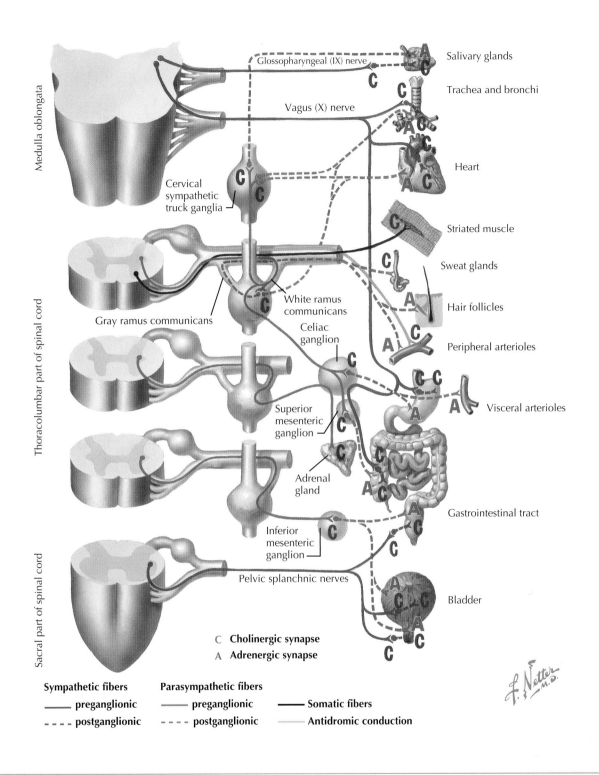

Medulla oblongata

Glossopharyngeal (IX) nerve

Vagus (X) nerve

Cervical sympathetic truck ganglia

Thoracolumbar part of spinal cord

Gray ramus communicans

White ramus communicans

Celiac ganglion

Superior mesenteric ganglion

Adrenal gland

Inferior mesenteric ganglion

Pelvic splanchnic nerves

Sacral part of spinal cord

Salivary glands

Trachea and bronchi

Heart

Striated muscle

Sweat glands

Hair follicles

Peripheral arterioles

Visceral arterioles

Gastrointestinal tract

Bladder

C **Cholinergic synapse**

A **Adrenergic synapse**

Sympathetic fibers	**Parasympathetic fibers**	
—— preganglionic	—— preganglionic	—— **Somatic fibers**
- - - postganglionic	- - - postganglionic	—— **Antidromic conduction**

9.40 CHOLINERGIC AND ADRENERGIC SYNAPSES

The autonomic nervous system is a two-neuron chain. All preganglionic neurons, sympathetic and parasympathetic, use ACh as the principal neurotransmitter in synapses on ganglion cells. These cholinergic (C) synapses activate mainly nicotinic receptors on the ganglion cells. Postganglionic parasympathetic neurons use ACh at synapses with target tissue, activating mainly muscarinic receptors. Postganglionic sympathetic neurons use mainly norepinephrine (adrenergic responses; A), to activate both alpha and beta receptors on target tissues. Although ACh and norepinephrine are the principal neurotransmitters used by autonomic neurons, many colocalized neuropeptides and other neuromediators are also present, including neuropeptide Y, substance P, somatostatin, enkephalins, histamine, glutamate, and others.

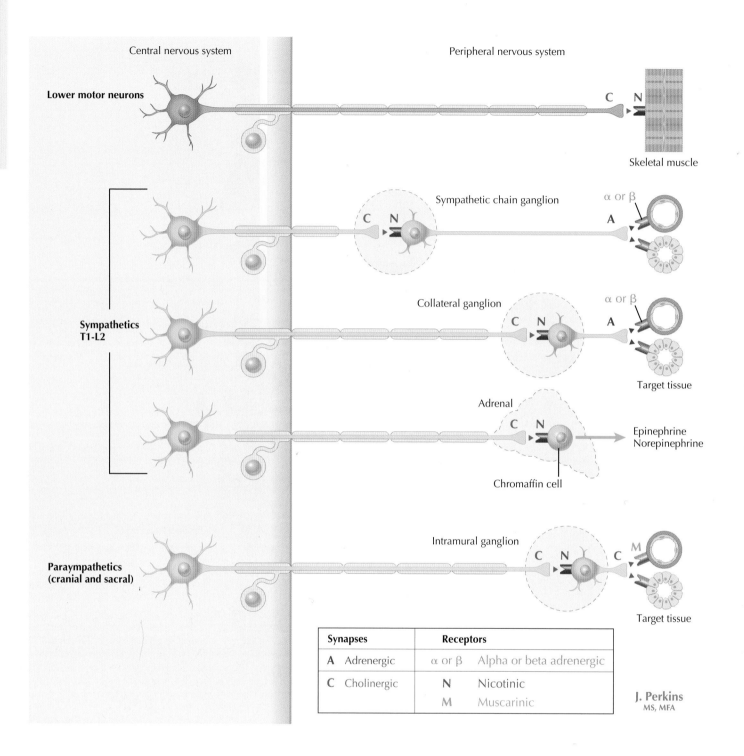

Synapses		Receptors	
A	Adrenergic	α or β	Alpha or beta adrenergic
C	Cholinergic	N	Nicotinic
		M	Muscarinic

J. Perkins
MS, MFA

9.41 SCHEMATIC OF CHOLINERGIC AND ADRENERGIC DISTRIBUTION TO MOTOR AND AUTONOMIC STRUCTURES

All preganglionic neurons of both the SNS and the PsNS use ACh as their neurotransmitter. All ganglion cells possess mainly nicotinic receptors for fast response to cholinergic release from preganglionic axons. However, additional muscarinic receptors and dopamine receptors on ganglion cells help to mediate longer term excitability. The postganglionic sympathetic nerves use mainly norepinephrine as their neurotransmitter, and target structures in the periphery possessing different subsets of alpha and beta adrenergic receptors for response to norepinephrine. Some postganglionic nerve fibers to sweat glands use ACh as their neurotransmitter. Postganglionic parasympathetic nerves use ACh as their neurotransmitter, and target structures in the periphery possessing mainly muscarinic receptors for response to ACh.

Trigeminal (V) nerve { Sensory root / Motor root / Ganglion }

Internal carotid artery and plexus

Facial (VII) nerve

Vestibulocochlear (VIII) nerve

Glossopharyngeal (IX) nerve

Vagus (X) nerve

Greater petrosal nerve
Deep petrosal nerve
Nerve of pterygoid canal
Oculomotor (III) nerve
Maxillary nerve
Ophthalmic nerve
Nasociliary nerve

Nasociliary nerve root
Sympathetic root } of ciliary ganglion
Oculomotor nerve root
Ciliary ganglion
Long and short ciliary nerves
Pterygopalatine nerves

Posterior lateral nasal nerves

Mandibular nerve
Internal carotid nerve
Chorda tympani
Superior laryngeal nerve
Superior cervical sympathetic trunk ganglion

Pterygopalatine ganglion
Otic ganglion
Greater and lesser palatine nerves
Lingual nerve
Submandibular ganglion
Inferior alveolar nerve

Vagus (X) nerve
Internal carotid artery
Cervical sympathetic trunk

Pharyngeal plexus
Maxillary artery and plexus
External carotid artery and plexus
Carotid sinus branch of glossopharyngeal nerve

Middle meningeal artery and plexus
Facial artery and plexus

Superior cervical cardiac branch of vagus neve
Carotid sinus
Common carotid artery and plexus
Superior cervical sympathetic cardiac nerve

9.42 AUTONOMIC DISTRIBUTION TO THE HEAD AND NECK: MEDIAL VIEW

Autonomic nerve distribution to the head and neck includes components of both the SNS and the PsNS. The parasympathetic components are associated with CNs III (ciliary ganglion); VII (pterygopalatine, submandibular ganglia); and IX (otic ganglion). The vagus nerve and its associated ganglia do not innervate effector tissue in the head and neck, although they are present in the neck. Sympathetic components are associated with the superior cervical ganglion and, to a lesser extent, the middle cervical ganglion. The geniculate ganglion (CN VII); petrosal ganglion (CN IX); and nodose ganglion (CN X) process taste information. They are sometimes thought of as autonomic afferents, but they are not components of the autonomic efferent nervous system.

CLINICAL POINT

The oculomotor (III nerve) parasympathetic distribution to the eye forms a vital link in one of the most important reflexes in neurology, the pupillary light reflex. Light shone into one eye provides an afferent signal that is processed by the retina, resulting in ganglion cell activation and axonal projections to the pretectum. The pretectum, through direct and contralateral connections via the posterior commissure, stimulates the nucleus of Edinger-Westphal bilaterally. This system,

via connections in the ciliary ganglion, distributes to the pupillary constrictor muscle, resulting in constriction of the ipsilateral (direct) and contralateral (consensual) pupils. The pupillary light reflex is particularly important in someone with a head injury, intracranial bleed, or space-occupying mass in whom possible brain herniation is suspected. The third nerve may be trapped and compressed against the free edge of the tentorium cerebelli, resulting in failure of the ipsilateral pupil to constrict and disruption of the pupillary light reflex

The superior cervical ganglion (SCG) is the most rostral component of the sympathetic chain. It supplies structures in the head and neck, including the pupillary dilator muscle, blood vessels, sweat glands, pineal gland, thymus gland, and superior tarsal (Muller's) muscle. The T1–T2 intermediolateral cell column in the spinal cord (preganglionic sympathetic neurons) innervates the SCG; this ganglion then distributes noradrenergic fibers to the pupillary dilator muscle, resulting in dilation of the pupil. When CN III is damaged (e.g., by compression during transtentorial herniation), the actions of the sympathetic SCG are unopposed, resulting in a fixed (unresponsive to the pupillary light reflex), dilated pupil. In circumstances in which the SCG or its central innervation is damaged (e.g., apical lung tumor, Horner's syndrome), the ipsilateral pupil cannot dilate and the pupil is constricted (miotic).

A pupil that constricts when light is shone into one eye and paradoxically appears to dilate when light is shone into the other eye (swinging flashlight test) indicates an afferent (CN II) defect, with the paradoxical dilation occurring as the result of recovery from the initial constriction because of the unresponsiveness of the damaged CN II.

Interior carotid nerve

Glossopharyngeal (IX) nerve

Vagus (X) nerve (*cut*)

Superior cervical sympathetic trunk ganglion

Gray rami communicantes

Subclavian artery

Pharyngeal plexus

Superior pharyngeal branch of vagus nerve

Exterior carotid artery and plexus

Superior laryngeal nerve

Interior carotid artery and carotid sinus branch of glossopharyngeal nerve

Carotid body

Carotid sinus

Superior cervical cardiac branch of vagus nerve

Superior cervical sympathetic cardiac nerve

Phrenic nerve

Middle cervical sympathetic trunk ganglion

Common carotid artery and plexus

Middle cervical sympathetic cardiac nerve

Vertebral ganglion

Vertebral artery and plexus

Recurrent laryngeal nerve

Cervicothoracic (stellate) ganglion

Ansa subclavia

Vagus (X) nerve (*cut*)

Inferior cervical sympathetic cardiac nerve

Thoracic sympathetic and vagal cardiac nerves

9.43 AUTONOMIC DISTRIBUTION TO THE HEAD AND NECK: LATERAL VIEW

The parasympathetic nerve fibers to the head and neck regulate pupillary constriction and accommodation for near vision (CN III, ciliary ganglion to pupillary constrictor muscle and ciliary muscle); tear production (CN VII, pterygopalatine ganglion to lacrimal glands); and salivation (CN VII, submandibular ganglion to submandibular and sublingual glands and CN IV, otic ganglion to parotid gland). The sympathetic nerve fibers to the head and neck derive mainly from the SCG, with synapses to the pupillary dilator muscle, sweat glands, vascular smooth muscle, and the thymus gland.

CLINICAL POINT

Blood flow to the brain, derived from the two internal carotid arteries and the two vertebral arteries, is highly regulated. The brain requires moment-to-moment delivery of oxygen and glucose to maintain cerebral activity and generate the adenosine triphosphate needed for the high energy demands of neurons. Blood flow to the brain is autoregulated; several levels of superimposed control derive from metabolic and neural regulatory systems. (1) Autoregulation may be based on smooth muscle responsiveness to stretch and on endothelial cell response to vasoactive secretory products. (2) Superimposed on autoregulation is metabolic control that is based on blood gases (oxygen, carbon dioxide) and on metabolic products stimulated by neuronal activity (nitric oxide, adenosine, lactate, some ions). (3) A third level of regulation derives from neural regulation. The superior cervical ganglion sends noradrenergic (colocalized with neuropeptide Y) sympathetic vasoconstrictor fibers along the vasculature, and the sphenopalatine ganglion sends acetylcholinergic (colocalized with vasoactive intestinal peptide; VIP) vasodilator fibers along the vasculature. The trigeminal ganglion also distributes substance P (colocalized with calcitonin gene-related peptide) vasodilator fibers along the vasculature; these fibers can be activated by pain. Some central regions, such as the fastigial nucleus of the cerebellum and the rostral ventrolateral medulla, can regulate the activation of some of these neural circuits to the cerebral vasculature, influencing blood flow to the brain.

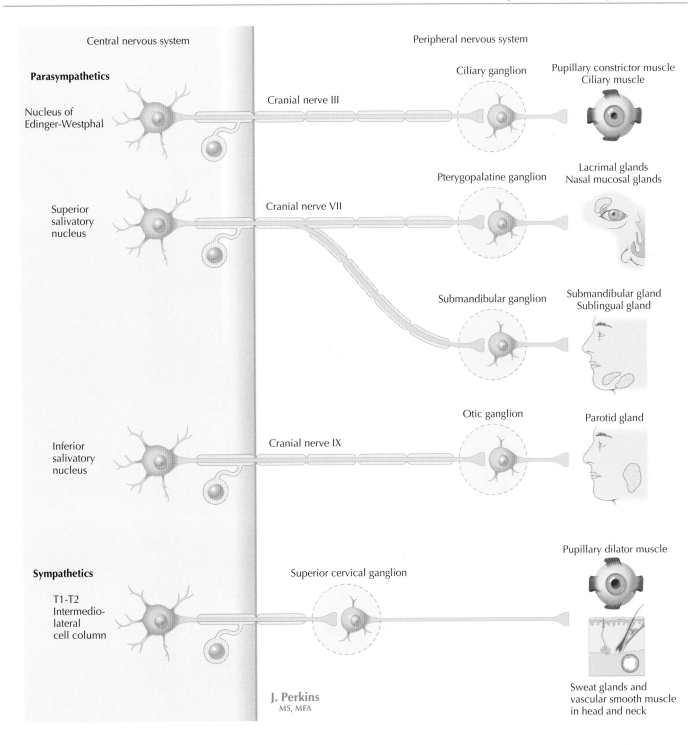

J. Perkins
MS, MFA

9.44 SCHEMATIC OF AUTONOMIC DISTRIBUTION TO THE HEAD AND NECK

Autonomic innervation to the head and neck is derived from parasympathetic neurons in the brain stem, including the nucleus of Edinger-Westphal (CN III), the superior salivatory nucleus (CN VII), and the inferior salivatory nucleus (CN IX), and from sympathetic neurons in the T1–T2 intermediolateral cell column in the spinal cord. The associated ganglia and target (effector) tissue are illustrated.

CLINICAL POINT

The superior and inferior salivatory nuclei provide important parasympathetic regulatory control over salivation. The superior salivatory nucleus innervates (via CN VII) the submandibular ganglion, which supplies the submandibular and sublingual glands; the inferior salivatory nucleus innervates (via CN IX) the otic ganglion, which supplies the parotid gland. These parasympathetic fibers stimulate secretion of saliva. In addition, sympathetic innervation from the superior cervical ganglion activates contraction of the myoepithelial cells of the salivary ducts. Salivation is important as an initial phase of the digestion process; it prepares food for swallowing, aids in speaking, and contains mediators and immunoglobulins that provide an initial protective barrier against potentially dangerous organisms that gain access to the oral cavity.

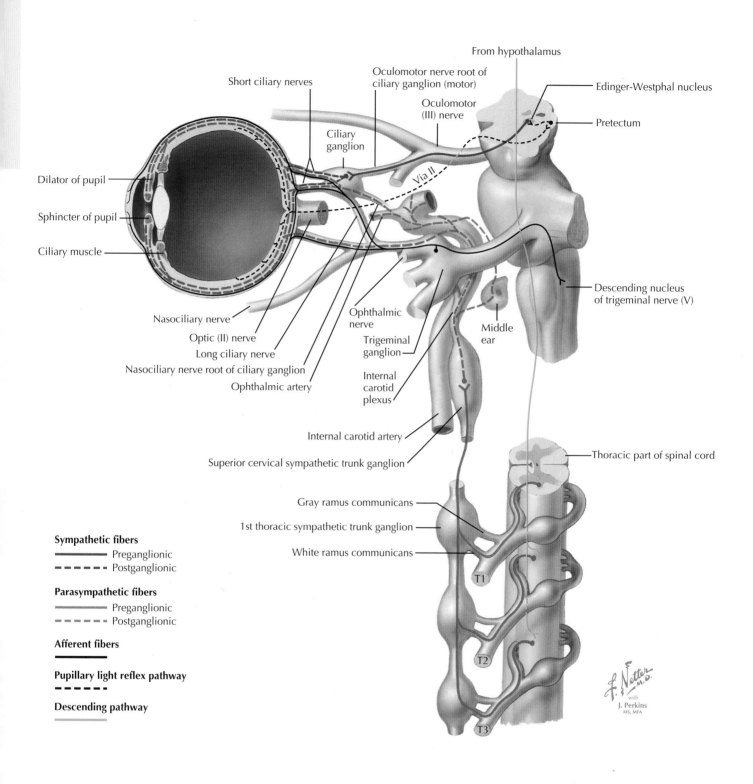

Short ciliary nerves

Oculomotor nerve root of
ciliary ganglion (motor)

From hypothalamus

Edinger-Westphal nucleus

Oculomotor
(III) nerve

Pretectum

Ciliary
ganglion

Dilator of pupil

Via II

Sphincter of pupil

Ciliary muscle

Descending nucleus
of trigeminal nerve (V)

Nasociliary nerve

Ophthalmic
nerve

Optic (II) nerve

Middle
ear

Long ciliary nerve

Trigeminal
ganglion

Nasociliary nerve root of ciliary ganglion

Ophthalmic artery

Internal
carotid
plexus

Internal carotid artery

Superior cervical sympathetic trunk ganglion

Thoracic part of spinal cord

Gray ramus communicans

1st thoracic sympathetic trunk ganglion

White ramus communicans

T1

T2

T3

Sympathetic fibers
——— Preganglionic
– – – – – Postganglionic

Parasympathetic fibers
——— Preganglionic
– – – – – Postganglionic

Afferent fibers
———

Pupillary light reflex pathway
– – – –

Descending pathway
———

9.45 AUTONOMIC DISTRIBUTION TO THE EYE

Parasympathetic preganglionic nerve fibers from the Edinger-Westphal nucleus innervate the ciliary ganglion, which supplies the ciliary muscle (aiding in accommodation to near vision) and the pupillary constrictor muscle (constricting the pupil). Sympathetic preganglionic nerve fibers from the T1–T2 intermediolateral cell column innervate the superior cervical ganglion, which supplies the dilator muscle of the pupil. The pupillary light reflex is a major reflex in neurological testing. The afferent limb is activated by light shone in either eye via CN II and processed through the pretectum to the Edinger-Westphal nucleus on both sides (via the posterior commissure); the efferent limb consists of autonomic parasympathetic outflow to the pupillary constrictor muscles of both sides.

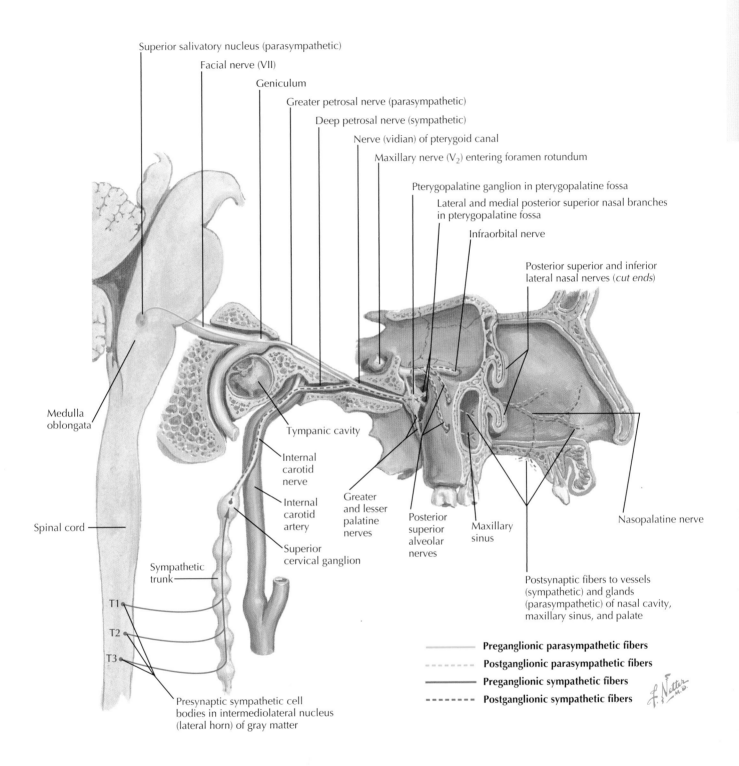

Superior salivatory nucleus (parasympathetic)

Facial nerve (VII)

Geniculum

Greater petrosal nerve (parasympathetic)

Deep petrosal nerve (sympathetic)

Nerve (vidian) of pterygoid canal

Maxillary nerve (V₂) entering foramen rotundum

Pterygopalatine ganglion in pterygopalatine fossa

Lateral and medial posterior superior nasal branches in pterygopalatine fossa

Infraorbital nerve

Posterior superior and inferior lateral nasal nerves (*cut ends*)

Medulla oblongata

Tympanic cavity

Internal carotid nerve

Internal carotid artery

Greater and lesser palatine nerves

Posterior superior alveolar nerves

Maxillary sinus

Nasopalatine nerve

Spinal cord

Sympathetic trunk

Superior cervical ganglion

Postsynaptic fibers to vessels (sympathetic) and glands (parasympathetic) of nasal cavity, maxillary sinus, and palate

T1

T2

T3

Presynaptic sympathetic cell bodies in intermediolateral nucleus (lateral horn) of gray matter

——————— **Preganglionic parasympathetic fibers**

- - - - - - - **Postganglionic parasympathetic fibers**

——————— **Preganglionic sympathetic fibers**

- - - - - - - **Postganglionic sympathetic fibers**

9.46 AUTONOMIC INNERVATION OF THE NASAL CAVITY

Parasympathetic preganglionic neurons in the superior salivatory nucleus innervate the pterygopalatine ganglion. Sympathetic preganglionic neurons from the T1–T2 intermediolateral cell column innervate the SCG. The pterygopalatine ganglion supplies secretory glands, and the SCG supplies blood vessels with postganglionic nerve fibers in the nasal cavity, maxillary sinus, and palate.

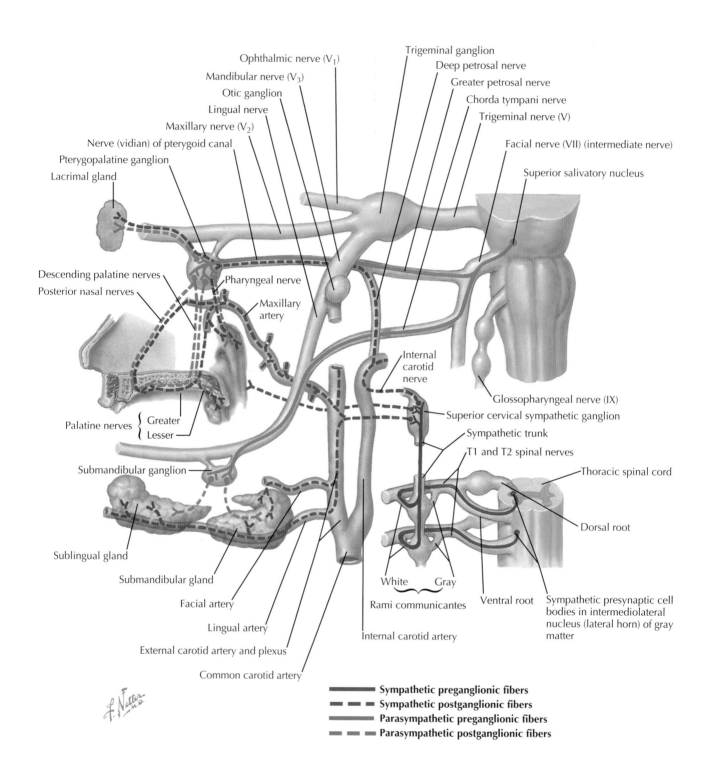

Ophthalmic nerve (V₁)

Mandibular nerve (V₃)

Otic ganglion

Lingual nerve

Maxillary nerve (V₂)

Nerve (vidian) of pterygoid canal

Pterygopalatine ganglion

Lacrimal gland

Trigeminal ganglion

Deep petrosal nerve

Greater petrosal nerve

Chorda tympani nerve

Trigeminal nerve (V)

Facial nerve (VII) (intermediate nerve)

Superior salivatory nucleus

Descending palatine nerves

Posterior nasal nerves

Pharyngeal nerve

Maxillary artery

Internal carotid nerve

Glossopharyngeal nerve (IX)

Superior cervical sympathetic ganglion

Sympathetic trunk

T1 and T2 spinal nerves

Thoracic spinal cord

Palatine nerves { Greater / Lesser

Submandibular ganglion

Sublingual gland

Submandibular gland

Facial artery

Lingual artery

External carotid artery and plexus

Common carotid artery

White   Gray

Rami communicantes

Internal carotid artery

Ventral root

Dorsal root

Sympathetic presynaptic cell bodies in intermediolateral nucleus (lateral horn) of gray matter

━━━━ **Sympathetic preganglionic fibers**
╍ ╍ ╍ **Sympathetic postganglionic fibers**
━━━━ **Parasympathetic preganglionic fibers**
╍ ╍ ╍ **Parasympathetic postganglionic fibers**

9.47 SCHEMATIC OF THE PTERYGOPALATINE AND SUBMANDIBULAR GANGLIA

The pterygopalatine and submandibular ganglia, innervated by the superior salivatory nucleus via CN VII, supply the lacrimal glands and nasal mucosal glands as well as the submandibular and sublingual salivary glands, respectively, with postganglionic parasympathetic cholinergic nerve fibers.

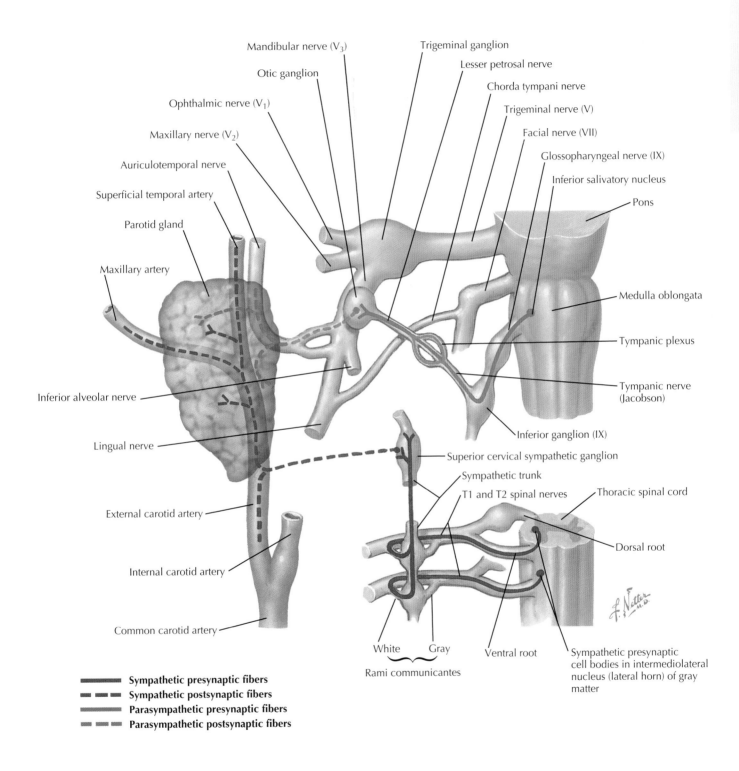

Mandibular nerve (V$_3$)
Otic ganglion
Ophthalmic nerve (V$_1$)
Maxillary nerve (V$_2$)
Auriculotemporal nerve
Superficial temporal artery
Parotid gland
Maxillary artery
Inferior alveolar nerve
Lingual nerve
External carotid artery
Internal carotid artery
Common carotid artery

Trigeminal ganglion
Lesser petrosal nerve
Chorda tympani nerve
Trigeminal nerve (V)
Facial nerve (VII)
Glossopharyngeal nerve (IX)
Inferior salivatory nucleus
Pons
Medulla oblongata
Tympanic plexus
Tympanic nerve (Jacobson)
Inferior ganglion (IX)
Superior cervical sympathetic ganglion
Sympathetic trunk
T1 and T2 spinal nerves
Thoracic spinal cord
Dorsal root
White   Gray
Rami communicantes
Ventral root
Sympathetic presynaptic cell bodies in intermediolateral nucleus (lateral horn) of gray matter

Sympathetic presynaptic fibers
Sympathetic postsynaptic fibers
Parasympathetic presynaptic fibers
Parasympathetic postsynaptic fibers

9.48 SCHEMATIC OF THE OTIC GANGLION

The otic ganglion, innervated by the inferior salivatory nucleus via CN IX, supplies the parotid salivary gland with postganglionic parasympathetic cholinergic nerve fibers.

Internal carotid nerve

Cervical sympathetic trunk ganglia

Cervical cardiac nerves

Gray ramus communicans

Brachial plexus

White ramus communicans

Upper thoracic sympathetic trunk ganglia

Thoracic sympathetic cardiac and aortic nerves

Intercostal nerves

Lower thoracic sympathetic trunk ganglia

Thoracic splanchnic nerves

Upper lumbar sympathetic trunk ganglia

Fibers direct to vessels

Lower lumbar and sacral sympathetic trunk ganglia

Sympathetic rami to lumbar and sacral plexuses and nerves to lower limb

Sympathetic fibers

——— preganglionic

- - - - postganglionic

9.49 INNERVATION OF THE LIMBS

Autonomic innervation to the limbs derives from the SNS. Preganglionic sympathetic nerve fibers from the thoracolumbar intermediolateral cell column supply sympathetic chain ganglia. These ganglia send postganglionic noradrenergic nerve fibers through the gray rami communicantes into the peripheral nerves to supply vascular smooth muscle (vasomotor fibers), sweat glands (sudomotor fibers), and arrector pili muscles associated with hair follicles (pilomotor fibers). Smooth muscle fibers of blood vessels in the viscera also are supplied with postganglionic sympathetic nerve fibers.

Cervicothoracic (stellate) ganglion

Ansa subclavia

Right sympathetic trunk

Cervical cardiac nerves (sympathetic and vagal)

Thoracic sympathetic cardiac nerves

Right vagus nerve (*cut*)

Thoracic vagal branches to pulmonary and cardiac plexuses

5th intercostal nerve (anterior ramus of 5th thoracic spinal nerve)

Gray and white rami communicantes

5th thoracic sympathetic trunk ganglion

Right greater thoracic splanchnic nerve

Sympathetic branch to esophageal plexus

Thoracic duct

Thoracic aortic plexus

Right lesser thoracic splanchnic nerve

Right lowest thoracic splanchnic nerve

Diaphragm (*pulled down*)

Azygos vein (*cut*)

Inferior vena cava (*cut*)

Cervicothoracic (stellate) ganglion

Cervical cardiac nerves (sympathetic and vagal)

Left vagus nerve (*cut*)

Left recurrent laryngeal nerve

Thoracic cardiac nerves (sympathetic and vagal)

Branches to anterior and posterior pulmonary plexuses

Cardiac plexus

Left sympathetic trunk

Thoracic aorta plexus

Esophageal plexus

Left greater thoracic splanchnic nerve

Left lesser thoracic splanchnic nerve

Anterior vagal trunk

Diaphragm (*pulled down*)

9.50 THORACIC SYMPATHETIC CHAIN AND SPLANCHNIC NERVES

The sympathetic chain is a collection of sympathetic ganglia that receive input from the thoracolumbar preganglionic nerve fibers derived from the spinal cord. The ganglia, interconnected by nerve trunks, are located in a paravertebral array from the neck to the coccygeal region. Postganglionic noradrenergic nerve fibers from the sympathetic chain supply effector tissue in the periphery. Some preganglionic nerve fibers do not synapse as they travel through the sympathetic chain. They continue along the splanchnic nerves to synapse in collateral ganglia, which supply noradrenergic innervation to effector tissue in the viscera.

CLINICAL POINT

The sympathetic chain (paravertebral ganglia) extends from the neck to the pelvis, whereas collateral (prevertebral) ganglia are present along the great vessels and distribute to internal target organs. These ganglia are supplied by preganglionic cholinergic fibers from the T1–L2 intermediolateral cell column (lateral horn), the chain ganglia via white rami communicantes, and the collateral ganglia via splanchnic nerves. A spinal cord crush injury above the T1 level damages the central regulation of the sympathetic preganglionic neurons and the parasympathetic S2–S4 preganglionic neurons. Initially the patient experiences a spinal shock syndrome, with hypotension (worse on standing), loss of sweating, loss of piloerection, paralysis of bladder function (neurogenic bladder), gastric dilatation, and paralytic ileus. As the process of spinal cord injury resolves to a permanent state and spinal shock recedes, the autonomic equivalent of spasticity (hyper-responsiveness) may result, accompanied by spikes in blood pressure and a spastic bladder.

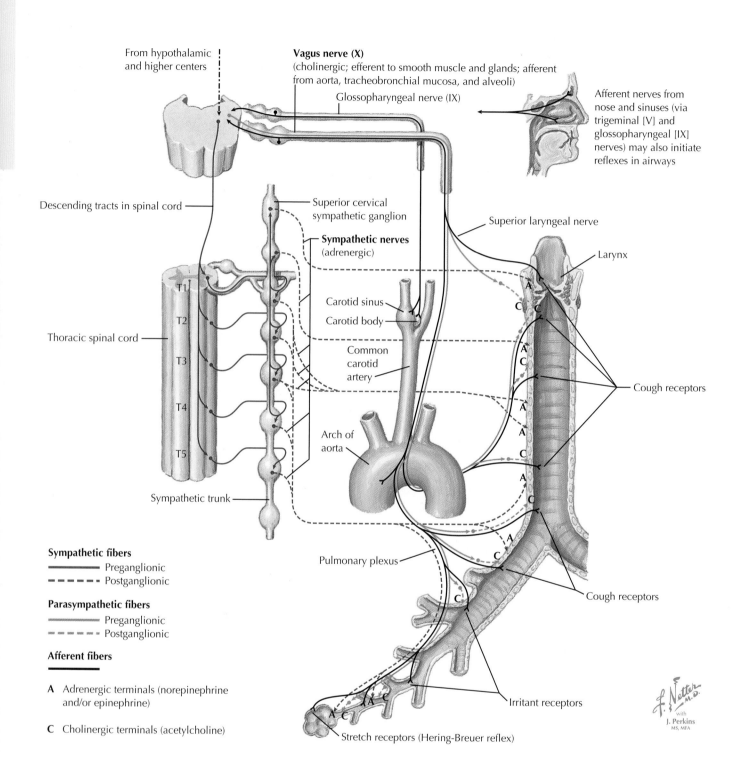

From hypothalamic and higher centers

Vagus nerve (X)
(cholinergic; efferent to smooth muscle and glands; afferent from aorta, tracheobronchial mucosa, and alveoli)

Glossopharyngeal nerve (IX)

Afferent nerves from nose and sinuses (via trigeminal [V] and glossopharyngeal [IX] nerves) may also initiate reflexes in airways

Descending tracts in spinal cord

Superior cervical sympathetic ganglion

Sympathetic nerves
(adrenergic)

Superior laryngeal nerve

Larynx

Thoracic spinal cord

T1
T2
T3
T4
T5

Carotid sinus

Carotid body

Common carotid artery

Cough receptors

Arch of aorta

Sympathetic trunk

Sympathetic fibers
——————— Preganglionic
- - - - - - - Postganglionic

Parasympathetic fibers
——————— Preganglionic
- - - - - - - Postganglionic

Afferent fibers

A Adrenergic terminals (norepinephrine and/or epinephrine)

C Cholinergic terminals (acetylcholine)

Pulmonary plexus

Cough receptors

Irritant receptors

Stretch receptors (Hering-Breuer reflex)

9.51 INNERVATION OF THE TRACHEOBRONCHIAL TREE

Both sympathetic (noradrenergic) and parasympathetic (cholinergic) innervation supplies smooth muscle of the tracheobronchial tree. Sympathetics derive from the sympathetic chain, and parasympathetics derive from vagal autonomic input to local intramural ganglia. Sympathetic influences result in bronchodilation and parasympathetic influences result in bronchoconstriction. Some medications for asthma use a sympathomimetic compound; others use a parasympathetic blocker. Additional neuropeptidergic innervation, some as colocalized or independent autonomic fibers and some as primary afferent fibers, also distributes along the epithelium and among the alveoli, where it can influence innate immune reactivity and the production of inflammatory mediators.

Dorsal vagal nucleus Solitary tract nucleus

Superior cervical sympathetic trunk ganglion

Superior cervical sympathetic cardiac nerve

Middle cervical sympathetic trunk ganglion

Middle cervical sympathetic cardiac nerve

Vertebral ganglion

Ansa subclavia

Cervicothoracic (stellate) ganglion

Ventral ramus of T1 (intercostal nerve)

Inferior cervical sympathetic cardiac nerve

2nd thoracic sympathetic trunk ganglion

Thoracic vagal cardiac branch

White rami communicantes

4th thoracic sympathetic trunk ganglion

Medulla oblongata

Vagus nerves

Superior cervical vagal cardiac branches

Inferior cervical vagal cardiac branches

Ascending connections

T1

T2

T3

T4

Gray ramus communicans

Thoracic sympathetic cardiac nerves

Cardiac plexus

Sympathetic fibers
——— Preganglionic
- - - - - Postganglionic

Afferent fibers
————

Parasympathetic fibers
——— Preganglionic
- - - - - Postganglionic

Afferent fibers
————

9.52 INNERVATION OF THE HEART

Sympathetic noradrenergic nerve fibers (derived from chain ganglia) and parasympathetic cholinergic nerve fibers (derived from cardiac intramural ganglia innervated by the vagus nerve) supply the atria, ventricles, sinoatrial node, and atrioventricular node and bundle. Sympathetic noradrenergic nerve fibers also distribute along the great vessels and the coronary arteries. Sympathetic fibers increase the force and rate of cardiac contraction, increase cardiac output, and dilate the coronary arteries. Parasympathetic fibers decrease the force and rate of cardiac contraction and decrease cardiac output.

CLINICAL POINT
Both sympathetic noradrenergic and parasympathetic cholinergic vagal postganglionic fibers innervate the heart. Cardiovascular autonomic

neuropathies sometimes occur in diabetes and other disorders. Vagal nerve damage can result in sustained tachycardia; excessive vagal activity can provoke bradycardia, atrial fibrillation or flutter, ventricular fibrillation, or paroxysmal tachycardia. Loss of sympathetic innervation of the heart results in severe exercise intolerance, painless myocardial ischemia, cardiomyopathy, and possibly sudden death. In studies of cardiac failure, the increased reflex drive on sympathetic cardiac nerves in an attempt to increase cardiac output results in accelerated release of norepinephrine, which produces highly toxic oxidative metabolites (free radicals) that are taken up by the noradrenergic nerve endings (through the high-affinity uptake carriers) and produce a dying-back sympathetic neuropathy, leaving the heart further denervated. In experimental models in dogs, either a norepinephrine-specific uptake inhibitor (desmethylimipramine) or potent antioxidants (vitamins C and E) can prevent this free-radical autodestructive process.

Right sympathetic trunk

Thoracic duct

Right greater and lesser thoracic splanchnic nerves

Right phrenic nerve

Right inferior phrenic artery and plexus

Right greater and lesser thoracic splanchnic nerves

Right adrenal plexus

Right aorticorenal ganglion

Right lowest thoracic splanchnic nerve

Right renal artery and plexus

Right sympathetic trunk

Gray and white rami communicantes

Cisterna chyli

3rd lumbar sympathetic trunk ganglion

Gray ramus communicans

Lumbar splanchnic nerves

Right ureter and plexus

Right testicular artery and plexus

Sacral part of right sympathetic trunk

Anterior and posterior vagal trunks

Celiac plexus and ganglia

Left greater and lesser thoracic spanchnic nerves

Superior mesenteric ganglion

Left aorticorenal ganglion

Left lowest thoracic splanchnic nerve

Left sympathetic trunk

Intermesenteric (abdominal aortic) plexus

Inferior mesenteric ganglion

Inferior mesenteric artery and plexus

Left colic artery and plexus

Left common iliac artery and plexus

Superior rectal artery and plexus

Superior hypogastric plexus (presacral nerve)

Hypogastric nerves to right and left inferior hypogastric (pelvic) plexuses

Left sacral plexus

9.53 ABDOMINAL NERVES AND GANGLIA

Abundant sympathetic nerves are present in the abdomen and pelvis and are associated with innervation of the gastrointestinal and urogenital systems, associated vessels, the peritoneum, and the adrenal gland. The lumbar portion of the sympathetic chain and its branches and the splanchnic nerves and their collateral ganglia (celiac, superior and inferior mesenteric, hepatic, aorticorenal, adrenal, superior hypogastric, and others) innervate smooth muscle, glands, lymphoid tissue, and metabolic cells in the abdomen and pelvis. Most of the collateral ganglia (plexuses) also contain parasympathetic contributions from the vagus nerve and associated ganglia.

CLINICAL POINT

The collateral ganglia (celiac, superior and inferior mesenteric, hepatic, aorticorenal, adrenal, superior hypogastric) and the lumbar sympathetic chain supply sympathetic innervation to the abdomen and pelvis. Parasympathetic vagal fibers and their associated intramural ganglia provide parasympathetic innervation. The importance of this innervation is illustrated by the relatively unusual disorder known as dysautonomic polyneuropathy, which is a postganglionic polyneuropathy of both sympathetic and parasympathetic nerves, most likely the result of autoimmune reactivity. The affected individual develops orthostatic hypotension, unresponsive pupillary light reflexes, paralytic ileus and constipation, bladder dysfunction, and diminished sweating, peripheral vasoconstriction, and piloerection.

Anterior view

Esophagus

Recurrent laryngeal nerves

Right recurrent laryngeal nerve

Ansa subclavia

3rd intercostal nerve

Gray and white rami communicantes

3rd thoracic sympathetic ganglion

Thoracic sympathetic trunk

Right greater splanchnic nerve

Sympathetic fibers along left inferior phrenic artery

Branch of posterior vagal trunk to celiac plexus

Greater splanchnic nerve

Sympathetic fibers along esophageal branch of left gastric artery

Celiac plexus and ganglia

Superior ganglion of vagus nerve

Superior cervical sympathetic ganglion

Inferior ganglion of vagus nerve

Pharyngeal branch of vagus nerve

Vagus nerve (X)

Superior laryngeal nerve

Cervical sympathetic trunk

Middle cervical sympathetic ganglion

Cervical (sympathetic and vagal) cardiac nerves

Vertebral ganglion of cervical sympathetic trunk

Ansa subclavia

Branch to esophagus and recurrent nerve from stellate ganglion

Cervicothoracic (stellate) ganglion

Left recurrent laryngeal nerve

Thoracic (vagal and sympathetic) cardiac branches

Cardiac plexus

Pulmonary plexuses

Esophageal plexus (anterior portion)

Branches to esophageal plexus from sympathetic trunk, greater splanchnic nerve and thoracic aortic plexus

Left greater splanchnic nerve

Anterior vagal trunk

Vagal branch to hepatic plexus via lesser omentum

Principal anterior vagal branch to lesser curvature of stomach

Vagal branch to fundus and body of stomach

Posterior view

Esophageal plexus (posterior portion)

Posterior vagal trunk

Vagal branch to celiac plexus

Posterior vagal branch to lesser curvature

Vagal branch to fundus and cardiac part of stomach

9.54 NERVES OF THE ESOPHAGUS

The sensory stimuli that initiate swallowing derive mainly from CN IX (some also from CNs V and X) and are mediated through nucleus solitarius in the medulla. Food passes through the cricopharyngeal sphincter at the proximal esophagus; this sphincter is controlled by the vagal nerve fibers derived from the dorsal motor nucleus of CN X. Movement of food through the esophagus is regulated by vagal nerve fibers derived from the dorsal motor nucleus of CN X, which synapse on neurons within the myenteric plexus of the esophagus. This plexus directly controls peristalsis through the esophagus by alternately relaxing and then contracting the muscles of the esophagus. Food then moves into the stomach through the lower esophageal sphincter, which relaxes when nitric oxide and VIP are released from some neurons of the myenteric plexus.

Right 6th thoracic sympathetic trunk ganglion

7th intercostal nerve

White and gray rami communicantes

Spinal ganglion and ventral root of 8th thoracic spinal nerve

Right greater and lesser thoracic splanchnic nerves

Celiac ganglia and plexus

Celiac trunk

Right lowest thoracic splanchnic nerve

Common hepatic artery

Right gastric artery

Superior mesenteric ganglion

Aorticorenal ganglia

Renal artery

Left 7th thoracic sympathetic trunk ganglion

Esophageal plexus

Aortic plexus

Left greater thoracic splanchnic nerve

Posterior vagal trunk and celiac branch

Anterior vagal trunk and celiac branch

Left gastric artery

Splenic artery

Short gastric arteries

Left gastroepiploic artery

Gastroduodenal artery

Right gastroepiploic artery

Superior mesenteric artery

Inferior pancreaticoduodenal artery

Sympathetic fibers	Parasympathetic fibers	
—— Preganglionic	—— Preganglionic	**——— Afferent fibers**
- - - Postganglionic	- - - Postganglionic	

9.55 INNERVATION OF THE STOMACH AND PROXIMAL DUODENUM

The stomach and proximal duodenum receive abundant sympathetic innervation from the celiac and superior mesenteric ganglia and, to a lesser extent, from the thoracic sympathetic trunk ganglia. The celiac and superior mesenteric ganglia receive their preganglionic input from the greater and lesser thoracic splanchnic nerves. Parasympathetic fibers distribute to the stomach and proximal duodenum from the celiac branches of the vagus nerve. Sympathetic fibers decrease peristalsis and secretomotor activities. Parasympathetic fibers increase peristalsis and secretomotor activity (such as gastrin and hydrochloric acid) and relax associated sphincters.

CLINICAL POINT
Diabetic neuropathy may be accompanied by delayed gastric emptying. The patient may experience nausea and vomiting, premature satiety, and large fluctuations in blood glucose. Weight loss may be noted. Approaches for treatment include parasympathetic agonists that stimulate gastric emptying and dopamine antagonists that remove the dopaminergic inhibition of gastric emptying. Delayed gastric emptying may also be accompanied by dysfunction of esophageal motility, resulting in dysphagia.

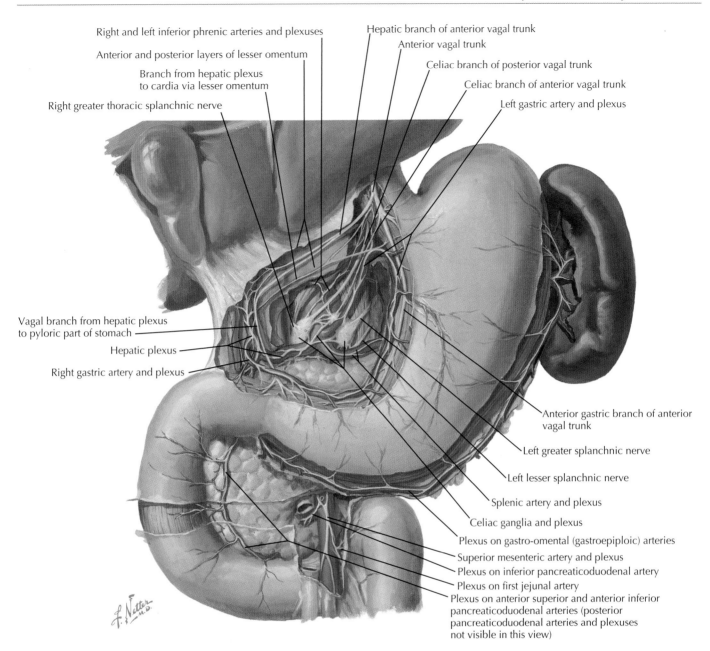

Right and left inferior phrenic arteries and plexuses

Anterior and posterior layers of lesser omentum

Branch from hepatic plexus
to cardia via lesser omentum

Right greater thoracic splanchnic nerve

Hepatic branch of anterior vagal trunk

Anterior vagal trunk

Celiac branch of posterior vagal trunk

Celiac branch of anterior vagal trunk

Left gastric artery and plexus

Vagal branch from hepatic plexus
to pyloric part of stomach

Hepatic plexus

Right gastric artery and plexus

Anterior gastric branch of anterior
vagal trunk

Left greater splanchnic nerve

Left lesser splanchnic nerve

Splenic artery and plexus

Celiac ganglia and plexus

Plexus on gastro-omental (gastroepiploic) arteries

Superior mesenteric artery and plexus

Plexus on inferior pancreaticoduodenal artery

Plexus on first jejunal artery

Plexus on anterior superior and anterior inferior
pancreaticoduodenal arteries (posterior
pancreaticoduodenal arteries and plexuses
not visible in this view)

F. Netter
M.D.

9.56 NERVES OF THE STOMACH AND DUODENUM

Parasympathetic and sympathetic nerve fibers distribute to the stomach and proximal duodenum through specific splanchnic nerves and branches of the vagus nerve. Sympathetic fibers decrease peristalsis and secretomotor activities. Parasympathetic fibers increase peristalsis and secretomotor activity (such as gastrin and hydrochloric acid) and relax associated sphincters.

CLINICAL POINT

Obesity may occur for a variety of reasons. The stomach expands, neural satiety signals do not provide effective feedback to the brain, and compulsive eating can overcome normal appetitive control mechanisms. In situations in which diet and exercise are ineffective for weight control and when diabetes and other serious comorbidities are life-threatening for a morbidly obese individual, bariatric surgery is an option. The Roux-en-Y gastric bypass procedure takes the distal 90% of the stomach, the duodenum, and approximately 20 cm of the proximal jejunum off-line; the digestive tract then consists of the esophagus and a very small proximal stomach pouch that is connected with the remaining jejunum (the off-line jejunum is anastomosed farther downstream). This procedure markedly reduces the stomach's capacity, slows gastric emptying, and produces deliberate partial malabsorption. Long-term data indicate extensive and permanent weight loss in many subjects (more than 70% of needed weight loss) and common reversal of diabetes, hypertension, sleep apnea, and many of the comorbid conditions that accompany morbid obesity. In addition, a striking alteration in the secretion of a variety of gastrointestinal hormones, inflammatory mediators, and other mediators has been noted. Autonomic and somatic neural signals are altered, central set-points related to appetitive behavior are reset, and changes in morbidity and mortality rates have been observed. The Roux-en-Y procedure is not without risks and complications, and chronic supplementation of nutrients such as calcium, iron, and B vitamins is required. Underlying psychopathology may lead to circumvention of the effectiveness of the procedure.

9.57 INNERVATION OF THE SMALL AND LARGE INTESTINES

Autonomic innervation of the small and large intestines is supplied by extrinsic sympathetic and parasympathetic fibers. Sympathetic innervation derives from the T5–L2 intermediolateral cell column of the spinal cord and distributes to collateral ganglia (superior and inferior mesenteric, celiac). Parasympathetic innervation derives from the vagus nerve and from the S2–S4 intermediate gray of the spinal cord; it distributes to intramural ganglia and plexuses via CN X and pelvis splanchnic nerves. Sympathetic nerve fibers generally decrease peristalsis and secretomotor functions (i.e., decreased fluid secretion). Parasympathetic nerve fibers generally increase peristalsis, relax involuntary sphincters, and increase secretomotor activities. The extrinsic innervation of the intestines is integrated with the intrinsic (enteric) innervation. Autonomic gastrointestinal neuropathies such as those seen in diabetes most commonly result in constipation, requiring treatment with pharmacological agents and high-fiber agents. However, diabetic diarrhea also is common and may require treatment to slow secretomotor function.

Recurrent branch of left inferior phrenic artery and plexus to esophagus

Anterior vagal trunk

Posterior vagal trunk

Hepatic branch of anterior vagal trunk (courses in lesser omentum, *removed here*)

Celiac branches of anterior and posterior vagal trunks

Inferior phrenic arteries and plexuses

Left gastric artery and plexus

Hepatic plexus

Greater splanchnic nerves

Right gastric artery and plexus (*cut*)

Celiac ganglia and plexus

Gastroduodenal artery and plexus

Lesser splanchnic nerves

Least splanchnic nerves

Aorticorenal ganglia

Superior mesenteric ganglion

Intermesenteric (aortic) plexus

Inferior pancreaticoduodenal arteries and plexuses

Superior mesenteric artery and plexus

Middle colic artery and plexus (*cut*)

Right colic artery and plexus

Ileocolic artery and plexus

Superior mesenteric artery and plexus

Peritoneum (*cut edge*)

Mesenteric branches

Mesoappendix (contains appendicular artery and nerve plexus)

9.58 NERVES OF THE SMALL INTESTINE

This figure shows the anatomy of the extrinsic innervation of the small intestine by the splanchnic and vagal nerves and their associated plexuses.

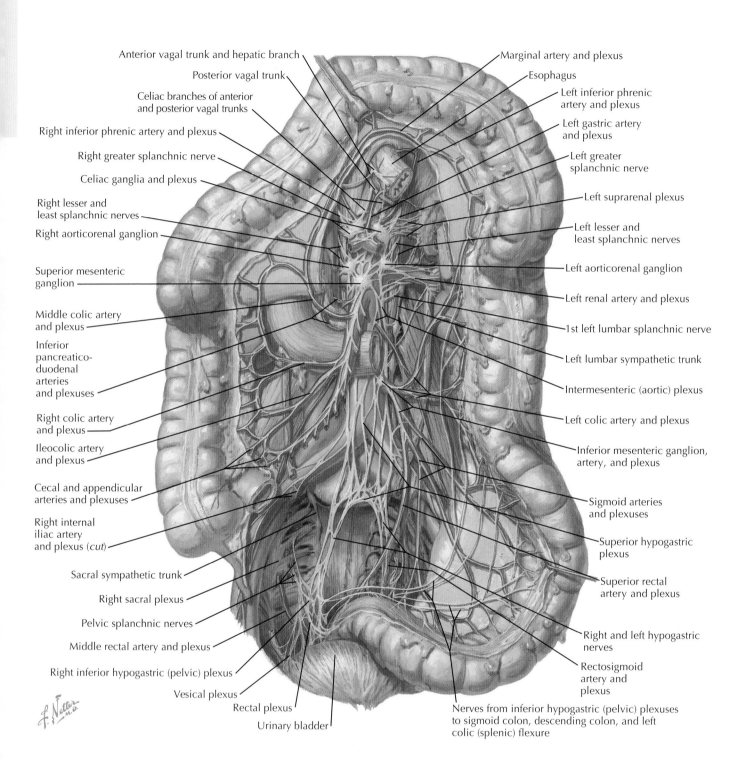

Anterior vagal trunk and hepatic branch

Posterior vagal trunk

Celiac branches of anterior and posterior vagal trunks

Right inferior phrenic artery and plexus

Right greater splanchnic nerve

Celiac ganglia and plexus

Right lesser and least splanchnic nerves

Right aorticorenal ganglion

Superior mesenteric ganglion

Middle colic artery and plexus

Inferior pancreatico-duodenal arteries and plexuses

Right colic artery and plexus

Ileocolic artery and plexus

Cecal and appendicular arteries and plexuses

Right internal iliac artery and plexus (cut)

Sacral sympathetic trunk

Right sacral plexus

Pelvic splanchnic nerves

Middle rectal artery and plexus

Right inferior hypogastric (pelvic) plexus

Vesical plexus

Rectal plexus

Urinary bladder

Marginal artery and plexus

Esophagus

Left inferior phrenic artery and plexus

Left gastric artery and plexus

Left greater splanchnic nerve

Left suprarenal plexus

Left lesser and least splanchnic nerves

Left aorticorenal ganglion

Left renal artery and plexus

1st left lumbar splanchnic nerve

Left lumbar sympathetic trunk

Intermesenteric (aortic) plexus

Left colic artery and plexus

Inferior mesenteric ganglion, artery, and plexus

Sigmoid arteries and plexuses

Superior hypogastric plexus

Superior rectal artery and plexus

Right and left hypogastric nerves

Rectosigmoid artery and plexus

Nerves from inferior hypogastric (pelvic) plexuses to sigmoid colon, descending colon, and left colic (splenic) flexure

9.59 NERVES OF THE LARGE INTESTINE

This figure shows the anatomy of the extrinsic innervation of the large intestine by the splanchnic and vagal nerves and their associated plexuses.

Subserous plexus

Longitudinal intramuscular plexus

Myenteric (Auerbach's) plexus

Circular intramuscular plexus

Submucosal (Meissner's) plexus

Periglandular plexus

Lumen
Mucosa and mucosal glands
Muscularis mucosae
Glands
Submucosa
Circular muscle layer
Intermuscular stroma
Longitudinal muscle
Subserous connective tissue
Visceral peritoneum

Myenteric plexus lying on longitudinal muscular layer. Fine secondary bundles crossing meshes (duodenum of guinea pig, Champy-Coujard, osmic stain, × 20)

Group of multipolar neurons, type II, in ganglion of myenteric plexus (ileum of cat, Bielschowsky, silver stain, × 200)

Submucous plexus (ascending colon of guinea pig, stained by Golgi impregnation, × 20)

9.60 ENTERIC NERVOUS SYSTEM: LONGITUDINAL VIEW

The enteric nervous system is made up of approximately 100 million neurons arranged principally in submucosal (Meissner's) and myenteric (Auerbach's) plexuses; it provides intrinsic innervation to the small and large intestines. Neurons of this system interconnect with one another and with neuronal processes of the autonomic nervous system, although most neuronal components of this network are free of autonomic influence. The enteric plexuses regulate peristaltic responses (which can proceed without extrinsic innervation), pacemaker activity, and other automated secretory processes.

The myenteric plexus controls primarily motility; the submucosal plexus controls primarily fluid secretion and absorption. More than 20 distinct neurotransmitters have been identified in enteric neurons (e.g., ACh, substance P, serotonin, VIP, somatostatin, nitric oxide). ACh and substance P are excitatory to smooth muscle, whereas VIP and nitric oxide are inhibitory. Extrinsic autonomic innervation helps to coordinate these enteric plexuses and circuits; optimal functioning of the gastrointestinal tract requires coordinated interactions among endocrine, paracrine, and neurocrine mediators. Disturbance of extrinsic innervation by a neuropathy can result in disorders of motility such as constipation or diarrhea.

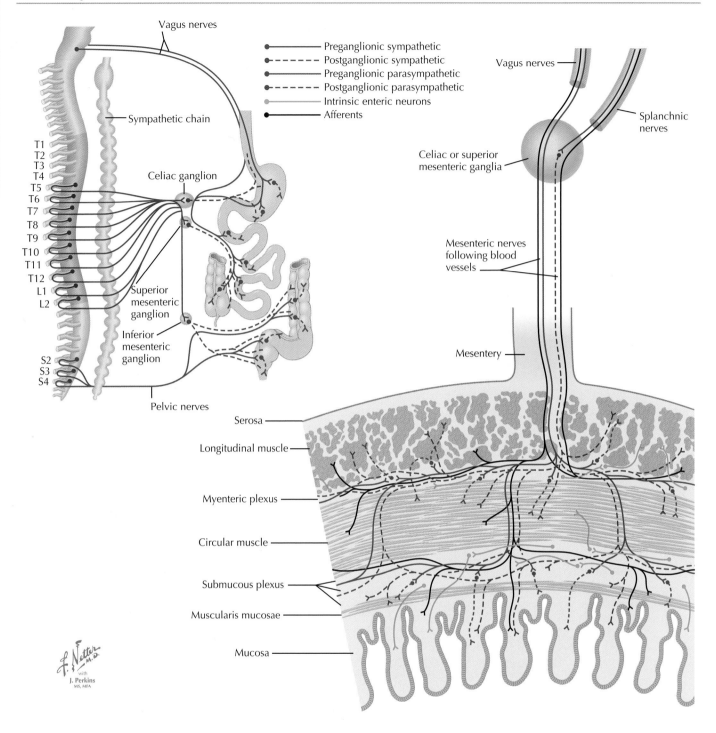

Vagus nerves

Preganglionic sympathetic
Postganglionic sympathetic
Preganglionic parasympathetic
Postganglionic parasympathetic
Intrinsic enteric neurons
Afferents

Sympathetic chain

Vagus nerves

Splanchnic nerves

Celiac ganglion

Celiac or superior mesenteric ganglia

T1
T2
T3
T4
T5
T6
T7
T8
T9
T10
T11
T12
L1
L2

Superior mesenteric ganglion

Mesenteric nerves following blood vessels

Inferior mesenteric ganglion

S2
S3
S4

Pelvic nerves

Mesentery

Serosa

Longitudinal muscle

Myenteric plexus

Circular muscle

Submucous plexus

Muscularis mucosae

Mucosa

9.61 ENTERIC NERVOUS SYSTEM: CROSS-SECTIONAL VIEW

In the myenteric and the submucosal plexuses, some neurons are innervated by sympathetic nerve fibers from the sympathetic chain and collateral ganglia and by vagal or pelvis splanchnic parasympathetic nerve fibers; other neurons are independent of autonomic regulation. Autonomic postganglionic nerve fibers and intrinsic neuropeptidergic nerve fibers also supply macrophages, T lymphocytes, plasma cells, and other cells of the immune system with innervation. This provides a regulatory network that modulates the host defenses of the gastrointestinal tract and the immune reactivity of gut-associated lymphoid tissue.

CLINICAL POINT

The intrinsic neuronal clusters that form the enteric nervous system derive from the neural crest. If these neural crest derivatives fail to migrate properly into the colon, as occurs in a developmental abnormality called Hirschsprung's disease (chronic megacolon), the intrinsic circuitry for peristalsis, pacemaker activity, and other gut functions cannot occur. The vagus nerve and sympathetic innervation from the pelvic splanchnic nerves cannot coordinate the activity of the colon in the absence of its enteric components. Therefore, megacolon (intestinal obstruction) results from absent peristalsis and loss of smooth muscle tone of the colon. Distention and hypertrophy of the colon may ensue.

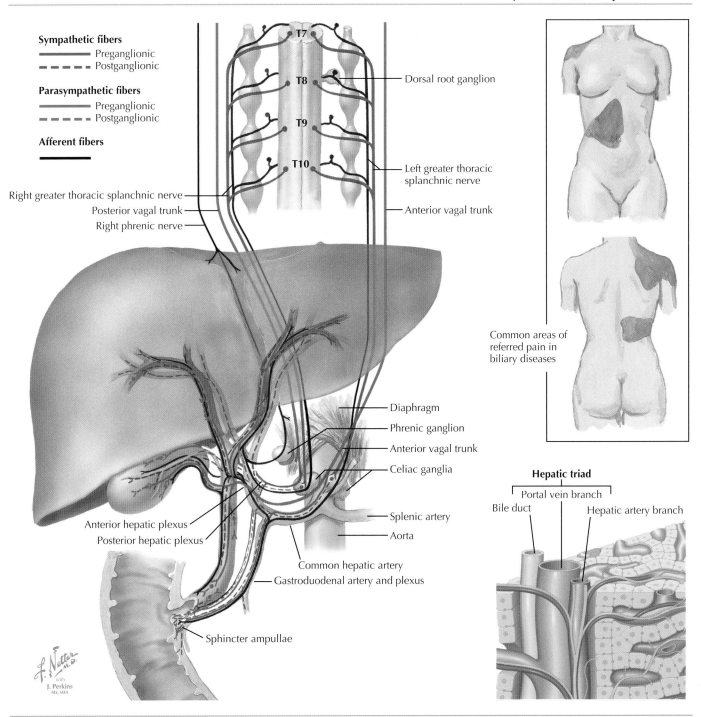

Sympathetic fibers
— Preganglionic
--- Postganglionic

Parasympathetic fibers
— Preganglionic
--- Postganglionic

Afferent fibers
—

T7
T8 — Dorsal root ganglion
T9
T10 — Left greater thoracic splanchnic nerve

Right greater thoracic splanchnic nerve
Posterior vagal trunk
Right phrenic nerve

Anterior vagal trunk

Diaphragm
Phrenic ganglion
Anterior vagal trunk
Celiac ganglia

Splenic artery
Aorta

Anterior hepatic plexus
Posterior hepatic plexus

Common hepatic artery
Gastroduodenal artery and plexus

Sphincter ampullae

Common areas of referred pain in biliary diseases

Hepatic triad
Portal vein branch
Bile duct
Hepatic artery branch

9.62 AUTONOMIC INNERVATION OF THE LIVER AND BILIARY TRACT

Sympathetic nerve fibers to the liver derive from T7–T10 of the spinal cord and distribute mainly via the celiac ganglion and its associated plexus. Parasympathetic nerve fibers to the liver derive from the abdominal vagus nerve. Postganglionic noradrenergic sympathetic nerve fibers end directly adjacent to hepatocytes; norepinephrine released from these nerve fibers initiates glycogenolysis and hyperglycemia for fight-or-flight responses and induces gluconeogenesis. Autonomic innervation helps to regulate vascular, secretory, and phagocytic processes in the liver. The gallbladder, especially the sphincter ampullae and the sphincter of the choledochal duct, is also supplied by autonomic nerve fibers. The sympathetic nerve fibers cause contraction of the sphincters and dilation of the gallbladder; the parasympathetic nerve fibers cause opening of the sphincters and contraction of the gallbladder.

CLINICAL POINT

Postganglionic sympathetic noradrenergic nerves to the liver can trigger glycogenolysis and gluconeogenesis, providing glucose as fuel for sympathetic arousal. Chronic activation of the SNS, with increased secretion of norepinephrine, can drive glucose levels, provoke insulin secretion, increase free-radical formation, increase platelet aggregation, and initiate other actions that are beneficial in an emergency but problematic when present chronically. These connections may be one route by which chronic stressors intersect with metabolic syndrome, diminish antiviral and antitumor immunity, and increase the risk for a variety of chronic diseases, including hypertension, cardiovascular disease and stroke, some cancers, and type II diabetes. Autonomic neuropathy to the gallbladder can result in atonic smooth muscle responses, with the development of gallstones (especially in individuals with hypercholesterolemia) and diarrhea.

Common areas of
pancreatic pain

Right symptomatic trunk

Right greater thoracic
splanchnic nerve

Posterior vagal trunk

Spinal sensory (dorsal root) ganglion

Left sympathetic trunk

Thoracic part of spinal cord

Left greater splanchnic nerve

Anterior vagal trunk

T5
T6
T7
T8
T9

Celiac ganglia

Splenic artery

Celiac trunk

Superior
mesenteric
ganglion

Superior mesenteric artery and plexus

Sympathetic fibers
Presynaptic
Postsynaptic

Parasympathetic fibers
Presynaptic
Postsynaptic

Afferent fibers

**Schema of intrinsic
nerve supply**

9.63 AUTONOMIC INNERVATION OF THE PANCREAS

Secretion by the pancreas is under both neural and endocrine control. Pancreatic exocrine glands and endocrine cells (islets of Langerhans) are innervated by parasympathetic subdiaphragmatic vagal nerve fibers via intramural ganglia and by sympathetic nerve fibers derived from T5–T9 intermediolateral spinal cord gray via the celiac ganglion. Although only a small anatomical component of the pancreas (1%), the endocrine pancreas secretes several vital endocrine products, including glucagon (a fuel-mobilizing hormone); insulin (a fuel-storing hormone); somatostatin (a suppressor of glucagons and insulin secretion); and pancreatic polypeptide (an inhibitor of the secretion of enzymes and HCO_3^-, the bicarbonate ion, by the exocrine pancreas). ACh supplied by the parasympathetic fibers stimulates insulin secretion by islet cells, and norepinephrine secretion by the sympathetic fibers (as well as epinephrine by the adrenal medulla) inhibits insulin secretion from the islet cells. ACh stimulates a variety of hormones. Secretin acts on ductal cells of the pancreas to stimulate secretion of fluid with a high HCO_3^- content. Cholecystokinin is secreted by I cells in response to fats in the duodenum and upper jejunum and acts on aciner cells to stimulate the secretion of enzymes.

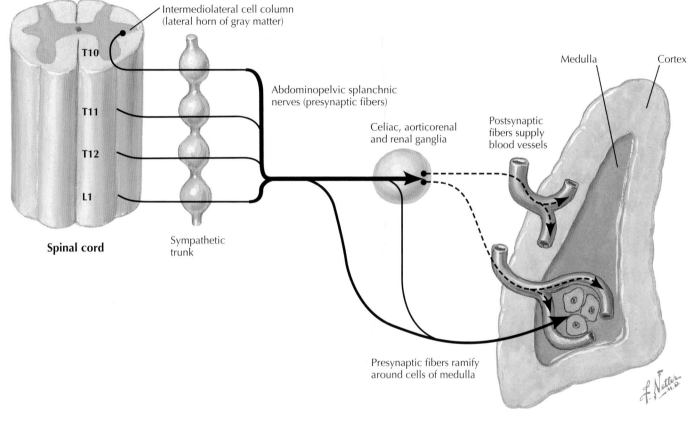

Intermediolateral cell column
(lateral horn of gray matter)

T10

T11

T12

L1

Spinal cord

Sympathetic trunk

Abdominopelvic splanchnic
nerves (presynaptic fibers)

Celiac, aorticorenal
and renal ganglia

Postsynaptic
fibers supply
blood vessels

Medulla

Cortex

Presynaptic fibers ramify
around cells of medulla

Suprarenal gland

9.64 SCHEMATIC OF INNERVATION OF THE ADRENAL GLAND

Sympathetic preganglionic nerve fibers from neurons in the T10–L1 intermediolateral cell column pass through the sympathetic chain, travel in splanchnic nerves, and directly innervate adrenal medullary chromaffin cells. These chromaffin cells are of neural crest origin and function as sympathetic ganglion cells.

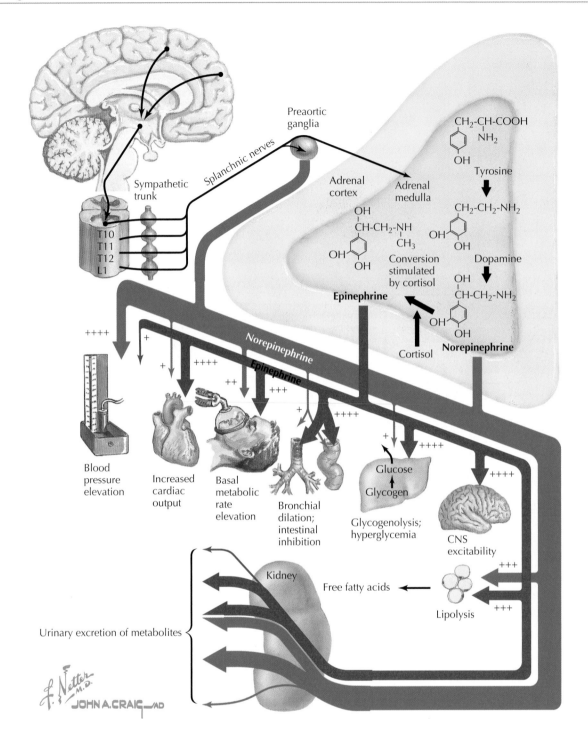

9.65 INNERVATION OF THE ADRENAL GLAND

The adrenal medullary chromaffin cells act as modified sympathetic ganglion cells, which are innervated by preganglionic sympathetic nerve fibers from T10 to L1 intermediolateral cells of the spinal cord. An adrenal portal system conveys blood directly from the adrenal cortex to the adrenal medulla. Cortisol, derived from action of the hypothalamo-pituitary-adrenal axis, bathes the chromaffin cells in very high concentrations, inducing the enzyme phenylethanolamine-N-methyl-transferase, which is responsible for the synthesis of epinephrine. Approximately 70% to 80% of the adrenal medullary output of catecholamines is epinephrine; the remaining output is norepinephrine. Both epinephrine and norepinephrine can be taken up into sympathetic postganglionic noradrenergic nerve terminals at any site throughout the body by the high-affinity uptake carrier and can be subsequently released. A sympathetic arousal response that generates the secretion of epinephrine from the adrenal medulla will therefore provide altered catecholamine content (higher epinephrine) because of high-affinity uptake in nerve terminals throughout the body; subsequent release of this epinephrine modifies the usual sympathetic balance of alpha versus beta receptor stimulation on target organs for a brief period.

Gray and white rami communicantes

L2

Right sympathetic trunk
and its 3rd lumbar ganglion

L3

Gray rami communicantes

L4

Right and left hypogastric nerves

1st sacral sympathetic trunk ganglion

Gray rami communicantes

L5

Sacral part of sympathetic trunk

S1

Sacral plexus

S2

S3

S4

S5

Pelvic splanchnic nerves
(sacral parasympathetic outflow)

Pudendal nerve

Right inferior hypogastric (pelvic) plexus

2nd lumbar sympathetic trunk ganglion

Intermesenteric (abdominal aortic) plexus

Inferior mesenteric ganglion

Lumbar splanchnic nerves

Inferior mesenteric artery and plexus

Superior hypogastric
plexus (presacral nerve)

Superior rectal artery and plexus

Nerves from inferior hypogastric
plexuses to sigmoid
and descending colon

Right ureter and ureteral plexus

Seminal vesicle

Ductus deferens

Vesical plexus

Inferior rectal plexus

Prostatic plexus

Cavernous plexus

Dorsal nerve of penis

9.66 AUTONOMIC PELVIC NERVES AND GANGLIA

Sympathetic nerve fibers supply the pelvis through the sympathetic trunk ganglia and the superior hypogastric plexus. These fibers travel along visceral and vascular nerves to the colon, ureters, and great vessels, such as the inferior mesenteric and common iliac vessels. Parasympathetic nerve fibers arise from the S2–S4 intermediate gray of the spinal cord and travel via the pelvic splanchnic nerves to distribute with the branches of the inferior hypogastric plexus. The parasympathetic ganglia are intramural, in or adjacent to the wall of the organ innervated.

CLINICAL POINT

The pelvic nerves and ganglia contain both sympathetic and parasympathetic components. The sympathetic trunk ganglia and superior hypogastric plexus distribute sympathetic nerve fibers to pelvic viscera, and S2–S4 intermediate gray neurons send pelvic splanchnic nerves via the inferior hypogastric plexuses to end in intramural ganglia that supply the pelvic viscera. Of particular functional importance is the autonomic distribution to the bladder and reproductive organs. Lesions in these pelvic autonomic nerves can occur with diabetes, demyelinating diseases, and mass lesions. Damage to pelvic parasympathetic nerves can produce a flaccid bladder with overflow incontinence and can cause erectile impotence in males. It should be noted that both parasympathetic and sympathetic autonomic nerves play roles in sexual function. Parasympathetic nerves are essential for proper erectile function, and sympathetic nerves play a role in ejaculation and may also contribute to erectile function; beta-adrenergic blockers sometimes have the side effect of erectile impotence.

Anterior vagal trunk

Posterior vagal trunk

Greater splanchnic nerve

Celiac ganglia and plexus

Lesser splanchnic nerve

Superior mesenteric ganglion

Least splanchnic nerve

Aorticorenal ganglion

Renal plexus and ganglion

2nd lumbar splanchnic nerve

Renal and upper ureteric branches from intermesenteric plexus

Intermesenteric (aortic) plexus

Testicular (ovarian) artery and plexus

Inferior mesenteric ganglion

Sympathetic trunk and ganglion

Middle ureteric branch

Superior hypogastric plexus

Sacral splanchnic nerves (branches from upper sacral sympathetic ganglia to hypogastric plexus)

Gray ramus communicans

Hypogastric nerves

Sacral plexus

Pudendal nerve

Pelvic splanchnic nerves

Inferior hypogastric (pelvic) plexus with periureteric loops and branches to lower ureter

Rectal plexus

Vesical plexus

Prostatic plexus

9.67 NERVES OF THE KIDNEYS, URETERS, AND URINARY BLADDER

This schematic demonstrates the nerves that distribute to the kidneys, ureters, and urinary bladder.

Sympathetic fibers
—————— Preganglionic
- - - - - Postganglionic

Parasympathetic fibers
—————— Preganglionic
- - - - - Postganglionic

Afferent fibers
——————

Solitary tract nucleus

Gray ramus communicans

White ramus communicans

Ventral ramus of T11 (intercostal nerve)

Sympathetic trunk ganglia

1st lumbar splanchnic nerve

Renal artery and plexus

Sacral plexus

Pelvic splanchnic nerves

Dorsal vagal nucleus
Medulla oblongata

Vagus (X) nerve
Spinal ganglion
Descending fibers
Ascending fibers

T10

Spinal cord (T10 to L1)

T11

T12

L1

Lesser thoracic splanchnic nerve

Lowest thoracic splanchnic nerve

Celiac plexus

Aorticorenal ganglion

Renal ganglion

Intermesenteric plexus

Superior hypogastric plexus (presacral nerve)

Hypogastric nerve

S2

S3

S4

Inferior hypogastric (pelvic) plexus

9.68 INNERVATION OF THE KIDNEYS AND UPPER URETER

Sympathetic innervation of the kidneys and upper ureter arises from the T10–L1 intermediolateral cell column preganglionic neurons in the spinal cord and travels through lower thoracic and upper lumbar splanchnic nerves to synapse in the celiac or aorticorenal ganglia. Noradrenergic postganglionic fibers travel in fascicles that accompany the upper ureteric, renal, pelvic, calyceal, and segmental branches of the renal vessels. Parasympathetic nerve fibers are distributed to renal ganglia by the vagus nerve and pelvic splanchnic nerves via a longer course through other plexuses. The sympathetic nerve fibers stimulate renin secretion (and the renin-angiotensin-aldosterone system); decrease the glomerular filtration rate; stimulate proximal tubule and collecting duct sodium chloride reabsorption (further elevating blood pressure); and stimulate contraction of the ureters. Parasympathetic nerve fibers cause relaxation of smooth muscle in the pelvis, the calyces, and the upper ureter and, when accompanied by decreased sympathetic activation, may lead to a decrease in blood pressure.

9.69 INNERVATION OF THE URINARY BLADDER AND LOWER URETER

The sympathetic innervation of the bladder and lower ureter derives mainly from the L1–L2 preganglionic neurons in the spinal cord and travels through sacral splanchnic nerves to the hypogastric plexus. Parasympathetic innervation derives from the S2–S4 intermediate gray of the spinal cord and distributes to intramural ganglia in the wall of the bladder via pelvic splanchnic nerves. Sympathetic nerve fibers relax the detrusor muscle and contract the trigone and the internal sphincter. Parasympathetic nerve fibers contract the detrusor muscle and relax the trigone and the internal sphincter, thus stimulating emptying of the bladder. Sensory nerves also are present in the bladder; when the bladder is stretched because it is full, these nerves can initiate the sensation of the need to empty the bladder.

CLINICAL POINT

Parasympathetic nerve damage, particularly in diabetic neuropathy, results in initial problems of incomplete emptying of the bladder, dribbling, and urinary stasis sufficient to increase the likelihood of infection. Later in the course of parasympathetic damage, a flaccid bladder with incomplete emptying and incontinence can occur. Sensory neuropathy also can result in an enlarged bladder caused by incomplete emptying because of the inability of the patient to sense fullness and by the decreased sense of urgency for urination.

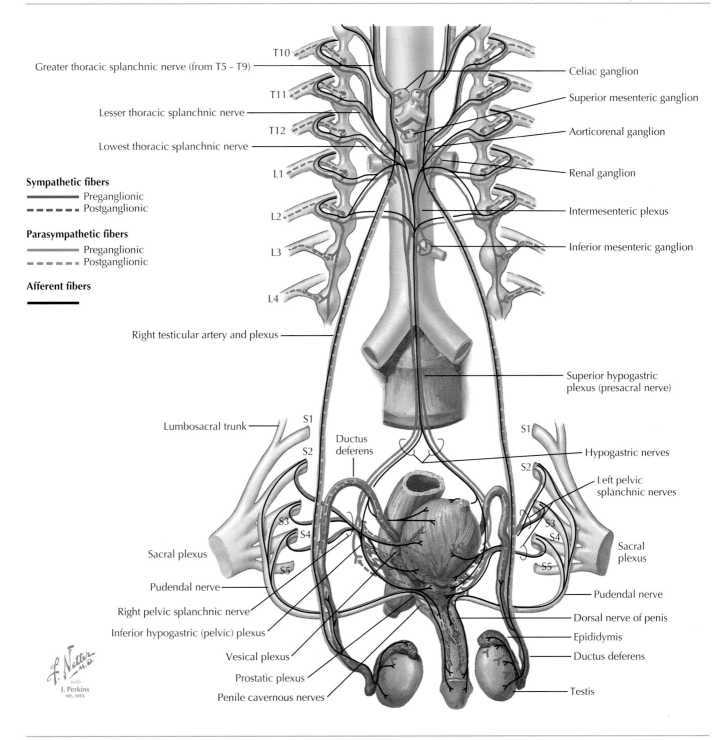

Greater thoracic splanchnic nerve (from T5 - T9)

T10

T11

Lesser thoracic splanchnic nerve

T12

Lowest thoracic splanchnic nerve

L1

Sympathetic fibers
Preganglionic
Postganglionic

L2

Parasympathetic fibers
Preganglionic
Postganglionic

L3

Afferent fibers

L4

Right testicular artery and plexus

Celiac ganglion

Superior mesenteric ganglion

Aorticorenal ganglion

Renal ganglion

Intermesenteric plexus

Inferior mesenteric ganglion

Superior hypogastric plexus (presacral nerve)

Lumbosacral trunk

S1

S2

Ductus deferens

S1

S2

Hypogastric nerves

Left pelvic splanchnic nerves

S3

S4

S3

S4

Sacral plexus

S5

S5

Sacral plexus

Pudendal nerve

Right pelvic splanchnic nerve

Inferior hypogastric (pelvic) plexus

Vesical plexus

Prostatic plexus

Penile cavernous nerves

Pudendal nerve

Dorsal nerve of penis

Epididymis

Ductus deferens

Testis

9.70 INNERVATION OF THE MALE REPRODUCTIVE ORGANS

Sympathetic innervation to the male reproductive organs derives from T10–L2 intermediolateral cell column neurons and reaches the hypogastric plexus via thoracic and upper lumbar splanchnic nerves. Parasympathetic innervation derives from the S2–S4 intermediate gray of the spinal cord and travels to the inferior hypogastric plexus via pelvic splanchnic nerves. Sympathetic nerve fibers cause contraction of the vas deferens and prostatic capsule and contract the sphincter to the bladder, which prevents retrograde ejaculation. Sympathetic nerve fibers also contribute to vascular responses in the penile corpora cavernosa that are related to erection; beta-receptor blockade can result in erectile dysfunction. Parasympathetic nerve fibers regulate the vascular dilation that initiates and maintains penile erection. Sympathetic and parasympathetic nerve fibers must work together to optimize sexual and reproductive function.

CLINICAL POINT

Parasympathetic nerve damage may lead to autonomic erectile dysfunction. Some individuals taking beta blockers might have similar responses. However, erectile function also depends extensively on psychological, perceptive, and sensory factors in addition to the need for coordinated autonomic function. Pharmacological compounds that enhance erectile function influence vascular responses through the production of nitric oxide to promote erection; these drugs may interact adversely with alpha-blockers used to treat benign prostatic hypertrophy and other conditions, resulting in hypotensive responses that are potentially fatal.

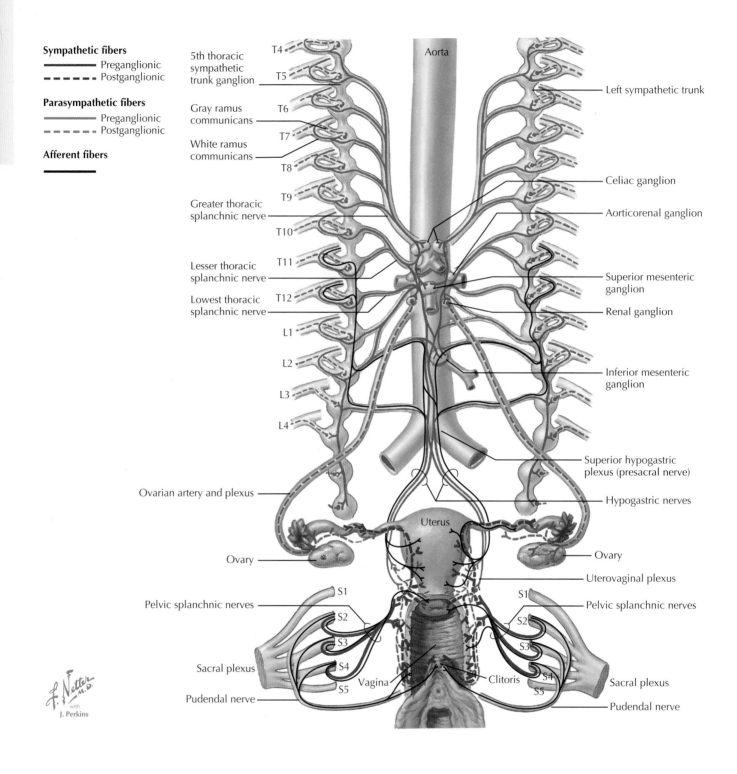

Sympathetic fibers
——— Preganglionic
‑ ‑ ‑ ‑ ‑ Postganglionic

Parasympathetic fibers
——— Preganglionic
‑ ‑ ‑ ‑ ‑ Postganglionic

Afferent fibers
———

5th thoracic sympathetic trunk ganglion

Gray ramus communicans

White ramus communicans

Greater thoracic splanchnic nerve

Lesser thoracic splanchnic nerve

Lowest thoracic splanchnic nerve

Ovarian artery and plexus

Ovary

Pelvic splanchnic nerves

Sacral plexus

Pudendal nerve

Aorta

Left sympathetic trunk

Celiac ganglion

Aorticorenal ganglion

Superior mesenteric ganglion

Renal ganglion

Inferior mesenteric ganglion

Superior hypogastric plexus (presacral nerve)

Hypogastric nerves

Uterus

Ovary

Uterovaginal plexus

Pelvic splanchnic nerves

Vagina

Clitoris

Sacral plexus

Pudendal nerve

9.71 INNERVATION OF THE FEMALE REPRODUCTIVE ORGANS

Autonomic nerves supplying the female reproductive organs have origins similar to those supplying their male counterparts. Sympathetic nerves can stimulate contraction of the uterus, but the extent of this action is determined also by hormonal receptor responsiveness and neurotransmitter receptor expression. Sympathetic nerve fibers also supply the vaginal arteries, the vestibular glands, and erectile tissue. Parasympathetic nerve fibers supply the muscular and mucous coats of the vagina and urethra, stimulate the erectile tissue of the vestibular bulb and corpora cavernosa of the clitoris, and supply the vestibular glands. Autonomic neuropathy affecting the nerves to female reproductive organs may result in dry, atrophic vaginal walls with very little lubrication, resulting in dyspareunia (painful intercourse).

10

SPINAL CORD

Nuclear cell columns   **Laminae of Rexed**

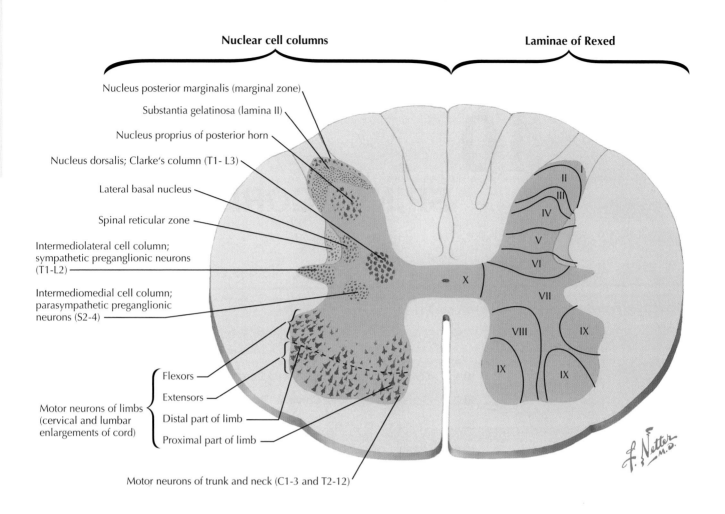

Nucleus posterior marginalis (marginal zone)

Substantia gelatinosa (lamina II)

Nucleus proprius of posterior horn

Nucleus dorsalis; Clarke's column (T1- L3)

Lateral basal nucleus

Spinal reticular zone

Intermediolateral cell column; sympathetic preganglionic neurons (T1-L2)

Intermediomedial cell column; parasympathetic preganglionic neurons (S2-4)

Flexors

Extensors

Distal part of limb

Proximal part of limb

Motor neurons of limbs (cervical and lumbar enlargements of cord)

Motor neurons of trunk and neck (C1-3 and T2-12)

10.1 CYTOARCHITECTURE OF THE SPINAL CORD GRAY MATTER

The spinal cord gray matter is located centrally in the interior of the spinal cord in a butterfly pattern. The gray matter is subdivided into three horns: (1) the dorsal horn, a site of major sensory processing; (2) the intermediate gray with a lateral horn, a site where preganglionic sympathetic (thoracolumbar) and parasympathetic (sacral) neurons reside and where interneuronal processing occurs; and (3) the ventral horn, a site where lower motor neurons (LMNs) reside and where converging reflex and descending control of LMNs occurs. Neuronal cell groups appear homogeneous in some regions of gray matter, intermixed with a presence of some discrete nuclei (e.g., Clarke's nucleus, substantia gelatinosa). Laminae of Rexed, an alternative system of cytoarchitectural classification established in the 1950s, subdivides the spinal cord gray matter into ten laminae. This system is used extensively for the dorsal horn and the intermediate gray, laminae I–VII, particularly in conjunction with anatomical details of nociceptive processing and for some reflex and cerebellar processing. Although these laminae have distinctive characteristics at each segmental level, they show some similarities across segmental levels. The absolute amount of spinal cord gray is more extensive in the cervical and lumbosacral enlargements of the spinal cord, which correspond to zones associated with limb innervation, than it is in upper cervical, thoracic, and sacral regions.

CLINICAL POINT

Classical descriptions of secondary sensory processing in the spinal cord describe neurons of lamina I (marginal zone) and lamina V of the dorsal horn as cells of origin for crossed projections into the spinothalamic/anterolateral system for the processing of pain and temperature sensation (protopathic modalities). Primary sensory large-diameter axons, carrying information about fine discriminative touch, vibratory sensation, and joint position sense (epicritic modalities), enter through the dorsal root entry zone and travel rostrally into the dorsal column system, bypassing synapses in the spinal cord; these axons terminate in their secondary sensory nuclei, gracilis and cuneatus, in the caudal medulla. According to this scheme, pure dorsal column lesions should result in the total loss of epicritic sensation on the ipsilateral side of the body below the level of the lesion. However, such lesions result in diminution of these epicritic sensations or in the inability to discriminate vibratory sensations of different frequencies, but not in the total loss of these modalities. Only with additional damage to the dorsolateral part of the lateral funiculus is the profound loss of epicritic sensation observed. This is because additional dorsal horn neurons receive primary sensory input related to epicritic sensation and send ipsilateral projections into the dorsolateral funiculus, providing additional contributions to lemniscal processing of fine discriminative modalities.

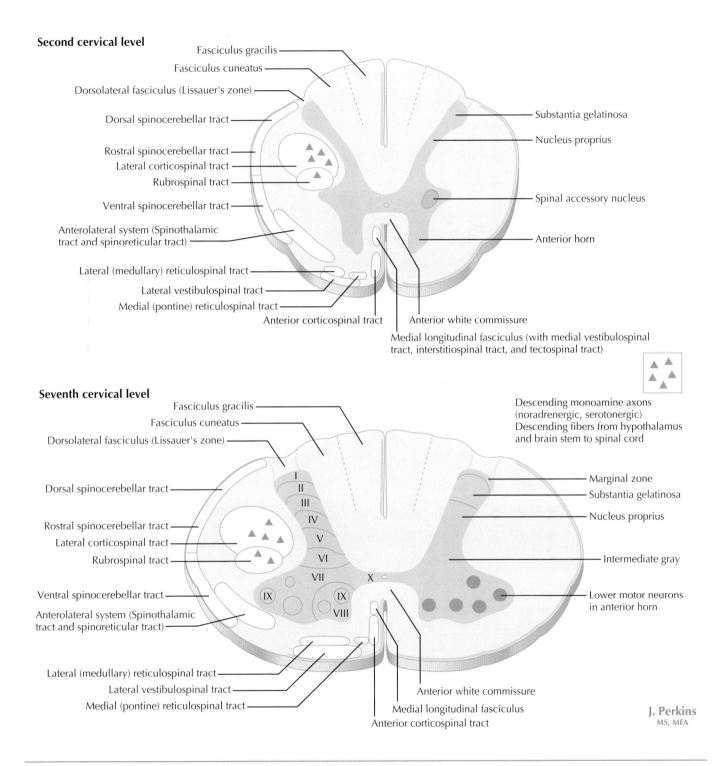

Second cervical level

Fasciculus gracilis

Fasciculus cuneatus

Dorsolateral fasciculus (Lissauer's zone)

Dorsal spinocerebellar tract

Rostral spinocerebellar tract

Lateral corticospinal tract

Rubrospinal tract

Ventral spinocerebellar tract

Anterolateral system (Spinothalamic tract and spinoreticular tract)

Lateral (medullary) reticulospinal tract

Lateral vestibulospinal tract

Medial (pontine) reticulospinal tract

Anterior corticospinal tract

Substantia gelatinosa

Nucleus proprius

Spinal accessory nucleus

Anterior horn

Anterior white commissure

Medial longitudinal fasciculus (with medial vestibulospinal tract, interstitiospinal tract, and tectospinal tract)

Seventh cervical level

Fasciculus gracilis

Fasciculus cuneatus

Dorsolateral fasciculus (Lissauer's zone)

Dorsal spinocerebellar tract

Rostral spinocerebellar tract

Lateral corticospinal tract

Rubrospinal tract

Ventral spinocerebellar tract

Anterolateral system (Spinothalamic tract and spinoreticular tract)

Lateral (medullary) reticulospinal tract

Lateral vestibulospinal tract

Medial (pontine) reticulospinal tract

Anterior corticospinal tract

Descending monoamine axons (noradrenergic, serotonergic) Descending fibers from hypothalamus and brain stem to spinal cord

Marginal zone

Substantia gelatinosa

Nucleus proprius

Intermediate gray

Lower motor neurons in anterior horn

Anterior white commissure

Medial longitudinal fasciculus

J. Perkins
MS, MFA

10.2 SPINAL CORD LEVELS: CERVICAL, THORACIC, LUMBAR, AND SACRAL

The organization of the gray matter into laminae of Rexed is retained throughout the spinal cord. The dorsal and ventral horns are larger and wider at levels of the cervical and lumbosacral enlargements. The lateral horn is present from L1 to T2. Some nuclei are found only in circumscribed regions, such as the intermediolateral cell column with preganglionic sympathetic neurons (T1–L2 lateral horn); Clarke's nucleus (C8–L2); and the parasympathetic preganglionic nucleus (S2–S4). The

white matter increases in absolute amount from caudal to rostral. The dorsal columns contain only fasciculus gracilis below T6; fasciculus cuneatus is added laterally above T6. The spinothalamic/spinoreticular anterolateral system increases from caudal to rostral. The descending upper motor neuron (UMN) pathways diminish from rostral to caudal. The lateral corticospinal pathway loses more than half of its axons as they synapse in the cervical segments; this tract then diminishes in size as it extends caudally.

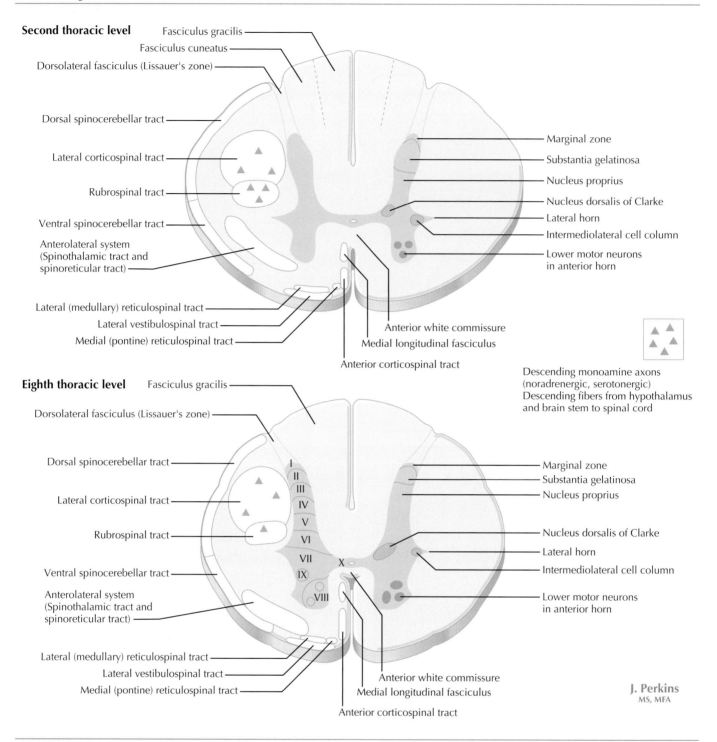

Second thoracic level
- Fasciculus gracilis
- Fasciculus cuneatus
- Dorsolateral fasciculus (Lissauer's zone)
- Dorsal spinocerebellar tract
- Lateral corticospinal tract
- Rubrospinal tract
- Ventral spinocerebellar tract
- Anterolateral system (Spinothalamic tract and spinoreticular tract)
- Lateral (medullary) reticulospinal tract
- Lateral vestibulospinal tract
- Medial (pontine) reticulospinal tract
- Anterior corticospinal tract
- Marginal zone
- Substantia gelatinosa
- Nucleus proprius
- Nucleus dorsalis of Clarke
- Lateral horn
- Intermediolateral cell column
- Lower motor neurons in anterior horn
- Anterior white commissure
- Medial longitudinal fasciculus

Descending monoamine axons (noradrenergic, serotonergic) Descending fibers from hypothalamus and brain stem to spinal cord

Eighth thoracic level
- Fasciculus gracilis
- Dorsolateral fasciculus (Lissauer's zone)
- Dorsal spinocerebellar tract
- Lateral corticospinal tract
- Rubrospinal tract
- Ventral spinocerebellar tract
- Anterolateral system (Spinothalamic tract and spinoreticular tract)
- Lateral (medullary) reticulospinal tract
- Lateral vestibulospinal tract
- Medial (pontine) reticulospinal tract
- Anterior corticospinal tract
- I, II, III, IV, V, VI, VII, IX, VIII, X
- Marginal zone
- Substantia gelatinosa
- Nucleus proprius
- Nucleus dorsalis of Clarke
- Lateral horn
- Intermediolateral cell column
- Lower motor neurons in anterior horn
- Anterior white commissure
- Medial longitudinal fasciculus

J. Perkins
MS, MFA

10.3 SPINAL CORD LEVELS: CERVICAL, THORACIC, LUMBAR, AND SACRAL (continued)

CLINICAL POINT

Damage to the lateral funiculus of the cervical spinal cord caused by demyelination, trauma, ischemia, or other causes can lead to disruption of (1) the descending lateral corticospinal tract and rubrospinal tract, resulting in ipsilateral spastic (long-term result) hemiplegia below the level of the lesion; and (2) the descending axons from the hypothalamus to the preganglionic sympathetic neurons in the intermediolateral cell column at the T1 and T2 segments of the cord. These preganglionic neurons supply the superior cervical ganglion, which provides postganglionic noradrenergic sympathetic innervation to the ipsilateral head. Disruption of these descending axons in the lateral funiculus or at any point distal in the sympathetic pathway can result

in Horner's syndrome, which consists of ipsilateral ptosis (because of effects on the superior tarsal muscle), miosis (because of effects on the pupillary dilator muscle), and anhidrosis (less sweat gland activity). Trauma that damages one entire side of the spinal cord at the cervical level produces the same symptoms (ipsilateral spastic paralysis with brisk reflexes, and ipsilateral Horner's syndrome) and also causes (1) flaccid paralysis of ipsilateral muscles innervated by LMNs damaged by the trauma; (2) loss of epicritic sensation (fine discriminative touch, vibratory sensation, joint position sense) ipsilaterally below the level of the trauma because of damage to the dorsal column and dorsolateral funiculus axons; and (3) loss of pain and temperature sensation contralaterally below the level of the lesion because of damage to the anterolateral system (spinothalamic/spinoreticular system). This collection of neurological deficits resulting from a hemisection lesion to the spinal cord is called a Brown-Séquard lesion.

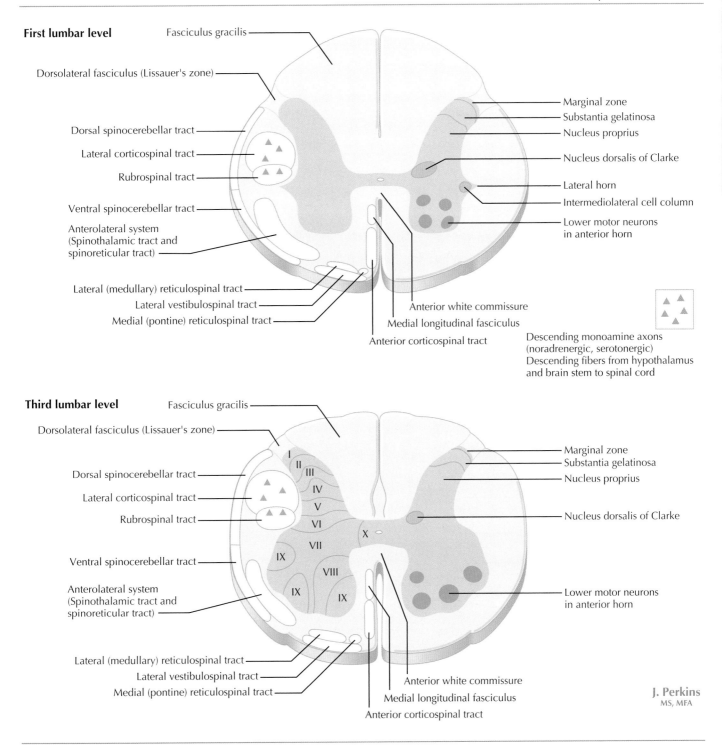

First lumbar level

Fasciculus gracilis

Dorsolateral fasciculus (Lissauer's zone)

Dorsal spinocerebellar tract

Lateral corticospinal tract

Rubrospinal tract

Ventral spinocerebellar tract

Anterolateral system
(Spinothalamic tract and
spinoreticular tract)

Lateral (medullary) reticulospinal tract

Lateral vestibulospinal tract

Medial (pontine) reticulospinal tract

Marginal zone

Substantia gelatinosa

Nucleus proprius

Nucleus dorsalis of Clarke

Lateral horn

Intermediolateral cell column

Lower motor neurons
in anterior horn

Anterior white commissure

Medial longitudinal fasciculus

Anterior corticospinal tract

Descending monoamine axons
(noradrenergic, serotonergic)
Descending fibers from hypothalamus
and brain stem to spinal cord

Third lumbar level

Fasciculus gracilis

Dorsolateral fasciculus (Lissauer's zone)

Dorsal spinocerebellar tract

Lateral corticospinal tract

Rubrospinal tract

Ventral spinocerebellar tract

Anterolateral system
(Spinothalamic tract and
spinoreticular tract)

Lateral (medullary) reticulospinal tract

Lateral vestibulospinal tract

Medial (pontine) reticulospinal tract

Marginal zone

Substantia gelatinosa

Nucleus proprius

Nucleus dorsalis of Clarke

Lower motor neurons
in anterior horn

Anterior white commissure

Medial longitudinal fasciculus

Anterior corticospinal tract

J. Perkins
MS, MFA

10.4 SPINAL CORD LEVELS: CERVICAL, THORACIC, LUMBAR, AND SACRAL (continued)

CLINICAL POINT

The central canal of the spinal cord is ordinarily a closed remnant of former neural tube development and in the adult does not convey or produce cerebrospinal fluid. However, a developmental defect may result in the formation of a syrinx in the central canal region of the spinal cord, either alone or in the presence of an obstruction of the foramen magnum (with Arnold-Chiari malformation). This condition, called syringomyelia, occurs mainly at a lower cervical or a thoracic level. The distinguishing feature is destruction of the axons in the anterior white commissure, resulting in a dissociated sensory loss of pain and temperature sensation at the levels of the syrinx, with preservation of epicritic sensation (dorsal columns and the dorsolateral funiculus are usually preserved). If the syrinx extends laterally, it most likely involves adjacent LMNs; this manifests as segmental weakness and muscle atrophy. Larger lesions may extend into the lateral funiculus and damage the descending UMN systems (the corticospinal and rubrospinal tracts), causing ipsilateral spastic paresis. Syringomyelia is sometimes accompanied by kyphoscoliosis and pain in the region of the neck and arms. The syrinx may extend to the brain stem (syringobulbia) and produce damage to lower brain stem structures.

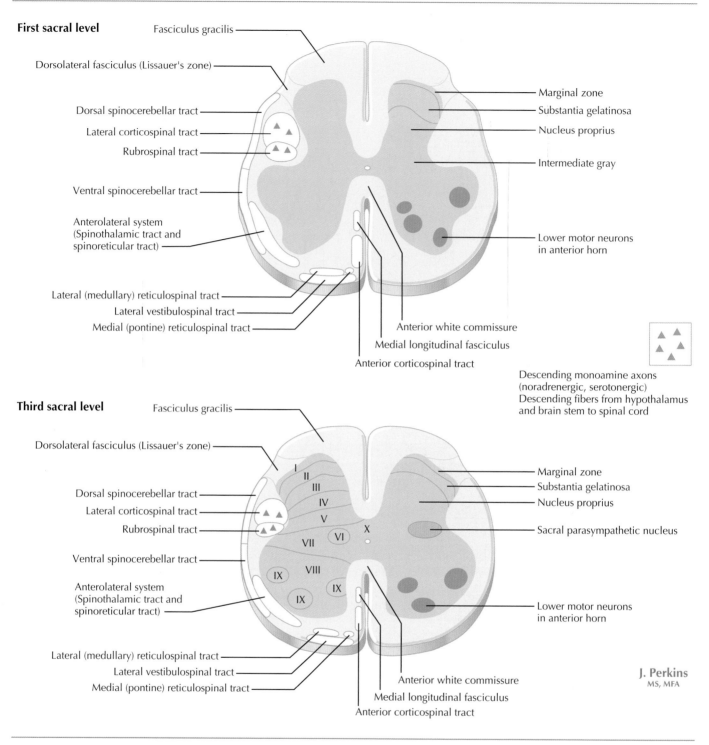

First sacral level

Fasciculus gracilis

Dorsolateral fasciculus (Lissauer's zone)

Dorsal spinocerebellar tract

Lateral corticospinal tract

Rubrospinal tract

Ventral spinocerebellar tract

Anterolateral system
(Spinothalamic tract and
spinoreticular tract)

Lateral (medullary) reticulospinal tract

Lateral vestibulospinal tract

Medial (pontine) reticulospinal tract

Marginal zone

Substantia gelatinosa

Nucleus proprius

Intermediate gray

Lower motor neurons
in anterior horn

Anterior white commissure

Medial longitudinal fasciculus

Anterior corticospinal tract

Descending monoamine axons
(noradrenergic, serotonergic)
Descending fibers from hypothalamus
and brain stem to spinal cord

Third sacral level

Fasciculus gracilis

Dorsolateral fasciculus (Lissauer's zone)

Dorsal spinocerebellar tract

Lateral corticospinal tract

Rubrospinal tract

Ventral spinocerebellar tract

Anterolateral system
(Spinothalamic tract and
spinoreticular tract)

Lateral (medullary) reticulospinal tract

Lateral vestibulospinal tract

Medial (pontine) reticulospinal tract

I
II
III
IV
V
VI
VII
VIII
IX
IX
IX
X

Marginal zone

Substantia gelatinosa

Nucleus proprius

Sacral parasympathetic nucleus

Lower motor neurons
in anterior horn

Anterior white commissure

Medial longitudinal fasciculus

Anterior corticospinal tract

J. Perkins
MS, MFA

10.5 SPINAL CORD LEVELS: CERVICAL, THORACIC, LUMBAR, AND SACRAL (continued)

CLINICAL POINT

A severe spinal cord crush injury damages local neurons and disrupts both the ascending and the descending tracts. Such a lesion at the lumbar level causes flaccid paralysis of muscles (with loss of tone and muscle stretch reflexes) at the damaged levels as the result of LMN injury and spastic paralysis of muscles (with increased tone and muscle stretch reflexes, possible clonus, and extensor plantar responses) in muscles supplied by LMNs below the level of the lesion as the result of damage to the UMN axons in the lateral funiculus. All sensation is lost below the level of the lesion because of disruption of both dorsal column and anterolateral axons, although some protopathic sensation may remain present, even in the case of a very extensive lesion. A severe crush injury also damages descending axons in both lateral funiculi that help to regulate bowel function, bladder function, and sexual function. The patient initially shows spinal shock syndrome, with unresponsive bowel and bladder; after recovery from spinal shock, a spastic bladder (small, stimulated to empty by reflex, with incontinence) occurs. In addition, voluntary control over erectile function in males is lost, but reflex erection caused by specific sensory stimuli may occur. Severe crush injury at higher levels (cervical) also can disrupt descending axons that regulate sympathetic outflow, resulting in dysregulated blood pressure, Horner's syndrome, and other autonomic symptoms.

A. Sagittal view - Cervical spine

— Pons

— Cerebellum

— Medulla

— Cisterna magna

— Subarachnoid space

— Cervical spinal cord

— Thoracic spinal cord

— Caudal lumbosacral spinal cord

— Lumbar cistern

— Cauda equina - nerve roots in subarachnoid space

B. Sagittal view - Lumbar spine

10.6 SPINAL CORD IMAGING

These two sagittal illustrations of the spinal cord are T2-weighted magnetic resonance images that reveal the spinal cord as a dark structure and the cerebrospinal fluid (subarachnoid space) as white. **A,** The cervical and thoracic spinal cord. **B,** The lumbosacral spinal cord and the long nerve roots coursing through the subarachnoid space (lumbar cistern) as the cauda equina. Some individual nerve roots can be seen in contrast to the white cerebrospinal fluid.

CLINICAL POINT

In adults, the sacral segments of the spinal cord are located at the T1 vertebral level. Trauma or a tumor at this specific vertebral level can result in conus medullaris syndrome, which includes paralysis of the muscles of the pelvic floor (LMN damage); a flaccid bladder with overflow incontinence (loss of both parasympathetic input and sensory fibers); constipation and diminished bowel function (loss of parasympathetic control); loss of erectile function (loss of parasympathetic control in males); and "saddle" anesthesia (loss of sensory processing). Pain is sometimes experienced in the gluteal or perineal region. If passing nerve roots of the cauda equina are also damaged, additional sensory and motor impairment of the legs may be seen.

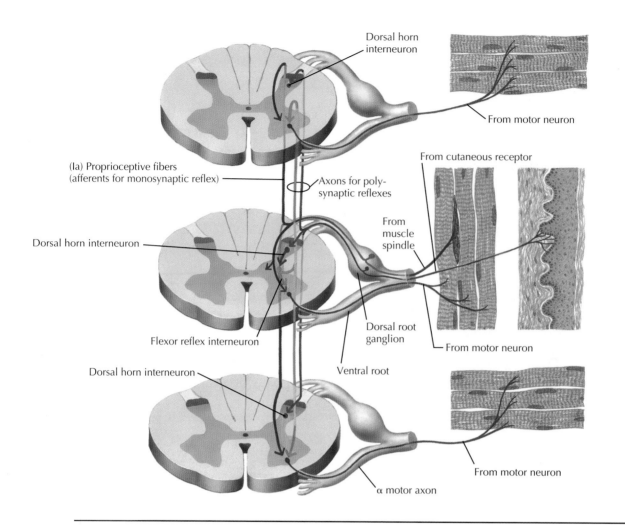

Dorsal horn interneuron

From motor neuron

(Ia) Proprioceptive fibers (afferents for monosynaptic reflex)

Axons for poly-synaptic reflexes

From cutaneous receptor

From muscle spindle

Dorsal horn interneuron

Flexor reflex interneuron

Dorsal root ganglion

From motor neuron

Dorsal horn interneuron

Ventral root

From motor neuron

α motor axon

Schematic representation of motor neurons

In cervical enlargement of spinal cord

Flexors

Extensors

In lumbar enlargement of spinal cord

Flexors

Extensors

10.7 SPINAL CORD LOWER MOTOR NEURON ORGANIZATION AND CONTROL

LMNs are located in the cervical, thoracic, lumbar, and sacral segments of the ventral (anterior) horn of the spinal cord. LMNs also have a medial to lateral and dorsal to ventral organization. LMNs supplying trunk musculature are found medially and ventrally; LMNs innervating more distal musculature are found dorsally and laterally. This organization also is apparent in the topography of UMN control of LMNs. UMNs from the corticospinal system that regulate fine hand and finger movements terminate on dorsal and lateral LMNs. UMNs from reticulospinal and vestibulospinal systems that regulate basic truncal tone and posture terminate on ventral and medial LMNs. Reflex pathways regulate LMN activity through monosynaptic (muscle stretch reflex Ia afferents) or polysynaptic (flexor or cutaneous reflex afferents) pathways. Superimposed on this organization is the descending UMN control and coordination of LMNs.

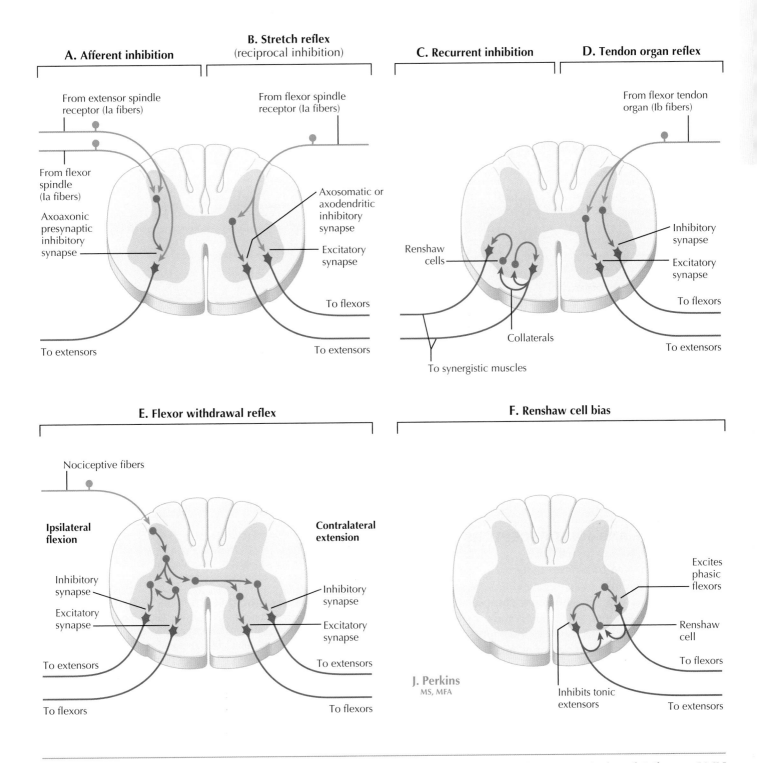

A. Afferent inhibition

From extensor spindle receptor (Ia fibers)

From flexor spindle (Ia fibers)

Axoaxonic presynaptic inhibitory synapse

To extensors

B. Stretch reflex
(reciprocal inhibition)

From flexor spindle receptor (Ia fibers)

Axosomatic or axodendritic inhibitory synapse

Excitatory synapse

To flexors

To extensors

C. Recurrent inhibition

Renshaw cells

Collaterals

To synergistic muscles

D. Tendon organ reflex

From flexor tendon organ (Ib fibers)

Inhibitory synapse

Excitatory synapse

To flexors

To extensors

E. Flexor withdrawal reflex

Nociceptive fibers

Ipsilateral flexion

Inhibitory synapse

Excitatory synapse

To extensors

To flexors

Contralateral extension

Inhibitory synapse

Excitatory synapse

To extensors

To flexors

F. Renshaw cell bias

Excites phasic flexors

Renshaw cell

To flexors

Inhibits tonic extensors

To extensors

J. Perkins
MS, MFA

10.8 SPINAL SOMATIC REFLEX PATHWAYS

In the muscle stretch reflex, Ia afferents excite the homonymous LMN pool directly and reciprocally inhibit the antagonist LMN pool via Ia inhibitory interneurons. The Golgi tendon organ reflex disynaptically inhibits the homonymous LMN pool and reciprocally excites the antagonist LMN pool. Flexor reflex responses excite a larger pool of LMNs through a great number of interneurons, with reciprocal inhibition of the appropriate antagonist LMNs, to bring about a protective withdrawal response from a noxious stimulus. These reflexes can extend throughout the entire spinal cord. When an LMN fires an action potential, it excites a Renshaw cell that inhibits that same LMN, thereby ensuring a clean slate for the next set of inputs to that LMN. Renshaw cells receive input from axon collaterals of both flexor and extensor LMNs and in turn exert an inhibitory bias that focuses particularly on the inhibition of extensor LMNs and reciprocal excitation of flexor LMNs. Thus, the Renshaw cells favor flexor movements and help to inhibit extensor movements.

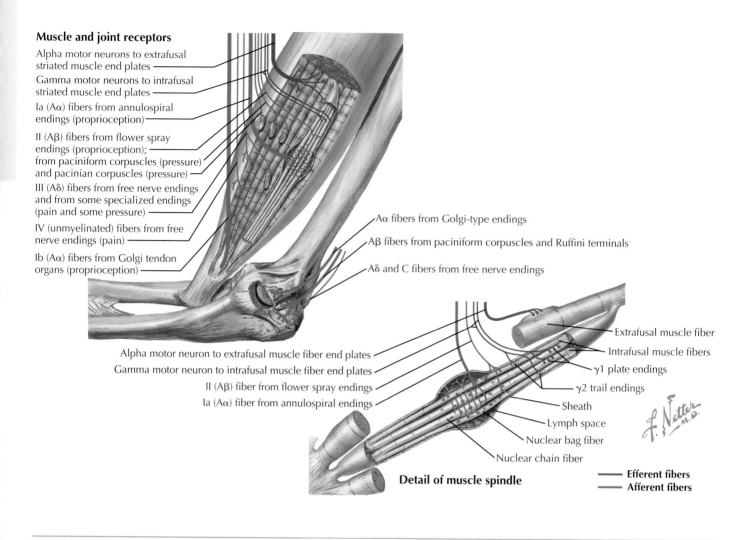

Muscle and joint receptors

Alpha motor neurons to extrafusal striated muscle end plates

Gamma motor neurons to intrafusal striated muscle end plates

Ia (Aα) fibers from annulospiral endings (proprioception)

II (Aβ) fibers from flower spray endings (proprioception); from paciniform corpuscles (pressure) and pacinian corpuscles (pressure)

III (Aδ) fibers from free nerve endings and from some specialized endings (pain and some pressure)

IV (unmyelinated) fibers from free nerve endings (pain)

Ib (Aα) fibers from Golgi tendon organs (proprioception)

Aα fibers from Golgi-type endings

Aβ fibers from paciniform corpuscles and Ruffini terminals

Aδ and C fibers from free nerve endings

Alpha motor neuron to extrafusal muscle fiber end plates

Gamma motor neuron to intrafusal muscle fiber end plates

II (Aβ) fiber from flower spray endings

Ia (Aα) fiber from annulospiral endings

Extrafusal muscle fiber

Intrafusal muscle fibers

γ1 plate endings

γ2 trail endings

Sheath

Lymph space

Nuclear bag fiber

Nuclear chain fiber

Detail of muscle spindle

—— Efferent fibers
—— Afferent fibers

10.9 MUSCLE AND JOINT RECEPTORS AND MUSCLE SPINDLES

Joints are innervated by a host of afferent receptors, including bare nerve endings, Golgi-type endings, paciniform endings, Ruffini-like endings, and other encapsulated endings. Golgi tendon organs innervate tendons and respond to stretch with increased discharge, causing disynaptic inhibition of the LMNs that contract the homonymous muscles. Muscle spindles are complex sensory receptors within muscles; they are arranged in parallel with the extrafusal (skeletal) muscle fibers. These receptors contain small intrafusal muscle fibers that are stretched when the skeletal muscle is stretched. The Ia afferent from the muscle spindle excites the homonymous LMN pool monosynaptically and responds to both the length and the velocity (change in length with respect to time) of the extrafusal muscle fiber. These muscle reflexes assist in maintaining homeostasis during contraction and help to regulate muscle tone during movement.

CLINICAL POINT

Skeletal muscles are supplied by both afferent (sensory) and efferent (motor) nerves and receptors. The sensory fibers are associated mainly with specialized sensory receptors, the muscle spindles. Muscle spindles are small, encapsulated sensory receptors that lie in parallel with the skeletal muscle fibers (extrafusal fibers). Each spindle contains nuclear bag fibers (innervated mainly by group Ia afferents) and nuclear chain fibers (innervated mainly by group II afferents). These afferents are responsive to the tension on the muscle spindle. The II afferents report mainly the lengths of the extrafusal fibers with which they are associated, whereas the Ia afferents report both the lengths and the velocities (dL/dt). In conjunction with the Ib afferents associated with Golgi tendon organs that report the force exerted on the tendon, Ia and group II muscle afferents provide continuous information to the CNS about the current state of the muscle and the projected changes occurring, based on the velocity response. The skeletal muscle fibers are supplied by motor axons derived from the alpha motor neurons in the ventral horn of the spinal cord. The muscle spindle's nuclear bag and chain fibers have small contractile fibers on either end by which they are anchored into the spindle. These contractile fibers (intrafusal fibers) are innervated by gamma (γ) LMNs whose cell bodies also are found in the ventral horn of the spinal cord. Descending UMN pathways generally activate both alpha and gamma LMNs (alpha-gamma coactivation), thereby achieving the shortening of the muscle spindle by the gamma LMNs in parallel with the shortening of the extrafusal fibers, keeping the muscle spindle in its dynamic range of sensory activity. Without such coactivation, the muscle spindle afferents would be silent in most ranges of extrafusal muscle contraction.

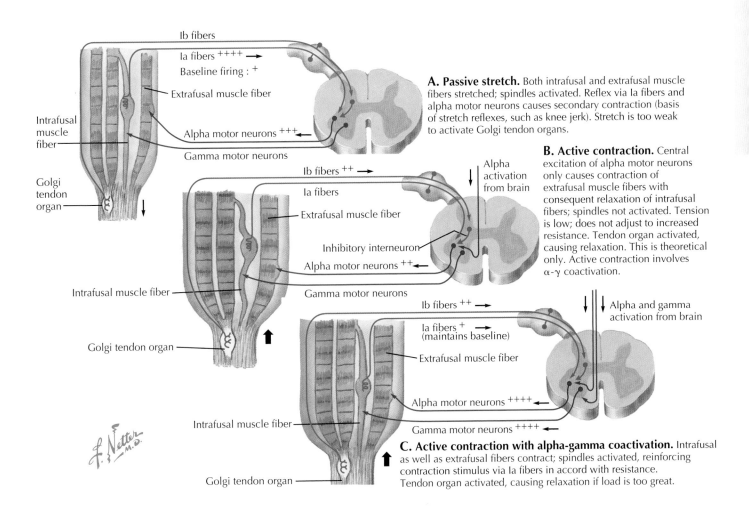

A. Passive stretch. Both intrafusal and extrafusal muscle fibers stretched; spindles activated. Reflex via Ia fibers and alpha motor neurons causes secondary contraction (basis of stretch reflexes, such as knee jerk). Stretch is too weak to activate Golgi tendon organs.

B. Active contraction. Central excitation of alpha motor neurons only causes contraction of extrafusal muscle fibers with consequent relaxation of intrafusal fibers; spindles not activated. Tension is low; does not adjust to increased resistance. Tendon organ activated, causing relaxation. This is theoretical only. Active contraction involves α-γ coactivation.

C. Active contraction with alpha-gamma coactivation. Intrafusal as well as extrafusal fibers contract; spindles activated, reinforcing contraction stimulus via Ia fibers in accord with resistance. Tendon organ activated, causing relaxation if load is too great.

10.10 THE MUSCLE STRETCH REFLEX AND ITS CENTRAL CONTROL VIA GAMMA MOTOR NEURONS

During passive stretch, a muscle stretch reflex excites homonymous LMNs, which results in muscle contraction to restore homeostasis. If active skeletal muscle contraction occurs without the activation of gamma LMNs, the muscle spindle "unloads" and the tension on the intrafusal fibers is reduced, resulting in diminished firing of both Ia and II afferents. However, when LMNs contract because of activity in the brain stem's UMNs or because of voluntary corticospinal activity, both alpha LMNs and gamma LMNs are activated together. This process, alpha-gamma coactivation, ensures that the tension on the muscle spindle (through the intrafusal innervation by gamma fibers) adjusts immediately, that is, as the extrafusal muscle contraction occurs (through alpha fiber innervation). Although alpha and gamma LMNs can be modulated separately by specific central neuronal circuits, in normal physiological circumstances they are coactivated. If gamma LMNs are differentially activated in pathological circumstances, increased muscle tone and spasticity may ensue.

CLINICAL POINT

The muscle stretch reflex, a mainstay of neurological diagnosis, depends upon the activity of afferents and efferents associated with the muscle spindle and the skeletal muscle (extrafusal) fibers. When a tendon is tapped with a reflex hammer (e.g., the patellar tendon), the skeletal muscle is briefly stretched, as are the muscle spindles lying in parallel with them. The stretch of the muscle spindle puts tension on the equatorial region of the nuclear bag fibers, resulting in a burst of action potentials from the associated Ia afferents. The Ia afferents synapse directly with alpha LMNs in the spinal cord ventral horn, resulting in contraction of the homonymous muscle (quadriceps) and restoration of homeostasis. The Ia afferents also synapse on Ia inhibitory interneurons in the spinal cord, producing reciprocal inhibition of the antagonist muscles (hamstrings). The excitability of the muscle spindles can determine the robustness of the Ia afferent response to stretch. If the muscle spindle is floppy (unloaded), no Ia afferent response is forthcoming when the related tendon is tapped, and no muscle contraction occurs; if the muscle spindle is on a hair-trigger of heightened responsiveness, as happens when the gamma LMNs are excessively activated, then a very brisk muscle contraction occurs when the related tendon is tapped. The latter situation may occur in cases of lesions in the UMNs of the spinal cord and brain, which may produce disinhibition of the dynamic gamma LMNs accompanied by hyperreflexia of the muscle stretch reflexes and spasticity of the involved muscles.

11

BRAIN STEM AND CEREBELLUM

Medulla-Spinal Cord Transition—Decussation of the Pyramids

Level of section

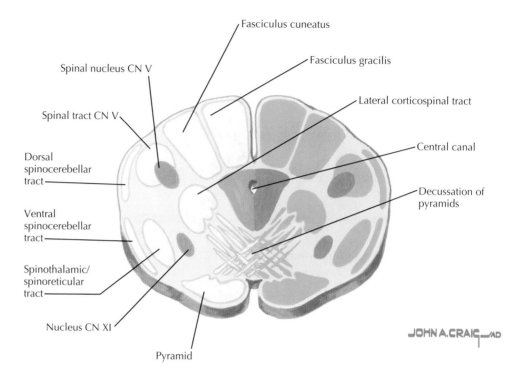

Fasciculus cuneatus

Fasciculus gracilis

Spinal nucleus CN V

Spinal tract CN V

Lateral corticospinal tract

Central canal

Dorsal spinocerebellar tract

Decussation of pyramids

Ventral spinocerebellar tract

Spinothalamic/ spinoreticular tract

Nucleus CN XI

Pyramid

JOHN A. CRAIG—MD

Labelled image available on www.studentconsult.com. If you have not registered for free access to this site, look for your pin code inside front cover.

BRAIN STEM CROSS-SECTIONAL ANATOMY

11.1 BRAIN STEM CROSS-SECTIONAL ANATOMY: SECTION 1

Illustrations of brain stem cross-sections (11.1 through 11.14) are arranged from caudal to rostral, from the spinal-medullary junction to the rostral mesencephalon-diencephalon junction;

T1-weighted magnetic resonance images of the brain stem and surrounding tissue are provided for each level. CN, cranial nerve.

Medulla–Level of the Dorsal Column Nuclei

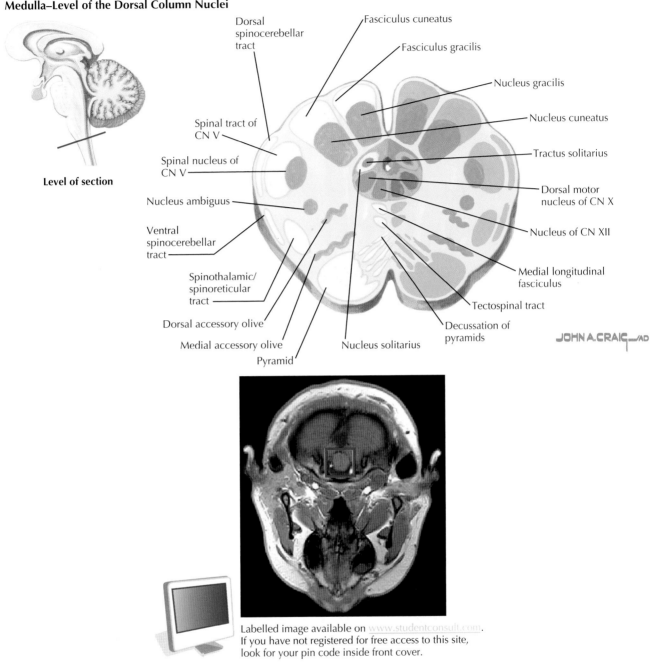

Level of section

Dorsal spinocerebellar tract

Fasciculus cuneatus

Fasciculus gracilis

Nucleus gracilis

Nucleus cuneatus

Spinal tract of CN V

Tractus solitarius

Spinal nucleus of CN V

Nucleus ambiguus

Dorsal motor nucleus of CN X

Ventral spinocerebellar tract

Nucleus of CN XII

Spinothalamic/ spinoreticular tract

Medial longitudinal fasciculus

Dorsal accessory olive

Tectospinal tract

Medial accessory olive

Nucleus solitarius

Decussation of pyramids

Pyramid

JOHN A.CRAIG—AD

Labelled image available on www.studentconsult.com.
If you have not registered for free access to this site,
look for your pin code inside front cover.

11.2 BRAIN STEM CROSS-SECTIONAL ANATOMY: SECTION 2

CLINICAL POINT

Several groups of LMNs are present in the lower brain stem, including those supplying the tongue (CN XII), the pharynx and larynx (nucleus ambiguus), and the face (CN VII). Neurodegeneration of these brain stem LMNs can occur in bulbar polio, amyotrophic lateral sclerosis, and other LMN diseases. The affected muscles are atrophic and flaccid. Such a condition is called bulbar palsy (or progressive bulbar paralysis), an LMN disorder, accompanied by loss of movement, tone, and reflexes. The tongue is weak and atrophic, and the patient cannot speak or vocalize (dysarthria or anarthria, not aphasia) and cannot swallow (dysphagia); as a consequence the patient may aspirate in an attempt to swallow. This LMN condition must be distinguished from UMN lesions which, when bilateral, can also result in dysphonia, dysphagia, and weakened bulbar muscles. This UMN condition is called pseudobulbar palsy or spastic bulbar palsy. In this condition, the muscles are not atrophic, and reflexes (jaw jerk and facial reflexes) are brisk. In amyotrophic lateral sclerosis, both LMN and UMN degeneration may occur progressively during the course of the disease. Because the LMNs are the final common pathway to the muscles, the LMN state usually progresses; once the LMNs have degenerated, continuing UMN damage does not make a difference functionally.

Medulla–Level of the Obex

Level of section

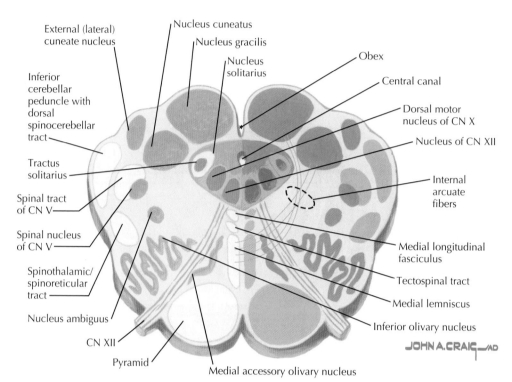

External (lateral) cuneate nucleus

Nucleus cuneatus

Nucleus gracilis

Nucleus solitarius

Obex

Central canal

Inferior cerebellar peduncle with dorsal spinocerebellar tract

Dorsal motor nucleus of CN X

Nucleus of CN XII

Internal arcuate fibers

Tractus solitarius

Spinal tract of CN V

Spinal nucleus of CN V

Spinothalamic/ spinoreticular tract

Nucleus ambiguus

CN XII

Pyramid

Medial accessory olivary nucleus

Medial longitudinal fasciculus

Tectospinal tract

Medial lemniscus

Inferior olivary nucleus

JOHN A. CRAIG—AD

Labelled image available on www.studentconsult.com. If you have not registered for free access to this site, look for your pin code inside front cover.

11.3 BRAIN STEM CROSS-SECTIONAL ANATOMY: SECTION 3

Medulla–Level of the Inferior Olive

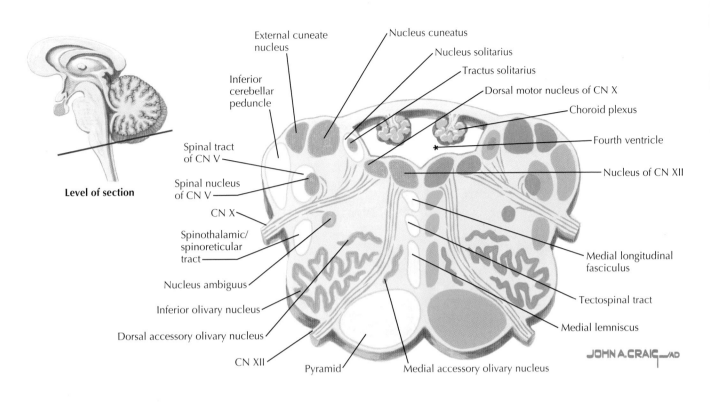

Level of section

External cuneate nucleus

Inferior cerebellar peduncle

Spinal tract of CN V

Spinal nucleus of CN V

CN X

Spinothalamic/spinoreticular tract

Nucleus ambiguus

Inferior olivary nucleus

Dorsal accessory olivary nucleus

CN XII

Pyramid

Nucleus cuneatus

Nucleus solitarius

Tractus solitarius

Dorsal motor nucleus of CN X

Choroid plexus

Fourth ventricle

Nucleus of CN XII

Medial longitudinal fasciculus

Tectospinal tract

Medial lemniscus

Medial accessory olivary nucleus

JOHN A. CRAIG—AD

Labelled image available on www.studentconsult.com.
If you have not registered for free access to this site,
look for your pin code inside front cover.

11.4 BRAIN STEM CROSS-SECTIONAL ANATOMY: SECTION 4

CLINICAL POINT

The medulla is supplied with blood by the paramedian and circumferential branches of the anterior spinal artery and the vertebral arteries. A major circumferential branch of the vertebral artery, the posterior inferior cerebellar artery supplies a lateral wedge of medulla with blood. A brain stem stroke or an infarct in a vertebral artery or in the posterior inferior cerebellar artery produces a complex of symptoms called the lateral medullary syndrome (Wallenberg syndrome), which is caused by damage to an array of nuclei and tracts. The patient can demonstrate (1) loss of pain and temperature sensation on the ipsilateral side of the face (descending nucleus and tract of V) and the contralateral side of the body (spinothalamic/spinoreticular system); (2) dysphagia and dysarthria (paralysis of ipsilateral pharyngeal and laryngeal muscles resulting from damage to the ipsilateral nucleus ambiguus); (3) ataxia of the limbs and falling to the ipsilateral side (inferior cerebellar peduncle and its afferent tracts); (4) vertigo with nausea, vomiting, and nystagmus (vestibular nuclei); and (5) ipsilateral Horner's syndrome, with ptosis, miosis, and anhidrosis (descending axons from the hypothalamus to the T1–T2 intermediolateral cell column of the spinal cord).

Medulla–Level of the CN X and the Vestibular Nuclei

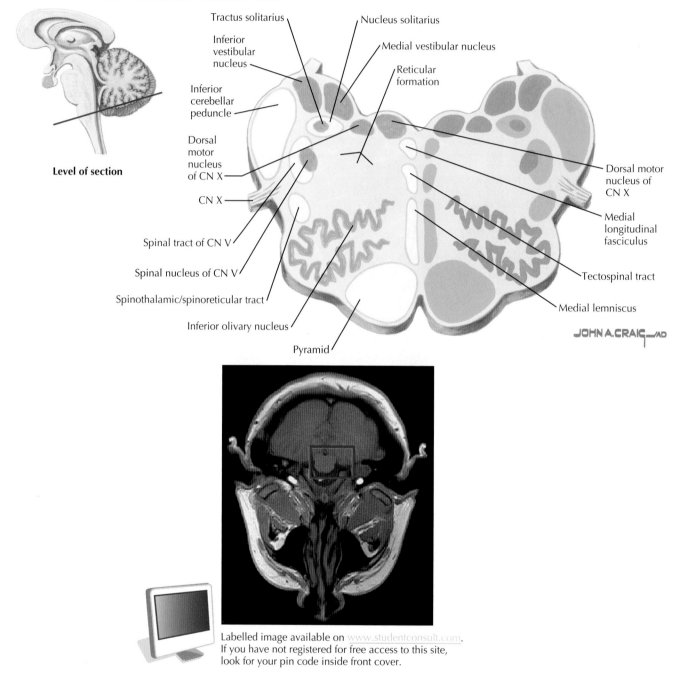

Level of section

Tractus solitarius

Nucleus solitarius

Inferior vestibular nucleus

Medial vestibular nucleus

Reticular formation

Inferior cerebellar peduncle

Dorsal motor nucleus of CN X

Dorsal motor nucleus of CN X

CN X

Medial longitudinal fasciculus

Spinal tract of CN V

Spinal nucleus of CN V

Tectospinal tract

Spinothalamic/spinoreticular tract

Medial lemniscus

Inferior olivary nucleus

Pyramid

JOHN A. CRAIG AD

Labelled image available on www.studentconsult.com. If you have not registered for free access to this site, look for your pin code inside front cover.

11.5 BRAIN STEM CROSS-SECTIONAL ANATOMY: SECTION 5

Medullo-Pontine Junction–Level of the Cochlear Nuclei

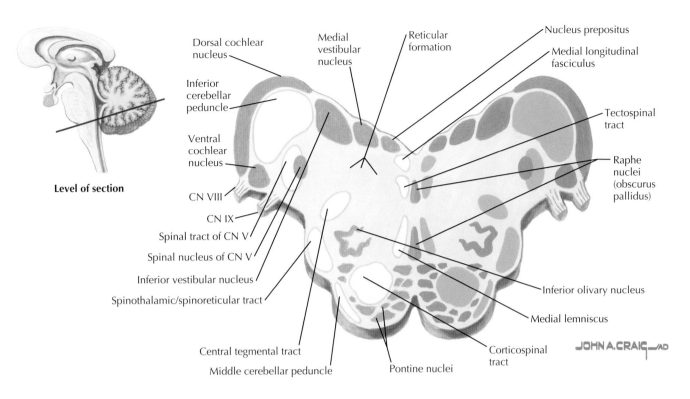

Level of section

Dorsal cochlear nucleus

Inferior cerebellar peduncle

Ventral cochlear nucleus

CN VIII

CN IX

Spinal tract of CN V

Spinal nucleus of CN V

Inferior vestibular nucleus

Spinothalamic/spinoreticular tract

Central tegmental tract

Middle cerebellar peduncle

Medial vestibular nucleus

Reticular formation

Pontine nuclei

Nucleus prepositus

Medial longitudinal fasciculus

Tectospinal tract

Raphe nuclei (obscurus pallidus)

Inferior olivary nucleus

Medial lemniscus

Corticospinal tract

JOHN A. CRAIG—AD

Labelled image available on www.studentconsult.com. If you have not registered for free access to this site, look for your pin code inside front cover.

11.6 BRAIN STEM CROSS-SECTIONAL ANATOMY: SECTION 6

CLINICAL POINT

Occlusion of a paramedian branch of the basilar artery in the lower pons results in medial inferior pontine syndrome. This vascular syndrome causes (1) contralateral hemiparesis (corticospinal system) and contralateral drooping of the lower face (corticobulbar fibers); (2) loss of fine, discriminative touch, vibratory sensation, and joint position sense on the contralateral body that is more severe in the upper extremity (medial lemniscus); (3) limb ataxia and gait ataxia (pontine nuclei and bilateral crossing connections going into the middle cerebellar peduncles); (4) paralysis of lateral gaze by the ipsilateral eye, with diplopia (abducens nerve, nucleus); (5) paralysis of conjugate gaze to ipsilateral side, with preservation of convergence (parapontine reticular formation); and (6) diplopia on attempted lateral gaze to the contralateral side, called internuclear ophthalmoplegia (medial longitudinal fasciculus).

Pons–Level of the Facial Nucleus

Level of section

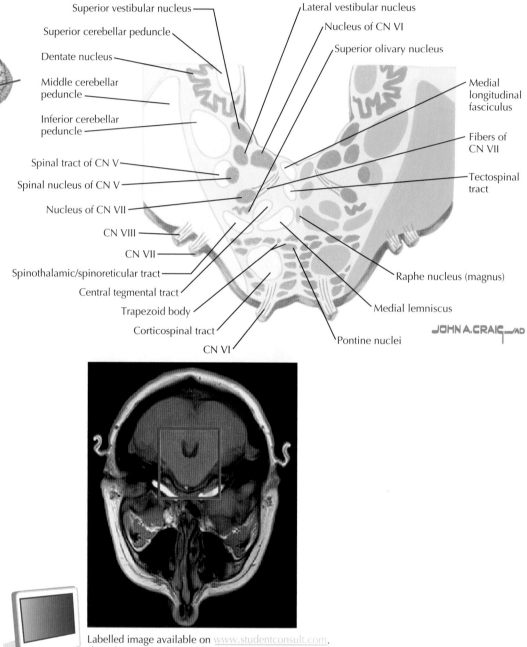

Superior vestibular nucleus

Superior cerebellar peduncle

Dentate nucleus

Middle cerebellar peduncle

Inferior cerebellar peduncle

Spinal tract of CN V

Spinal nucleus of CN V

Nucleus of CN VII

CN VIII

CN VII

Spinothalamic/spinoreticular tract

Central tegmental tract

Trapezoid body

Corticospinal tract

CN VI

Lateral vestibular nucleus

Nucleus of CN VI

Superior olivary nucleus

Medial longitudinal fasciculus

Fibers of CN VII

Tectospinal tract

Raphe nucleus (magnus)

Medial lemniscus

Pontine nuclei

JOHN A. CRAIG—AD

Labelled image available on www.studentconsult.com.
If you have not registered for free access to this site,
look for your pin code inside front cover.

11.7 BRAIN STEM CROSS-SECTIONAL ANATOMY: SECTION 7

Pons–Level of the Genu of the Facial Nerve

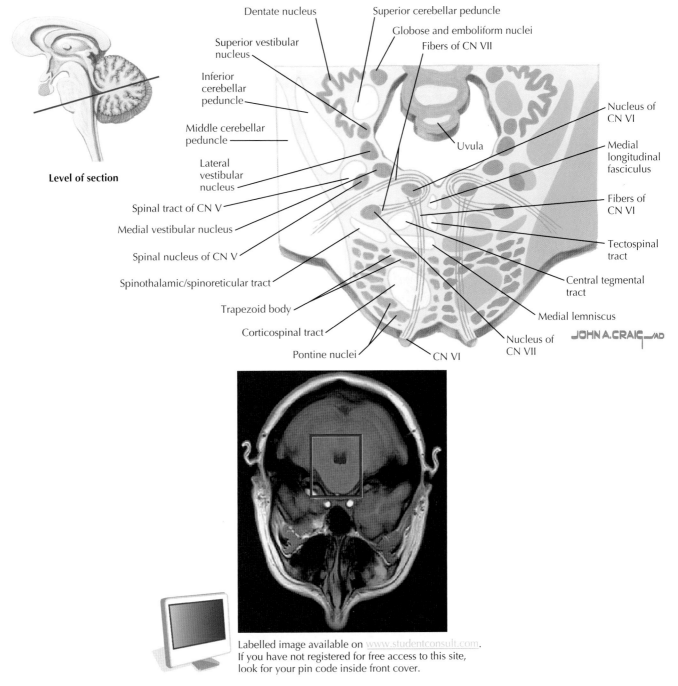

Level of section

Dentate nucleus

Superior cerebellar peduncle

Globose and emboliform nuclei

Fibers of CN VII

Superior vestibular nucleus

Inferior cerebellar peduncle

Middle cerebellar peduncle

Lateral vestibular nucleus

Spinal tract of CN V

Medial vestibular nucleus

Spinal nucleus of CN V

Spinothalamic/spinoreticular tract

Trapezoid body

Corticospinal tract

Pontine nuclei

Uvula

Nucleus of CN VI

Medial longitudinal fasciculus

Fibers of CN VI

Tectospinal tract

Central tegmental tract

Medial lemniscus

Nucleus of CN VII

CN VI

JOHN A. CRAIG—AD

Labelled image available on www.studentconsult.com.
If you have not registered for free access to this site,
look for your pin code inside front cover.

11.8 BRAIN STEM CROSS-SECTIONAL ANATOMY: SECTION 8

CLINICAL POINT

The pons is a common site for a hemorrhagic stroke. A pontine hemorrhage is commonly large and lethal. When not fatal, such a hemorrhage may result in the rapid progression of (1) total paralysis (quadriplegia); (2) decerebrate posturing (extensor posturing) caused by UMN damage to the corticospinal and rubrospinal systems, thereby disinhibiting the lateral vestibular nuclei; (3) coma; (4) paralysis of ocular movements; and (5) small but reactive pupils. A pontine hemorrhage that results in coma is commonly lethal. A large infarct in the basilar artery may produce the same clinical picture. Some small, lacunar infarcts also may occur in the pons; these infarcts may produce purely motor symptoms (contralateral UMN paresis at base of pons), ataxia, or both (cerebellar peduncles, pontine nuclei).

Pons–Level of Trigeminal Motor and Main Sensory Nuclei

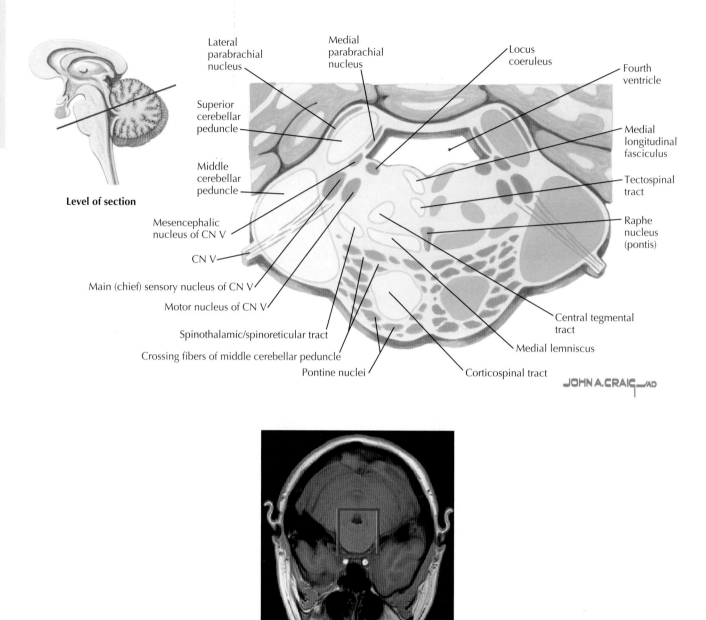

Level of section

Lateral parabrachial nucleus

Medial parabrachial nucleus

Locus coeruleus

Fourth ventricle

Superior cerebellar peduncle

Medial longitudinal fasciculus

Middle cerebellar peduncle

Tectospinal tract

Mesencephalic nucleus of CN V

Raphe nucleus (pontis)

CN V

Main (chief) sensory nucleus of CN V

Motor nucleus of CN V

Central tegmental tract

Spinothalamic/spinoreticular tract

Crossing fibers of middle cerebellar peduncle

Medial lemniscus

Pontine nuclei

Corticospinal tract

JOHN A. CRAIG ᴀᴅ

Labelled image available on www.studentconsult.com.
If you have not registered for free access to this site,
look for your pin code inside front cover.

11.9 BRAIN STEM CROSS-SECTIONAL ANATOMY: SECTION 9

CLINICAL POINT

A vascular lesion of circumferential branches of the basilar artery or the anterior inferior cerebellar artery can cause lateral pontine syndrome, which is characterized by (1) contralateral loss of sensation in the body, both epicritic and protopathic (medial lemniscus and anterolateral system); (2) loss of pain and temperature sensation on the contralateral face (ventral trigeminal lemniscus, located on dorsal surface of the medial lemniscus); (3) loss of fine, discriminative touch (main sensory nucleus of CN V) or impaired general sensation (CN V fibers) on the ipsilateral face; (4) ipsilateral paralysis of muscles of mastication (motor nucleus of CN V); (5) limb ataxia (middle and superior cerebellar peduncles); (6) paralysis of conjugate gaze to the ipsilateral side (parapontine reticular formation and its connections); and (7) other possible ipsilateral brain stem problems, depending on the extent of the vascular involvement, such as deafness or tinnitus (auditory nuclei or nerve fibers); vertigo and nystagmus (vestibular nuclei or nerve fibers); facial palsy (CN VII nucleus or nerve fibers); and Horner's syndrome (descending hypothalamo-spinal sympathetic connections).

Pons-Midbrain Junction–Level of CN IV and Locus Coeruleus

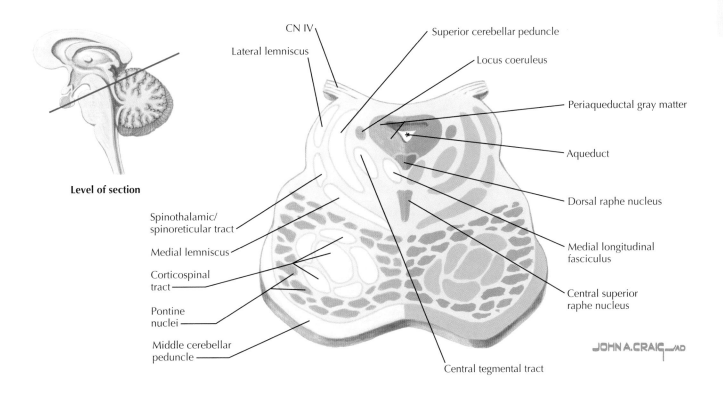

Level of section

CN IV
Lateral lemniscus
Superior cerebellar peduncle
Locus coeruleus
Periaqueductal gray matter
Aqueduct
Dorsal raphe nucleus
Spinothalamic/spinoreticular tract
Medial lemniscus
Corticospinal tract
Pontine nuclei
Middle cerebellar peduncle
Medial longitudinal fasciculus
Central superior raphe nucleus
Central tegmental tract

JOHN A. CRAIG—AD

Labelled image available on www.studentconsult.com.
If you have not registered for free access to this site,
look for your pin code inside front cover.

11.10 **BRAIN STEM CROSS-SECTIONAL ANATOMY: SECTION 10**

Midbrain–Level of the Inferior Colliculus

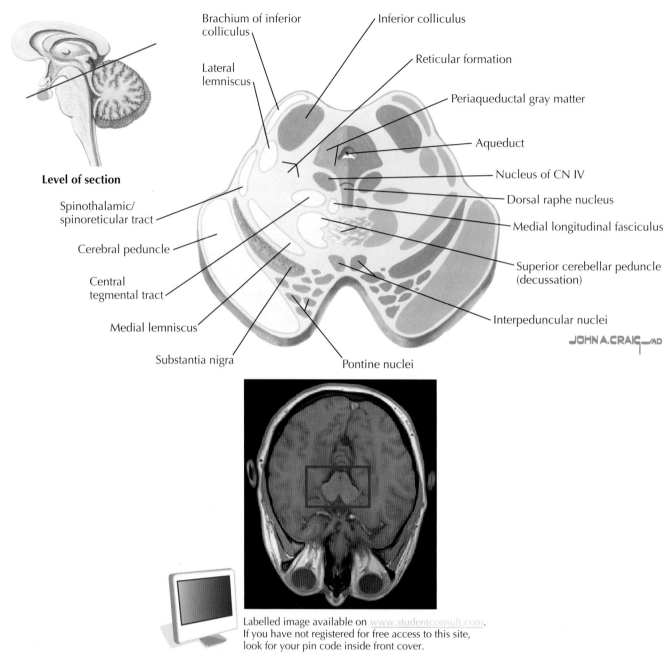

Level of section

- Brachium of inferior colliculus
- Lateral lemniscus
- Inferior colliculus
- Reticular formation
- Periaqueductal gray matter
- Aqueduct
- Nucleus of CN IV
- Dorsal raphe nucleus
- Medial longitudinal fasciculus
- Superior cerebellar peduncle (decussation)
- Interpeduncular nuclei
- Spinothalamic/ spinoreticular tract
- Cerebral peduncle
- Central tegmental tract
- Medial lemniscus
- Substantia nigra
- Pontine nuclei

JOHN A.CRAIG—AD

Labelled image available on www.studentconsult.com.
If you have not registered for free access to this site,
look for your pin code inside front cover.

11.11 BRAIN STEM CROSS-SECTIONAL ANATOMY: SECTION 11

CLINICAL POINT

A space-occupying lesion in the forebrain, such as a bleed (epidural or subdural hematoma), a tumor, or increased intracranial pressure resulting from a variety of causes, can cause herniation of the forebrain through the tentorium cerebelli. This transtentorial herniation displaces the thalamus and upper midbrain in a downward direction and causes a variety of changes in brain function. These changes are characterized by functions attributable to the remaining intact lower midbrain and more caudal structures, with loss of function of the upper midbrain and more rostral structures. Most conspicuous is a progressive deterioration of the state of consciousness, rapidly going from drowsiness to stupor to an unarousable state of coma; consciousness requires an intact brain stem reticular formation and at least one functioning cerebral hemisphere. When both hemispheres are nonfunctional, coma ensues. With the loss of activity in the corticospinal system and the rubrospinal system and removal of cortical influence on the other UMN pathways, a state of decerebration occurs (called decerebrate rigidity, although it is really spasticity, not true rigidity). The neck is extended (opisthotonus), the arms and legs are extended and rotated inward, and the hands, fingers, feet, and toes are flexed. Plantar responses are extensor. Cheyne-Stokes respiration is seen (crescendo-decrescendo breathing), followed at a slightly later stage of damage by shallow hyperventilation. The pupils are midsized and usually unresponsive because of compression of the third nerves against the free edge of the tentorium. Caloric testing or the doll's-eye maneuver shows no vertical eye movements (visual tectal damage), and the eyes do not move in a conjugate fashion.

Midbrain–Level of the Superior Colliculus

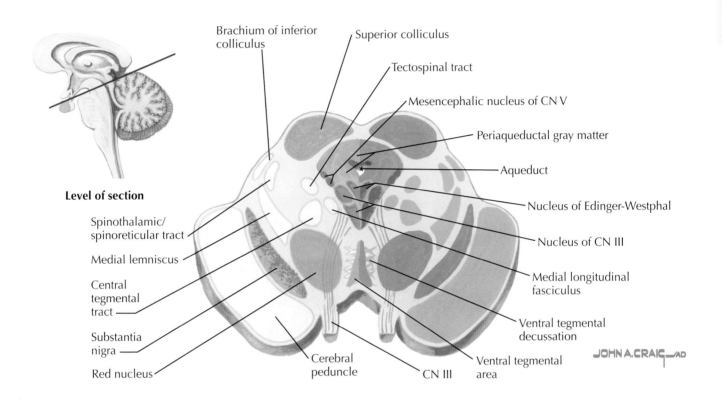

Brachium of inferior colliculus

Superior colliculus

Tectospinal tract

Mesencephalic nucleus of CN V

Periaqueductal gray matter

Aqueduct

Nucleus of Edinger-Westphal

Nucleus of CN III

Medial longitudinal fasciculus

Ventral tegmental decussation

Ventral tegmental area

CN III

Cerebral peduncle

Red nucleus

Substantia nigra

Central tegmental tract

Medial lemniscus

Spinothalamic/ spinoreticular tract

Level of section

JOHN A.CRAIG—AD

Labelled image available on www.studentconsult.com. If you have not registered for free access to this site, look for your pin code inside front cover.

11.12 BRAIN STEM CROSS-SECTIONAL ANATOMY: SECTION 12

Midbrain–Level of the Medial Geniculate Body

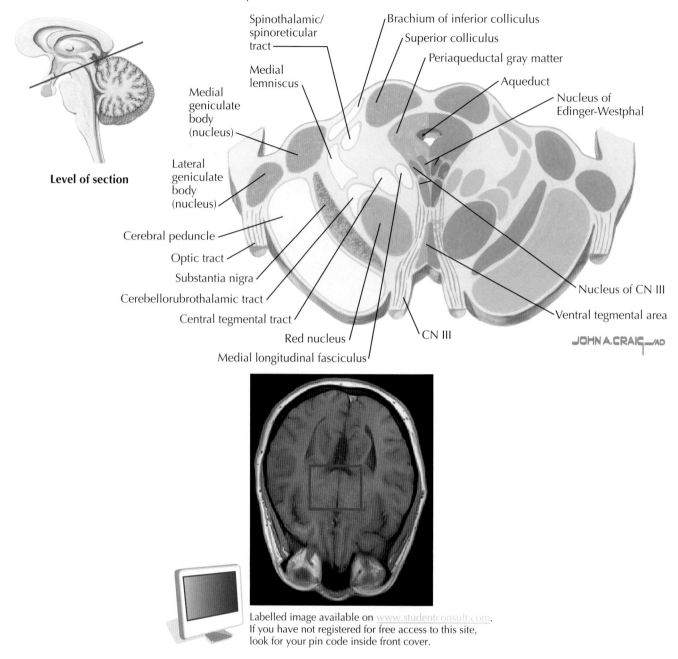

Level of section

Spinothalamic/spinoreticular tract

Medial lemniscus

Medial geniculate body (nucleus)

Lateral geniculate body (nucleus)

Cerebral peduncle

Optic tract

Substantia nigra

Cerebellorubrothalamic tract

Central tegmental tract

Red nucleus

Medial longitudinal fasciculus

Brachium of inferior colliculus

Superior colliculus

Periaqueductal gray matter

Aqueduct

Nucleus of Edinger-Westphal

Nucleus of CN III

Ventral tegmental area

CN III

JOHN A. CRAIG—AD

Labelled image available on www.studentconsult.com.
If you have not registered for free access to this site,
look for your pin code inside front cover.

11.13 BRAIN STEM CROSS-SECTIONAL ANATOMY: SECTION 13

CLINICAL POINT

Paramedian regions of the upper midbrain receive their blood supply mainly from branches of the posterior cerebral and posterior communicating arteries. A vascular lesion at this level (Weber's syndrome) results in damage to the exiting third nerve fibers, the medial and central portions of the cerebral peduncle, and some passing tracts. A supratentorial mass lesion also can cause lateral and downward compression of one cerebral peduncle and the third nerve against the free edge of the tentorium cerebelli, presenting a similar clinical picture. Compression of the cerebral peduncle with possible involvement of the red nucleus on the affected side produces contralateral hemiplegia, rapidly evolving to a spastic state with a plantar extensor response. A central (lower) facial palsy occurs because of damage to corticobulbar fibers, which travel in the cerebral peduncle. An ipsilateral oculomotor palsy also occurs, with the ipsilateral eye deviated laterally and the ipsilateral pupil fixed (unresponsive to light) and dilated because of unopposed actions of the sympathetics. If the lesion involves the substantia nigra, red nucleus, pallidothalamic fibers, or dentatorubral and dentatothalamic fibers, contralateral movement problems may occur, including akinesia, intention tremor, or choreoathetoid movements. Damage to these later structures, with their accompanying contralateral problems, may occur in isolation along with third-nerve damage caused by more distal vascular involvement of the paramedian branches to the upper midbrain (Benedict's syndrome).

Midbrain-Diencephalon Junction–Level of the Posterior Commissure

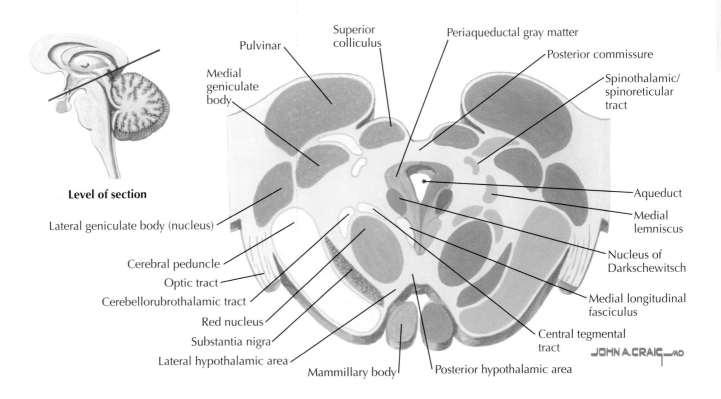

Level of section

Pulvinar

Medial geniculate body

Superior colliculus

Periaqueductal gray matter

Posterior commissure

Spinothalamic/ spinoreticular tract

Aqueduct

Medial lemniscus

Nucleus of Darkschewitsch

Medial longitudinal fasciculus

Central tegmental tract

Lateral geniculate body (nucleus)

Cerebral peduncle

Optic tract

Cerebellorubrothalamic tract

Red nucleus

Substantia nigra

Lateral hypothalamic area

Mammillary body

Posterior hypothalamic area

JOHN A.CRAIG—AD

Labelled image available on www.studentconsult.com. If you have not registered for free access to this site, look for your pin code inside front cover.

11.14 BRAIN STEM CROSS-SECTIONAL ANATOMY: SECTION 14

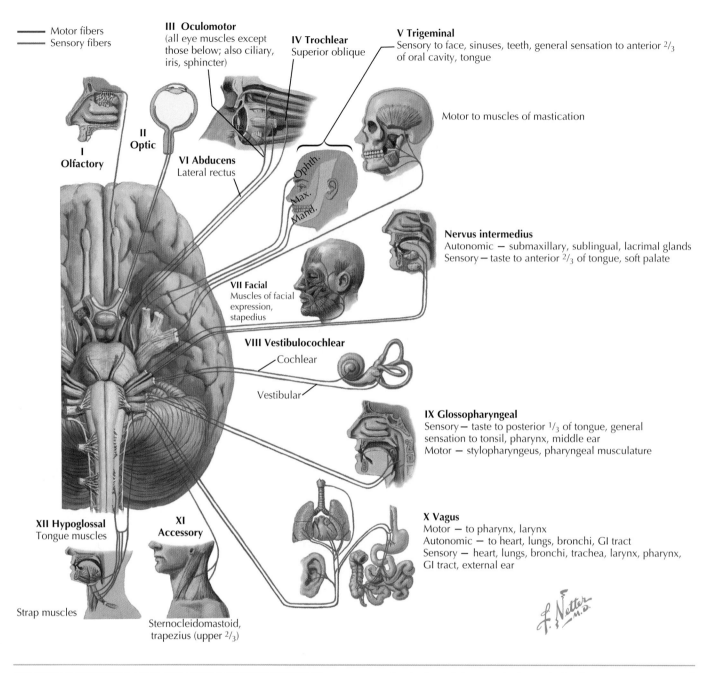

Motor fibers
Sensory fibers

III Oculomotor
(all eye muscles except those below; also ciliary, iris, sphincter)

IV Trochlear
Superior oblique

V Trigeminal
Sensory to face, sinuses, teeth, general sensation to anterior $^2/_3$ of oral cavity, tongue

Motor to muscles of mastication

II Optic

I Olfactory

VI Abducens
Lateral rectus

Ophth.
Max.
Mand.

Nervus intermedius
Autonomic — submaxillary, sublingual, lacrimal glands
Sensory — taste to anterior $^2/_3$ of tongue, soft palate

VII Facial
Muscles of facial expression, stapedius

VIII Vestibulocochlear
Cochlear
Vestibular

IX Glossopharyngeal
Sensory — taste to posterior $^1/_3$ of tongue, general sensation to tonsil, pharynx, middle ear
Motor — stylopharyngeus, pharyngeal musculature

XII Hypoglossal
Tongue muscles

XI Accessory

X Vagus
Motor — to pharynx, larynx
Autonomic — to heart, lungs, bronchi, GI tract
Sensory — heart, lungs, bronchi, trachea, larynx, pharynx, GI tract, external ear

Strap muscles

Sternocleidomastoid, trapezius (upper $^2/_3$)

CRANIAL NERVES AND CRANIAL NERVE NUCLEI

11.15 CRANIAL NERVES: SCHEMATIC OF DISTRIBUTION OF SENSORY, MOTOR, AND AUTONOMIC FIBERS

CNs I and II, both sensory, are tracts of the central nervous system (CNS) that are derived from the neural tube and myelinated by oligodendroglia. CNs III–XII emerge from the brain stem and supply sensory (CNs V, VII–X); motor (CNs III–VII and IX–XII); and autonomic (CNs III, VII, IX, X) nerve fibers to structures in the head and neck. All of the CNs that emerge from the brain stem distribute ipsilaterally to their target structures. With the exception of CN nucleus IV (trochlear) and some motor components of CN nucleus III (oculomotor), the CN nuclei are located ipsilateral to the point of emergence of the CN. The spinal accessory portion of CN XI emerges from motor neurons in the

rostral spinal cord; it ascends through the foramen magnum and then exits with CNs IX and X; thus it is considered a CN.

CLINICAL POINT

Multiple CNs can be affected by some pathological conditions, such as tumors and granulomas, brain stem infarcts, leptomeningeal carcinomatosis, and aneurysms. Extramedullary pathology affects mainly the sensory, motor, and autonomic components of the involved CNs: internal pathology in the brain stem also involves the long tracts. An aneurysm in the cavernous sinus may involve CNs III–VI. A large tumor in the middle cranial fossa in the retrosphenoid space may affect cranial nerves III–VI. A large tumor in the cerebellopontine angle involves CNs VII and VIII and sometimes expands to involve V and IX. Tumors and aneurysms in the jugular foramen may involve CNs IX, X, and XI. Granulomatous lesions such as sarcoids in the posterior retroparotid space may affect cranial nerves IX–XII as well as the sympathetic nerves to the head.

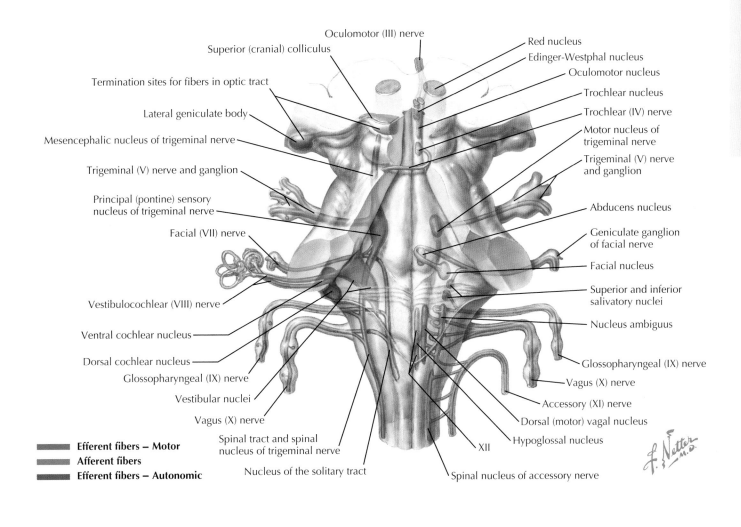

Oculomotor (III) nerve

Superior (cranial) colliculus

Termination sites for fibers in optic tract

Lateral geniculate body

Mesencephalic nucleus of trigeminal nerve

Trigeminal (V) nerve and ganglion

Principal (pontine) sensory nucleus of trigeminal nerve

Facial (VII) nerve

Vestibulocochlear (VIII) nerve

Ventral cochlear nucleus

Dorsal cochlear nucleus

Glossopharyngeal (IX) nerve

Vestibular nuclei

Vagus (X) nerve

Spinal tract and spinal nucleus of trigeminal nerve

Nucleus of the solitary tract

Red nucleus

Edinger-Westphal nucleus

Oculomotor nucleus

Trochlear nucleus

Trochlear (IV) nerve

Motor nucleus of trigeminal nerve

Trigeminal (V) nerve and ganglion

Abducens nucleus

Geniculate ganglion of facial nerve

Facial nucleus

Superior and inferior salivatory nuclei

Nucleus ambiguus

Glossopharyngeal (IX) nerve

Vagus (X) nerve

Accessory (XI) nerve

Dorsal (motor) vagal nucleus

Hypoglossal nucleus

XII

Spinal nucleus of accessory nerve

■■■ Efferent fibers – Motor
■■■ Afferent fibers
■■■ Efferent fibers – Autonomic

11.16 CRANIAL NERVES AND THEIR NUCLEI: SCHEMATIC VIEW FROM ABOVE

The LMNs of the brain stem are localized in a medial column (CN motor nuclei for III [oculomotor]; IV [trochlear]; VI [abducens]; and XII [hypoglossal]) and a lateral column (CN motor nuclei for V [trigeminal]; VII [facial]; IX and X [ambiguus]; and XI [spinal accessory]). Preganglionic parasympathetic nuclei are found medially in the Edinger-Westphal nucleus (CN III) and the dorsal (motor) vagal nucleus (CN X) and laterally in the superior (CN VII) and inferior (CN IX) salivatory nuclei. Secondary sensory nuclei include the main sensory and descending nuclei of CN V, the vestibular nuclei and cochlear nuclei (CN VIII), and the nucleus solitarius (CNs VII, IX, and X). The superior colliculus and the lateral geniculate body (nucleus) receive secondary sensory axonal projections from the optic tract; the inferior colliculus receives input from the cochlear nuclei and other accessory auditory nuclei. The nuclei gracilis and cuneatus, located in the medulla, receive input from dorsal root ganglion cells, which convey epicritic somatosensory modalities (fine, discriminative touch, vibratory sensation, joint position sense).

CLINICAL POINT

CNs I, II, V, and VII–X have primary afferent components. CN I, the olfactory nerve, is a CNS tract and terminates directly in limbic forebrain structures, unlike any other CNs. CN II, the optic nerve, also is a CNS tract; its retinal ganglion cells act as a secondary sensory nucleus, projecting to the thalamus (lateral geniculate body), superior colliculus, pretectum, suprachiasmatic nucleus of the hypothalamus, and other brain stem sites. CNs V and VII–X can be affected by peripheral nerve problems, such as demyelinating disease (Guillain-Barré syndrome), neuropathies (diabetic), tumors, vascular infarcts, traumas, and other pathology; these nerve problems generally result in loss of the specific sensory modality carried by that nerve. Secondary sensory CN nuclei associated with the peripheral CNs (III–XII) include the trigeminal nuclei (main sensory, descending [spinal] nucleus), nucleus solitarius, cochlear nuclei (dorsal and ventral), and vestibular nuclei (medial, lateral, inferior, superior). These nuclei can be damaged by vascular infarcts, tumors, and other pathology; such pathology often involves other central nuclei and long tracts and produces syndromes that clearly indicate CNS pathology (e.g., UMN damage). Involvement of some secondary sensory cranial nerve nuclei (e.g., the descending nucleus of CN V damaged by a posterior inferior cerebellar artery infarct) results in a dissociated loss of a specific set of modalities (pain and temperature) in the innervated territory (ipsilateral face); a trigeminal nerve lesion on one side results in total anesthesia in the innervated territory.

Medial dissection

Red nucleus

Oculomotor nerve (III)

Mesencephalic nucleus of trigeminal nerve

Trigeminal nerve (V) and ganglion

Principal sensory nucleus of trigeminal nerve

Motor nucleus of trigeminal nerve

Facial nerve (VII)

Vestibulocochlear nerve (VIII)

Abducens nerve (VI)

Glossopharyngeal nerve (IX)

Hypoglossal nerve (XII)

Vagus nerve (X)

Accessory nerve (XI)*

Olive

Spinal tract and spinal nucleus of trigeminal nerve

Accessory oculomotor (Edinger-Westphal) nucleus

Oculomotor nucleus

Trochlear nucleus

Trochlear nerve (IV)

Abducens nucleus

Internal genu of facial nerve

Facial nucleus

Vestibular nuclei

Anterior and posterior cochlear nuclei

Superior and inferior salivatory nuclei

Solitary tract nucleus

Posterior (dorsal) nucleus of vagus nerve (X)

Hypoglossal nucleus

Nucleus ambiguus

Spinal nucleus of accessory nerve

■ Efferent fibers
■ Afferent fibers
■ Mixed fibers

*Evidence suggests that the accessory nerve lacks a cranial root and has no connection to the vagus nerve. Verification of this finding awaits further investigation.

11.17 CRANIAL NERVES AND THEIR NUCLEI: SCHEMATIC LATERAL VIEW

CN III exits from the ventral and medial surface of the mid-brain. CN IV is the only CN to exit from the dorsal surface of the brain stem, in the midbrain near the pons-midbrain junction. CN V exits from the lateral surface of the mid pons. CN VI exits from the pons medially, just rostral to the medullo-pontine junction. CNs VII and VIII exit from the cerebello-pontine angle at the junction of the medulla and pons. CNs IX and X exit from the lateral part of the medulla and are joined by CN XI, which ascends through the foramen magnum. CN XII exits medially from the preolivary sulcus. These CN sites of entry and exit are important localizing features in the brain stem that permit regional localization of lesions resulting from vascular insults, tumors, and degenerative disorders.

CLINICAL POINT

The CN nuclei that contain LMNs are found in two longitudinal columns, including a medial column (CN nuclei III, IV, VI, and XII) and a lateral column (motor CN nuclei V, VII, and nucleus ambiguus). These LMN groups are found in the CNS and send axons into the peripheral nervous system to synapse on their appropriate groups of skeletal muscles using acetylcholine, and they exert important trophic influences on their innervated muscles. An LMN lesion (bulbar polio, amyotrophic lateral sclerosis, and other LMN palsies) results in total paralysis of the affected muscle; atrophy is caused by denervation, loss of tone, and loss of reflexes. Denervated muscles commonly demonstrate denervation hypersensitivity, with resultant fibrillation as seen on an electromyogram. As LMNs die (particularly conspicuous in amyotrophic lateral sclerosis) their agonal electrical responses occur as spontaneous discharges of individual motor units (an LMN and its innervated muscle fibers); each discharge produces a visible fasciculation (or twitch). With some LMN disorders such as polio, if enough neighboring LMNs survive, their axons can sprout and reinnervate previously denervated skeletal muscle fibers; this process must occur within approximately 1 year, or the atrophy becomes permanent. In UMN paralysis, in which the LMNs do not die, the affected muscle fibers are not denervated; reflexes are brisk, tone is increased with passive stretch (spasticity), and pathological reflexes (plantar extensor response) are seen.

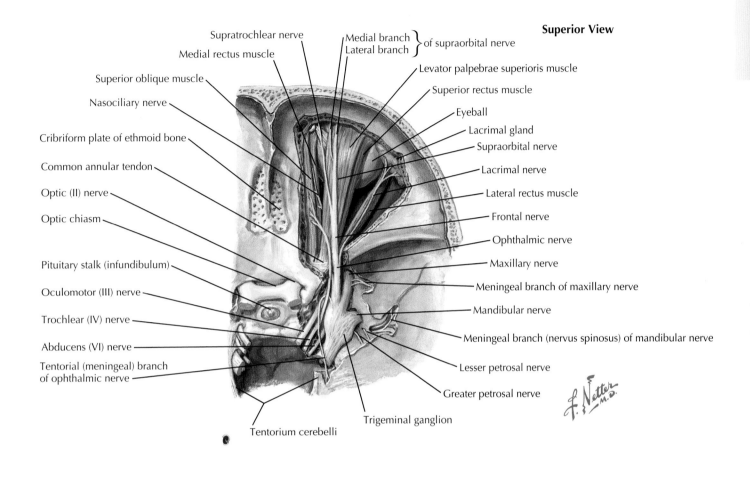

Superior View

Supratrochlear nerve

Medial rectus muscle

Superior oblique muscle

Nasociliary nerve

Cribriform plate of ethmoid bone

Common annular tendon

Optic (II) nerve

Optic chiasm

Pituitary stalk (infundibulum)

Oculomotor (III) nerve

Trochlear (IV) nerve

Abducens (VI) nerve

Tentorial (meningeal) branch
of ophthalmic nerve

Medial branch ⎫
Lateral branch ⎭ of supraorbital nerve

Levator palpebrae superioris muscle

Superior rectus muscle

Eyeball

Lacrimal gland

Supraorbital nerve

Lacrimal nerve

Lateral rectus muscle

Frontal nerve

Ophthalmic nerve

Maxillary nerve

Meningeal branch of maxillary nerve

Mandibular nerve

Meningeal branch (nervus spinosus) of mandibular nerve

Lesser petrosal nerve

Greater petrosal nerve

Trigeminal ganglion

Tentorium cerebelli

11.18 NERVES OF THE ORBIT

CN II carries visual information from the ipsilateral retina. Axons from the temporal hemiretinas remain ipsilateral, whereas axons from the nasal hemiretinas cross the midline in the optic chiasm. All axons then enter the optic tract. CNs III (from oculomotor nuclei), IV, and VI innervate the extrinsic muscles of the eye. Sensory portions of the ophthalmic division of V supply general sensation to the cornea and eyeball and provide the afferent limb of the corneal reflex. Motor fibers of CN VII innervate the orbicularis oculi muscle, closing the eye; these fibers constitute the efferent limb of the corneal reflex.

CLINICAL POINT

CN II (the optic nerve) is a CNS tract myelinated by oligodendroglia. It can be damaged by demyelinating disease (optic neuritis in multiple sclerosis), by optic nerve gliomas, by ischemic injury (central retinal artery), or by trauma (sphenoid fracture). The resultant defect is ipsilateral blindness or a scotoma (blind spot). The ipsilateral nature of the deficit rules out optic chiasm, optic tract, or central visual lesions. The retina also is CNS tissue and can undergo neurodegenerative changes. Macular degeneration involves damage to the cone-intensive regions of the retina (macula) and leads to the inability to read and the loss of acuity. Increased intracranial pressure can result in papilledema, a condition in which pressure pushes the optic nerve head inward (toward the center of the eyeball), producing a swollen appearance on ophthalmoscopy. This process takes 24 hours to occur after onset of intracranial pressure; the presence of papilledema is used diagnostically to identify intracranial pressure.

A. Superior view with extraocular muscles partially cut away

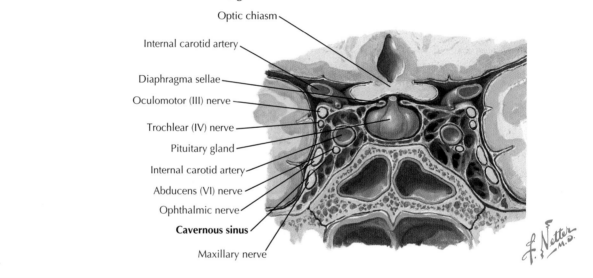

Supratrochlear nerve *(cut)*

Medial and lateral branches of supraorbital nerve *(cut)*

Infratrochlear nerve

Anterior ethmoidal nerve

Long ciliary nerves

Optic (II) nerve

Posterior ethmoidal nerve

Nasociliary nerve

Ophthalmic nerve

Trochlear (IV) nerve *(cut)*

Oculomotor (III) nerve

Abducens (VI) nerve

Levator palpebrae superioris muscle *(cut)*

Superior rectus muscle *(cut)*

Lacrimal nerve *(cut)*

Short ciliary nerves

Branch of oculomotor nerve to inferior oblique muscle

Ciliary ganglion

Motor (parasympathetic) root from oculomotor nerve

Sympathetic root from internal carotid plexus

Sensory root from nasociliary nerve

Branches to medial and inferior rectus muscles

Abducens (VI) nerve (to lateral rectus muscle)

Inferior division of oculomotor nerve

Superior division of oculomotor nerve

B. Coronal section through the cavernous sinus

Optic chiasm

Internal carotid artery

Diaphragma sellae

Oculomotor (III) nerve

Trochlear (IV) nerve

Pituitary gland

Internal carotid artery

Abducens (VI) nerve

Ophthalmic nerve

Cavernous sinus

Maxillary nerve

11.19 NERVES OF THE ORBIT (CONTINUED)

Parasympathetic preganglionic fibers from the nucleus of Edinger-Westphal distribute to the ciliary ganglion, which supplies the pupillary constrictor muscle and the ciliary muscle (accommodation for near vision). Preganglionic parasympathetic axons from the superior salivatory nucleus distribute to the pterygopalatine ganglion, which supplies the lacrimal gland (tear production). Sympathetic postganglionic nerve fibers from the superior cervical ganglion supply the pupillary dilator muscle and the superior tarsal muscle (damage results in mild ptosis). CNs III, IV, VI, and V (ophthalmic and maxillary divisions) traverse the cavernous sinus and are vulnerable to damage by cavernous sinus thrombosis.

CLINICAL POINT

The extraocular nerves can be damaged by trauma, vascular infarcts, tumors, aneurysms, pressure (compression of CN III against the free edge of the tentorium with transtentorial herniation), or other pathology. Oculomotor palsy (CN III) results in paralysis or weakness of the medial rectus, superior and inferior rectus, inferior oblique, and levator palpebrae superioris muscles. The most conspicuous deficit is the inability to adduct the ipsilateral eye, a lateral strabismus (resulting from unopposed action of the lateral rectus), and diplopia. Damage to the levator palpebrae superioris muscle results in profound ptosis of the ipsilateral eye. Lesions in CN III also disrupt the outflow from the Edinger-Westphal nucleus to the ciliary ganglion, producing a fixed (unresponsive) and dilated ipsilateral pupil.

A lesion in CN IV (trochlear) results in paralysis or weakness of the superior oblique muscle. This muscle is a depressor of the eye when it is directed nasally. Thus, a patient has difficulty walking down stairs and stepping off curbs and has trouble reading while lying down. The patient tries to compensate for a lesion in CN IV by turning the head away from the side of the lesion to avoid having to use the paralyzed muscle.

A lesion in CN VI (abducens) results in paralysis or weakness of the ipsilateral lateral rectus muscle, with a resultant medial strabismus and diplopia upon attempted lateral gaze.

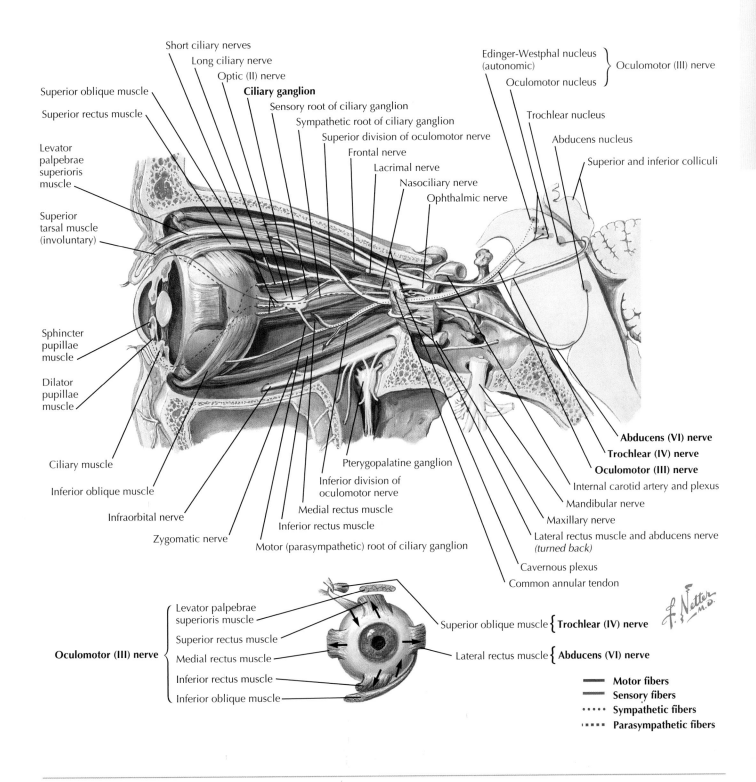

Short ciliary nerves
Long ciliary nerve
Optic (II) nerve
Ciliary ganglion
Sensory root of ciliary ganglion
Sympathetic root of ciliary ganglion
Superior division of oculomotor nerve
Frontal nerve
Lacrimal nerve
Nasociliary nerve
Ophthalmic nerve

Edinger-Westphal nucleus (autonomic)
Oculomotor nucleus } Oculomotor (III) nerve
Trochlear nucleus
Abducens nucleus
Superior and inferior colliculi

Superior oblique muscle
Superior rectus muscle
Levator palpebrae superioris muscle
Superior tarsal muscle (involuntary)
Sphincter pupillae muscle
Dilator pupillae muscle
Ciliary muscle
Inferior oblique muscle
Infraorbital nerve
Zygomatic nerve
Motor (parasympathetic) root of ciliary ganglion
Inferior division of oculomotor nerve
Medial rectus muscle
Inferior rectus muscle
Pterygopalatine ganglion

Abducens (VI) nerve
Trochlear (IV) nerve
Oculomotor (III) nerve
Internal carotid artery and plexus
Mandibular nerve
Maxillary nerve
Lateral rectus muscle and abducens nerve *(turned back)*
Cavernous plexus
Common annular tendon

Oculomotor (III) nerve {
Levator palpebrae superioris muscle
Superior rectus muscle
Medial rectus muscle
Inferior rectus muscle
Inferior oblique muscle

Superior oblique muscle { **Trochlear (IV) nerve**
Lateral rectus muscle { **Abducens (VI) nerve**

— Motor fibers
— Sensory fibers
···· Sympathetic fibers
ıııı Parasympathetic fibers

11.20 EXTRAOCULAR NERVES (III, IV, AND VI) AND THE CILIARY GANGLION: VIEW IN RELATION TO THE EYE

CN VI innervates the lateral rectus muscle; damage results in ipsilateral paralysis of lateral gaze. CN IV innervates the superior oblique muscle; damage results in inability to look in and down (most conspicuous when climbing stairs, stepping off a curb, reading in bed). CN III (oculomotor nuclei) innervates the medial rectus, superior rectus, inferior rectus, and inferior oblique muscles (damage results in paralysis of the ipsilateral medial gaze) and also innervates the levator palpebrae superioris muscle (damage results in profound ptosis). The ciliary ganglion gives rise to postganglionic parasympathetic axons that supply the pupillary constrictor muscle and the ciliary muscle; damage results in a fixed and dilated pupil that does not constrict for the pupillary light reflex and does not accommodate to near vision.

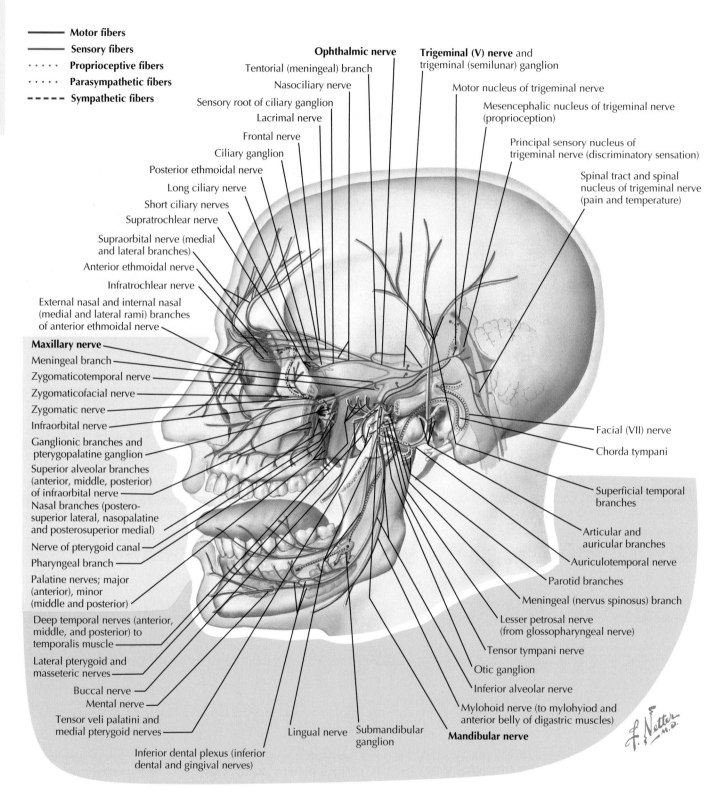

Motor fibers
Sensory fibers
· · · · Proprioceptive fibers
· · · · Parasympathetic fibers
- - - - Sympathetic fibers

Ophthalmic nerve
Tentorial (meningeal) branch
Nasociliary nerve
Sensory root of ciliary ganglion
Lacrimal nerve
Frontal nerve
Ciliary ganglion
Posterior ethmoidal nerve
Long ciliary nerve
Short ciliary nerves
Supratrochlear nerve
Supraorbital nerve (medial and lateral branches)
Anterior ethmoidal nerve
Infratrochlear nerve
External nasal and internal nasal (medial and lateral rami) branches of anterior ethmoidal nerve

Maxillary nerve
Meningeal branch
Zygomaticotemporal nerve
Zygomaticofacial nerve
Zygomatic nerve
Infraorbital nerve
Ganglionic branches and pterygopalatine ganglion
Superior alveolar branches (anterior, middle, posterior) of infraorbital nerve
Nasal branches (postero-superior lateral, nasopalatine and posterosuperior medial)
Nerve of pterygoid canal
Pharyngeal branch
Palatine nerves; major (anterior), minor (middle and posterior)
Deep temporal nerves (anterior, middle, and posterior) to temporalis muscle
Lateral pterygoid and masseteric nerves
Buccal nerve
Mental nerve
Tensor veli palatini and medial pterygoid nerves
Inferior dental plexus (inferior dental and gingival nerves)

Trigeminal (V) nerve and trigeminal (semilunar) ganglion
Motor nucleus of trigeminal nerve
Mesencephalic nucleus of trigeminal nerve (proprioception)
Principal sensory nucleus of trigeminal nerve (discriminatory sensation)
Spinal tract and spinal nucleus of trigeminal nerve (pain and temperature)

Facial (VII) nerve
Chorda tympani
Superficial temporal branches
Articular and auricular branches
Auriculotemporal nerve
Parotid branches
Meningeal (nervus spinosus) branch
Lesser petrosal nerve (from glossopharyngeal nerve)
Tensor tympani nerve
Otic ganglion
Inferior alveolar nerve
Mylohoid nerve (to mylohyoid and anterior belly of digastric muscles)
Mandibular nerve

Lingual nerve
Submandibular ganglion

Trigeminal Nerve (V)

11.21 **TRIGEMINAL NERVE (V)**

The trigeminal nerve (CN V) carries sensory information from the face, sinuses, teeth, and anterior portion of the oral cavity. It has three subdivisions: (1) ophthalmic—sensory innervation; (2) maxillary—sensory innervation; and (3) mandibular—sensory innervation and motor innervation of the masticatory muscles and tensor tympani muscles. Each of the subdivisions has a distinct distribution and sharp boundaries. Unlike the somatosensory dermatomes, which exhibit considerable overlap with nerve fibers of adjacent roots, the trigeminal subdivisions show no overlap at all. Damage to one of the subdivisions results in total anesthesia in the territory of sensory distribution.

Primary sensory axons from trigeminal (semilunar, gasserian) ganglion cells that process fine, discriminative touch (epicritic sensation) terminate in the main sensory nucleus of CN V and the rostral portion of the descending (spinal) nucleus of CN V. Axons that process pain and temperature sensation (protopathic sensation) terminate in the caudal and middle regions of the descending (spinal) nucleus of CN V. The trigeminal nerve also carries proprioceptive information from muscle spindles in muscles of mastication and extraocular muscles. Those primary sensory cell bodies are found in the mesencephalic nucleus of CN V within the CNS, the only example of primary sensory neurons residing in the CNS.

CLINICAL POINT

Trigeminal neuralgia (tic douloureux) involves sudden, brief (lasting less than a minute), excruciating paroxysms of pain, sometimes described as stabbing or lancinating, usually in the territory of one of the divisions of the trigeminal nerve. The maxillary and mandibular divisions are more common targets than the ophthalmic division, and the disorder is more common in older individuals. These episodes of pain may recur several times a day, with paroxysms experienced for weeks on end. Often there is a trigger point, at which mild stimuli such as light touch, chewing, or even talking can provoke an attack. During an attack, no loss of sensation occurs in the distribution of the affected branch. Trigeminal neuralgia can be idiopathic or symptomatic of other disorders. In some cases, compression of the trigeminal nerve root by a small aberrant branch of the superior cerebellar artery or another nearby artery is the suspected cause; in other cases a tumor, an inflammation, or a demyelinating plaque may precipitate such attacks. If trigeminal neuralgia occurs in the accompaniment of other progressive pathology, the neurological examination reveals sensory and motor deficits associated with the involved branch of the trigeminal nerve. Idiopathic trigeminal neuralgia usually can be treated with carbamazepine or other antiseizure and membrane-stabilizing agents, which sometimes permit the condition to regress. Surgical decompression of a compressing blood vessel may help. In other cases, the nerve root is ablated temporarily or permanently; the resultant functional deficit is often better tolerated than the excruciating paroxysms of pain.

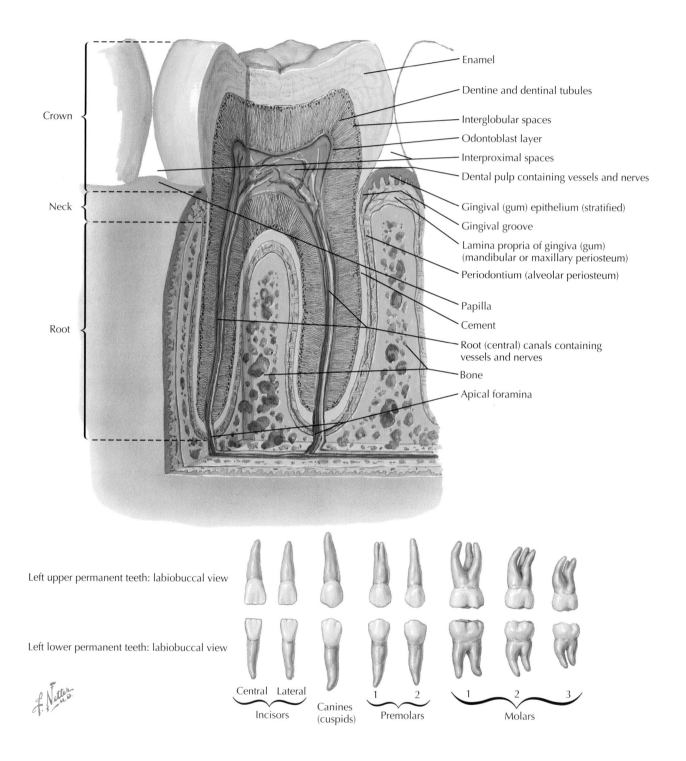

Crown

Neck

Root

Enamel

Dentine and dentinal tubules

Interglobular spaces

Odontoblast layer

Interproximal spaces

Dental pulp containing vessels and nerves

Gingival (gum) epithelium (stratified)

Gingival groove

Lamina propria of gingiva (gum)
(mandibular or maxillary periosteum)

Periodontium (alveolar periosteum)

Papilla

Cement

Root (central) canals containing
vessels and nerves

Bone

Apical foramina

Left upper permanent teeth: labiobuccal view

Left lower permanent teeth: labiobuccal view

Central Lateral

Incisors

Canines
(cuspids)

1   2

Premolars

1   2   3

Molars

11.22 INNERVATION OF THE TEETH

Sensory nerve fibers of the maxillary (upper teeth) and mandibular (lower teeth) subdivisions of the trigeminal nerve innervate the dental pulp of the teeth. With erosion of a lesion (decay) into the dental pulp or close to the dental pulp, these nerve fibers may become exquisitely sensitive to temperature changes (especially cold) or pressure (by edema or mechanical force), resulting in the sensation of severe pain.

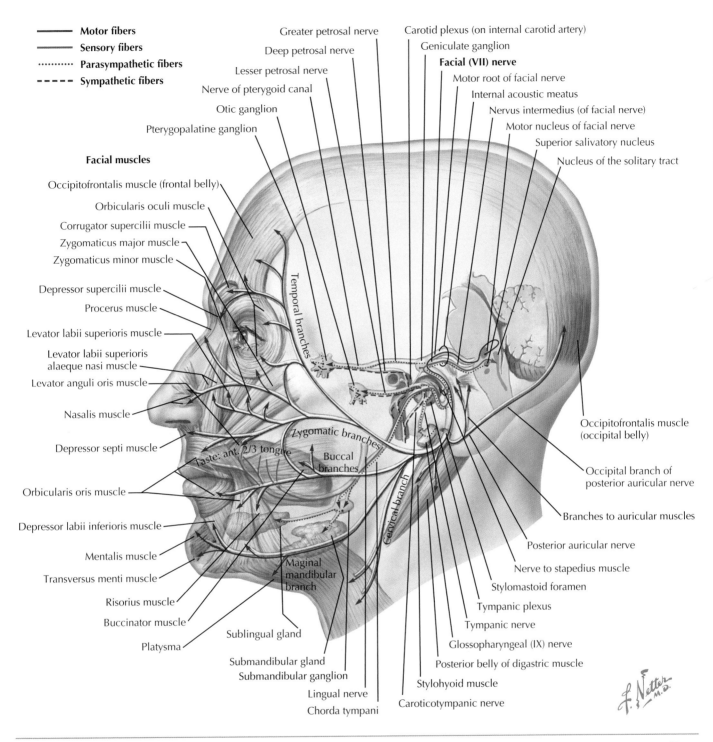

Motor fibers
Sensory fibers
Parasympathetic fibers
Sympathetic fibers

Greater petrosal nerve
Deep petrosal nerve
Lesser petrosal nerve
Nerve of pterygoid canal
Otic ganglion
Pterygopalatine ganglion

Carotid plexus (on internal carotid artery)
Geniculate ganglion
Facial (VII) nerve
Motor root of facial nerve
Internal acoustic meatus
Nervus intermedius (of facial nerve)
Motor nucleus of facial nerve
Superior salivatory nucleus
Nucleus of the solitary tract

Facial muscles
Occipitofrontalis muscle (frontal belly)
Orbicularis oculi muscle
Corrugator supercilii muscle
Zygomaticus major muscle
Zygomaticus minor muscle
Depressor supercilii muscle
Procerus muscle
Levator labii superioris muscle
Levator labii superioris alaeque nasi muscle
Levator anguli oris muscle
Nasalis muscle
Depressor septi muscle
Orbicularis oris muscle
Depressor labii inferioris muscle
Mentalis muscle
Transversus menti muscle
Risorius muscle
Buccinator muscle
Platysma

Temporal branches

Taste: ant. 2/3 tongue
Zygomatic branches
Buccal branches
Cervical branch
Maginal mandibular branch

Sublingual gland
Submandibular gland
Submandibular ganglion
Lingual nerve
Chorda tympani

Occipitofrontalis muscle (occipital belly)
Occipital branch of posterior auricular nerve
Branches to auricular muscles
Posterior auricular nerve
Nerve to stapedius muscle
Stylomastoid foramen
Tympanic plexus
Tympanic nerve
Glossopharyngeal (IX) nerve
Posterior belly of digastric muscle
Stylohyoid muscle
Caroticotympanic nerve

11.23 FACIAL NERVE (VII)

The facial nerve (VII) is a mixed nerve with motor, parasympathetic, and sensory components. The motor fibers distribute to the muscles of facial expression, including the scalp, the auricle, the buccinator, the stapedius, and the stylohyoid muscles, and to the posterior belly of the digastric muscle. Damage results in ipsilateral paralysis of facial expression, including the forehead (Bell's palsy); facial palsy caused by central corticobulbar lesions spare the upper face. Activation of the stapedius muscle dampens the ossicles in the presence of sustained loud noise; damage to

CN VII results in hyperacusis. Parasympathetic nerve fibers of CN VII from the superior salivatory nucleus distribute to the pterygopalatine ganglion, which innervates the lacrimal glands, and to the submandibular ganglion, which innervates the submandibular and sublingual salivary glands. Special sensory taste fibers from the anterior two thirds of the tongue (via the chorda tympani) and the soft palate (via the greater petrosal nerve), whose primary sensory cell bodies are located in the geniculate ganglion, convey that information to the rostral portion of nucleus solitarius in the medulla.

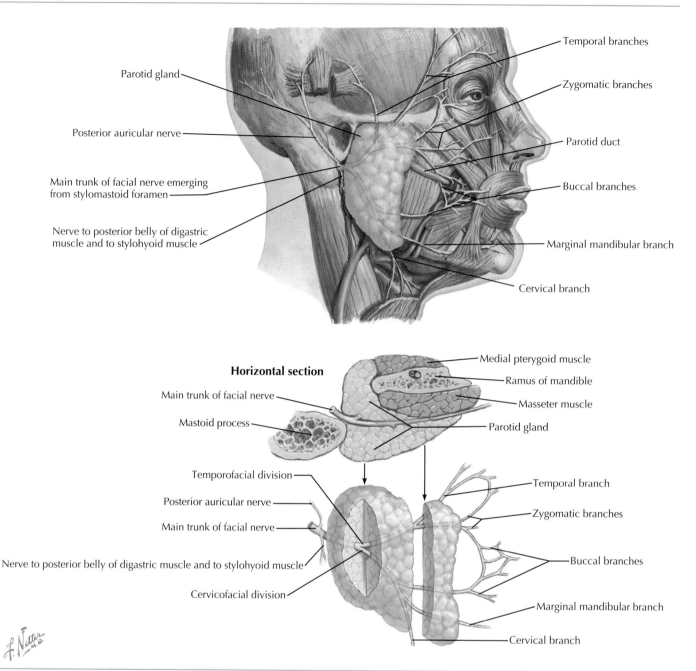

Parotid gland

Posterior auricular nerve

Main trunk of facial nerve emerging from stylomastoid foramen

Nerve to posterior belly of digastric muscle and to stylohyoid muscle

Temporal branches

Zygomatic branches

Parotid duct

Buccal branches

Marginal mandibular branch

Cervical branch

Horizontal section

Main trunk of facial nerve

Mastoid process

Medial pterygoid muscle

Ramus of mandible

Masseter muscle

Parotid gland

Temporofacial division

Posterior auricular nerve

Main trunk of facial nerve

Nerve to posterior belly of digastric muscle and to stylohyoid muscle

Cervicofacial division

Temporal branch

Zygomatic branches

Buccal branches

Marginal mandibular branch

Cervical branch

11.24 FACIAL NERVE BRANCHES AND THE PAROTID GLAND

The facial nerve and its branches directly penetrate the parotid gland. Surgical procedures in this region of the face, particularly those performed to remove mass lesions, may damage the facial nerve, resulting in facial palsy in affected muscles.

CLINICAL POINT

Bell's palsy, the most common disorder of CN VII, usually occurs acutely, over the course of a few hours to a day or so, and results in weak or paralyzed muscles on one side of the face. Some patients report previous retroauricular pain, decreased tearing, or hyperacusis for a day or two. The facial palsy involves all of the muscles on the affected side, unlike a central facial palsy resulting from a lesion in the contralateral genu of the internal capsule, which affects only the lower part of the face. In Bell's palsy, the ipsilateral forehead does not wrinkle, the eye cannot be closed, the face appears smooth, and the corner of the mouth droops. Viral infections (especially herpes simplex I) or inflammation may precipitate Bell's palsy; less commonly, Lyme disease, HIV, diabetes, sarcoidosis, or another infection may be the cause. Sensory loss is not part of the disorder, although loss of taste sensation on the anterior two thirds of the tongue, supplied by CN VII, may occur if the nerve is affected proximal to its merging with the chorda tympani. Involvement of the nerve to the stapedius muscle results in sensitivity to loud sounds (hyperacusis). Recovery can occur within a few weeks or months, particularly if only partial damage to the nerve has occurred and only some weakness has been present. With profound paralysis of facial muscles, the regenerative process may take as long as 2 years. During such a regenerative process, some regenerating nerve fibers may sprout to aberrant sites; former autonomic fibers that innervated salivary glands may be redirected to the lacrimal glands, resulting in "crocodile tears" or an abnormal gustatory-lacrimal reflex. Some aberrant regenerating facial nerve fibers may reach the wrong muscle fibers, resulting in tics, spasms, dyskinesias, or contractures.

Greater petrosal nerve

Spiral ganglion of cochlea

Geniculate ganglion of facial nerve

Cochlear part of vestibulocochlear nerve

Facial canal

Head of malleus

Motor root of facial nerve
and nervus intermedius

Tympanic cavity

Vestibulocochlear (VIII) nerve

Incus

Medulla oblongata

Chorda tympani

Ampulla of superior
semicircular duct

Ampulla of lateral
semicircular duct

Utricle

Ampulla of posterior
semicircular duct

Internal acoustic meatus

Saccule

Superior division } of vestibular part of
vestibulocochlear nerve
Inferior division

Medial
Inferior
Vestibular nuclei {
Superior
Lateral

Ventral } Cochlear nuclei
Dorsal

Vestibular ganglion

Vestibular part of vestibulocochlear nerve

Inferior cerebellar peduncle (to cerebellum)

11.25 VESTIBULOCOCHLEAR NERVE (VIII)

The vestibulocochlear nerve (CN VIII) arises from bipolar primary sensory neurons in the vestibular ganglion (Scarpa's ganglion) and the spiral (cochlear) ganglion. The peripheral process of the vestibular ganglion neurons innervates hair cells in the utricle and saccule that respond to linear acceleration (gravity) and in the ampullae of the semicircular ducts that respond to angular acceleration (movement). The utricle, the saccule, and the semicircular ducts provide neural signals for coordination and equilibration of position and for movement of the head and neck. The central processes of the vestibular ganglion cells terminate in vestibular nuclei (medial, lateral, superior, and inferior) in the medulla and pons and in the cerebellum. The peripheral processes of spiral ganglion cells innervate hair cells that lie along the cochlear duct in the organ of Corti. They convey hearing information via central axonal processes into the cochlear nuclei (dorsal and ventral). A lesion in CN VIII results in ipsilateral deafness, vertigo, and loss of equilibrium.

CLINICAL POINT

The vestibulocochlear nerve emerges from the ventrolateral margin of the brain stem near the junction of the medulla, pons, and cerebellum (the cerebellopontine angle). At this site, Schwann cell tumors of CN VIII, acoustic schwannomas, can arise, usually from the vestibular portion of CN VIII. Initial irritation of the vestibular division of CN VIII can result in vertigo, dizziness, nausea, and unsteadiness or spatial disorientation. These symptoms persist with nerve destruction. Initial irritation of the auditory division of CN VIII by a schwannoma may first produce tinnitus, followed by slow loss of hearing and the inability to determine the direction from which a sound is coming. As nerve destruction occurs, tinnitus diminishes and ipsilateral deafness ensues. Because of the proximity of CNs VII and VIII, acoustic schwannomas also often produce ipsilateral facial paralysis or palsy. The tumor may extend rostrally to the trigeminal nerve or caudally to the glossopharyngeal and vagus nerves and also may affect the adjacent brain stem and cerebellum. At this point, hydrocephalus and increased intracranial pressure can occur.

— Sensory fibers
— Motor fibers
······ Parasympathetic fibers

Tympanic nerve
Tympanic cavity and plexus
Stylomastoid foramen
Caroticotympanic nerve
Greater petrosal nerve
Deep petrosal nerve
Lesser petrosal nerve
Nerve of pterygoid canal
Pterygopalatine ganglion
Mandibular nerve
Otic ganglion
Auriculotemporal nerve
Parotid gland
Tubal branch of tympanic plexus
Auditory (eustachian) tube and pharyngeal opening
Stylopharyngeus muscle and nerve
Pharyngeal plexus

Geniculate ganglion of facial nerve
Inferior salivatory nucleus
Solitary tract nucleus
Spinal tract and descending (spinal) nucleus of trigeminal (V) nerve
Nucleus ambiguus
Glossopharyngeal (IX) nerve
Jugular foramen
Communication to auricular branch of vagus nerve
Superior and inferior ganglia of glossopharyngeal nerve
Communication to facial nerve
Superior cervical sympathetic ganglion
Vagus (X) nerve
Pharyngeal branch of vagus nerve
Sympathetic trunk

Taste and general sensation from posterior 1/3 of tongue: Taste to rostral solitary tract nucleus; general sensation to descending (spinal) nucleus of trigeminal (V) nerve

Carotid sinus branch of glossopharyngeal nerve
Internal carotid artery
Carotid body
Carotid sinus
Common carotid artery

Pharyngeal, tonsillar, and lingual branches of glossopharyngeal nerve

11.26 GLOSSOPHARYNGEAL NERVE (IX)

CN IX is a mixed nerve with motor, parasympathetic, and sensory components. Motor fibers from the nucleus ambiguus supply the stylopharyngeus muscle and may assist in the innervation of pharyngeal muscles for swallowing. Preganglionic axons from the inferior salivatory nucleus travel with CN IX to the otic ganglion, whose neurons innervate the parotid and mucous glands. Special sensory axons from the petrosal (inferior) ganglion carry information from taste buds on the posterior one third of the tongue (including numerous taste buds in the vallate papillae) and part of the soft palate. These axons terminate in the rostral portion of nucleus solitarius. Axons from additional primary sensory neurons in the inferior ganglion also carry general sensation from the posterior one third of the tongue and from the pharynx, the fauces, the tonsils, the tympanic cavity, the eustachian tube, and the mastoid cells. The central axon branches terminate in the descending (spinal) nucleus of CN V. The general sensory fibers from the pharynx provide the afferent limb of the gag reflex.

Additional primary sensory neurons innervate the carotid body (chemoreception of carbon dioxide) and the carotid sinus (baroceptors) and convey their central axons to the caudal nucleus solitarius (solitary tract nucleus). Primary sensory neurons in the superior ganglion innervate a small region behind the ear and convey general sensation into the descending nucleus of CN V.

CLINICAL POINT
The glossopharyngeal nerve can be affected by brief, excruciating paroxysms of pain (glossopharyngeal neuralgia) similar to those experienced in trigeminal neuralgia. The pain originates in the throat (tonsillar fossa) or sometimes the jaw and radiates to the ear. Some patients experience pain in the tongue, face, or jaw. The triggering activity is usually swallowing, coughing, sneezing, or yawning. If the irritative process activates glossopharyngeal afferents associated with brain stem vasomotor responses, the patient may experience bradycardia and syncope. The treatment of glossopharyngeal neuralgia is similar to treatment of trigeminal neuralgia. Successful treatment also has occurred surgically through decompression of a tortuous aberrant vessel.

Cranial root of accessory nerve (joins vagus nerve to supply muscles of larynx — except cricothyroid — via recurrent laryngeal nerve)

Nucleus ambiguus

Vagus (X) nerve

Spinal root of accessory nerve

Foramen magnum

Jugular foramen

Superior ganglion of vagus nerve

Accessory (XI) nerve

Internal branch of accessory nerve

Inferior ganglion of vagus nerve

1st spinal nerve (C1)

2nd spinal nerve (C2)

External branch of accessory nerve (to sternocleidomastoid and trapezius muscles)

Sternocleidomastoid muscle

3rd spinal nerve (C3)

4th spinal nerve (C4)

Trapezius muscle

— **Motor fibers**
— **Proprioceptive fibers**

11.27 ACCESSORY NERVE (XI)

The accessory nerve (CN XI) is a motor nerve with cranial and spinal portions. The cranial portion arises from LMNs at the caudal end of the nucleus ambiguus; the axons travel through an internal branch that distributes with the pharyngeal and laryngeal branches of the vagus nerve (CN X) and with nerves to the soft palate. These axons often are considered to be part of CN X. The spinal portion arises from LMNs in the lateral part of the upper four or five segments of the cervical spinal cord. The axons then emerge as rootlets from the lateral margin of the spinal cord, ascend behind the denticulate ligaments, and coalesce as a single nerve. This nerve then ascends through the foramen magnum and joins the vagus nerve to exit through the jugular foramen. The LMNs of the spinal accessory nerve supply the sternocleidomastoid muscle and the upper two thirds of the trapezius muscle. Damage to this division of CN XI results in weakness in head rotation and shoulder elevation.

CLINICAL POINT

The cranial portion of the accessory nerve is derived from the nucleus ambiguus and has been considered to be part of the vagal complex. The spinal accessory nerve derives from LMNs of the upper segments (C1–C4) of the cervical spinal cord; it ascends through the foramen magnum and emerges with cranial nerves IX and X through the jugular foramen. Tumors, meningitis, and trauma may damage CN XI, although these lesions commonly damage nerves IX and X as well. LMN disorders, such as polio or amyotrophic lateral sclerosis or compression of the foramen magnum as in Arnold-Chiari malformation, can damage the spinal accessory nerve on one side. This results in ipsilateral flaccid paralysis of the sternocleidomastoid muscle and the upper two thirds of the trapezius, causing atrophy and loss of tone. The patient has great difficulty turning his or her head to the opposite side (sternocleidomastoid). The shoulder hangs downward, with caudal and lateral displacement of the scapula, and the arm cannot be raised more than 90 degrees. In circumstances in which bilateral damage occurs to the spinal accessory nucleus (as in amyotrophic lateral sclerosis), the bilateral denervation of the sternocleidomastoid leaves the patient unable to hold up his or her head.

Vagus (X) Nerve

Glossopharyngeal (IX) nerve

Meningeal branch of vagus nerve

Auricular branch of vagus nerve

Auditory (eustachian) tube

Levator veli palatini muscle

Salpingopharyngeus muscle

Palatoglossus

Palatopharyngeus

Superior constrictor
muscle of pharynx

Stylopharyngeus muscle

Middle constrictor muscle of pharynx

Inferior constrictor muscle of pharynx

Cricothyroid muscle

Trachea

Esophagus

Right recurrent
laryngeal nerve

—— **Motor fibers**
═══ **Afferent fibers**
······ **Parasympathetic fibers**

Heart

Hepatic branch of anterior
vagal trunk (in lesser omentum)

Celiac branches (from anterior
and posterior vagal trunks
to celiac plexus)

Pyloric branch
from hepatic plexus

Liver

Gallbladder and bile ducts

Pancreas

Duodenum

Ascending colon

Cecum

Appendix

Dorsal (motor)
nucleus of CN X

Solitary tract nucleus

Spinal tract and spinal
nucleus of trigeminal
nerve

Nucleus ambiguus
(voluntary motor)

Cranial root
of accessory nerve

Vagus (X) nerve

Jugular foramen

Superior ganglion of vagus nerve

Inferior ganglion of vagus nerve

Pharyngeal branch of vagus nerve (motor to muscles
of pharynx and palate; sensory to lower pharynx)

Vagal branch to carotid sinus branch
of glossopharyngeal nerve

Pharyngeal plexus

Internal branch (sensory)
External branch (motor to cricothyroid muscle)

Superior laryngeal nerve

Superior cervical cardiac branch of vagus nerve

Inferior cervical cardiac branch of vagus nerve

Thoracic cardiac branch of vagus nerve

Left recurrent laryngeal nerve (motor to muscles
of larynx except cricothyroid; parasympathetic,
motor, and sensory to upper esophagus and trachea)

Pulmonary plexus

Cardiac plexus

Esophageal plexus

Anterior vagal trunk

Gastric branches of anterior vagal trunk

Vagal branches (parasympathetic
motor, secretomotor and sensory
fibers) accompany superior
mesenteric artery and its branches
to small intestine, cecum, appendix,
and colon, often as far as left colic
(splenic) flexure

Small intestine

Vagus Nerve (X)

11.28 VAGUS NERVE (X)

The vagus nerve (CN X) is a mixed nerve with motor, parasympathetic, and sensory components. LMN axons from neurons in the nucleus ambiguus in the medulla supply muscles of the soft palate, the pharynx, and the larynx and control speaking and swallowing. A lesion in these axons results in hoarseness, dysphagia, and decreased gag reflex (efferent limb). Preganglionic parasympathetic axons from neurons in the dorsal (motor) nucleus of CN X in the medulla distribute to intramural ganglia associated with thoracic and abdominal viscera and supply autonomic innervation to the heart, the lungs, and the gastrointestinal tract to the descending colon. Special sensory axons from the nodose (inferior) ganglion, which carry information from taste buds in the posterior pharynx (found mainly in children), send central branches to terminate in the rostral nucleus solitarius. Primary sensory axons from the inferior ganglion also convey general sensation from the larynx, the pharynx, and the thoracic and abdominal viscera and terminate mainly in the caudal nucleus solitarius. Primary sensory axons from the superior (jugular) ganglion convey general sensation from the external auditory meatus and terminate in the descending (spinal) nucleus of CN V.

CLINICAL POINT

The vagus nerve emerges from the lateral surface of the medulla and can be involved in both intracranial and extracranial pathology. Intracranially, this nerve can be damaged by a tumor, hematoma, vascular infarct, aneurysm, meningitis, and other disorders. Extracranially, the vagus nerve can be damaged by a tumor, aneurysm, trauma, or infectious process. Unilateral damage to the vagus nerve results in (1) drooping of the soft palate, with the intact contralateral soft palate pulled to the opposite side during phonation, accompanied by nasal speech; (2) hoarseness resulting from involvement of the nucleus ambiguus fibers that extend to the laryngeal muscles; (3) ipsilateral laryngeal anesthesia; and (4) tachycardia and arrhythmias in some instances.

Styloglossus muscle

Meningeal branch

Hypoglossal nucleus

Intrinsic musculature of tongue

Hypoglossal (XII) nerve
(in hypoglossal canal)

Inferior
longitudinal

Transverse
and vertical

Superior
longitudinal

Occipital condyle

Inferior ganglion of vagus nerve

Ventral rami of C1, C2, and C3
forming cervical plexus

Superior cervical sympathetic
trunk ganglion

Superior root (descendens
hypoglossi) of ansa cervicalis

Genioglossus muscle

Internal carotid artery

Geniohyoid muscle

Inferior root (descendens
hypoglossi) of ansa cervicalis

Hyoglossus muscle

Thyrohyoid muscle

Ansa cervicalis (ansa hypoglossi)

Omohyoid muscle (superior belly)

Internal jugular vein

Sternothyroid muscle

Omohyoid muscle (inferior belly)

Sternohyoid muscle

—————— **Motor fibers**

—————— **Sensory fibers**

11.29 HYPOGLOSSAL NERVE (XII)

The hypoglossal nerve (CN XII) is a motor nerve. LMNs in the hypoglossal nucleus of the caudal medulla exit from the ventral surface of the medulla in the preolivary sulcus (between the medullary pyramid and the inferior olive) to innervate the extrinsic muscles of the tongue (the hyoglossus, styloglossus, chondroglossus, and genioglossus muscles) and the intrinsic muscles of the tongue (the superior and inferior longitudinal, transverse, and vertical lingual muscles). Damage to this nerve leads to weakness of the ipsilateral tongue muscles; the tongue, when protruded, deviates toward the weak side because of the unopposed action of the innervated contralateral genioglossus muscle.

CLINICAL POINT

The hypoglossal nerve emerges from the ventral surface of the medulla just lateral to the medullary pyramids. The emerging hypoglossal nerve fibers can be damaged intracranially by a paramedian infarct (that also damages the pyramid and medial lemniscus, producing a so-called alternating hemiplegia) or can be damaged peripherally by a meningeal tumor, a metastatic tumor, or bony overgrowth or as an unwanted consequence of a carotid endarterectomy. Hypoglossal nerve damage on one side produces flaccid paralysis of the ipsilateral tongue musculature, accompanied by atrophy. An attempt to protrude the tongue results in deviation of the tongue toward the weak side because of the unopposed actions of the intact genioglossus muscle. As damage to CN XII progresses, fasciculations can be seen on the ipsilateral tongue up to the point where total denervation occurs.

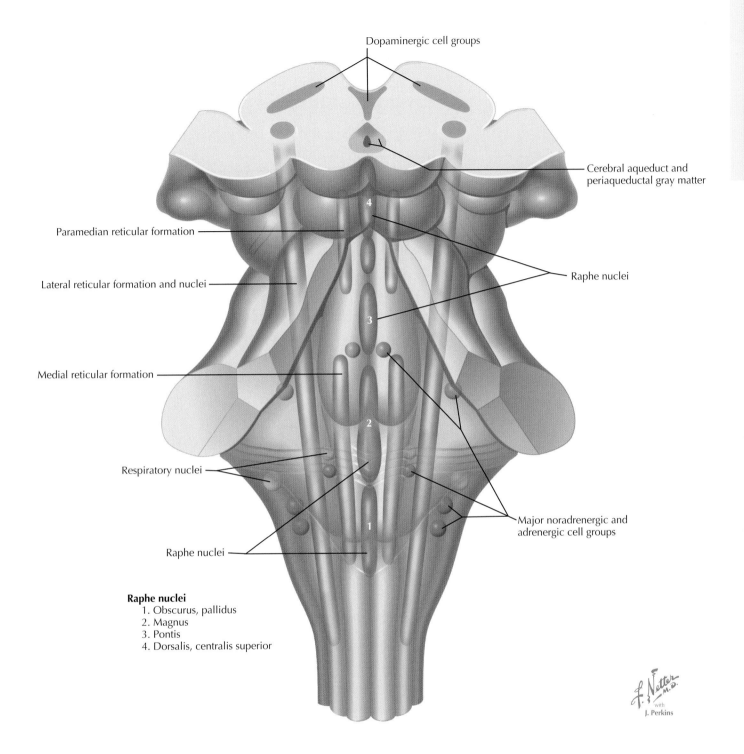

Dopaminergic cell groups

Cerebral aqueduct and periaqueductal gray matter

Paramedian reticular formation

Raphe nuclei

Lateral reticular formation and nuclei

Medial reticular formation

Respiratory nuclei

Major noradrenergic and adrenergic cell groups

Raphe nuclei

Raphe nuclei
1. Obscurus, pallidus
2. Magnus
3. Pontis
4. Dorsalis, centralis superior

RETICULAR FORMATION

11.30 RETICULAR FORMATION: GENERAL PATTERN OF NUCLEI IN THE BRAIN STEM

The reticular formation (RF), the neuronal core of the brain stem, consists of neurons with characteristic isodendritic morphology. The RF extends from the rostral spinal cord through the hypothalamus into the septal region. RF neurons are large cells with axonal arborizations that terminate at a distance from their cell bodies and dendritic tree; they are not interneurons. The major nuclei of the RF are found in a lateral zone (predominantly sensory functions), a medial zone (predominantly motor functions), and a column of raphe nuclei (serotonergic neurons). The serotonergic neurons exert mainly modulatory influences on their targets. The catecholaminergic neurons (locus coeruleus, tegmental noradrenergic, and adrenergic groups) in several regions of the RF have widespread projections and exert mainly modulatory influences on their targets. The dopaminergic neurons of the midbrain are included in this illustration, although some experts question whether they are RF neurons.

A. Thalamus and hypothalamus

Thalamus:
Intralaminar nuclei
Reticular nucleus of thalamus
Midline nuclei
Lateral hypothalamic area through septal nuclei

B. Midbrain

Lateral RF of the mid brain
Substantia nigra
Interpeduncular nucleus

Periaqueductal gray matter
Raphe nuclei (dorsal, central superior)
Ventral tegmental nucleus

C. Pons

Locus coeruleus
A5
Raphe nuclei (pontis)
Lateral RF

Parabrachial nucleus
Parapontine RF (lateral gaze center)
Pontine RF (pontis, caudalis, ovalis)

D. Medulla

Lateral RF
Medullary RF (gigantocellular)
Raphe nuclei (obscurus, pallidus, magnus)

A2
Respiratory nuclei
Rostral ventrolateral medulla (RVLM)
A1
Lateral reticular nucleus

E. Spinal cord–medullary junction

Lamina 7 - caudal RF

J. Perkins
MS, MFA

11.31 RETICULAR FORMATION: NUCLEI AND AREAS IN THE BRAIN STEM AND DIENCEPHALON

Many of the named nuclei of the RF are present in the medulla, the pons, and the midbrain. Important medial RF groups include the medullary (gigantocellular) and the pontine (caudal and rostral) RFs, which are involved in reticulospinal regulation of spinal cord LMNs; and the parapontine RF, also known as the horizontal (lateral) gaze center. Lateral RF areas and nuclei (such as the lateral reticular nucleus) are involved in polymodal sensory functions. RF respiratory and cardiovascular neurons are found in the medulla. Catecholaminergic neurons are found in the locus coeruleus and tegmental groups denoted here as Groups A1, A2, and A5 (norepinephrine-containing neurons). Raphe nuclei are found in the midline and in wings of cells that extend laterally. The core of the RF continues rostrally from the lateral regions of the brain stem into the lateral hypothalamic area and extends through the hypothalamus to the septal nuclei. Several thalamic nuclei (intralaminar, midline, and reticular nucleus of the thalamus) also are classified as part of the RF.

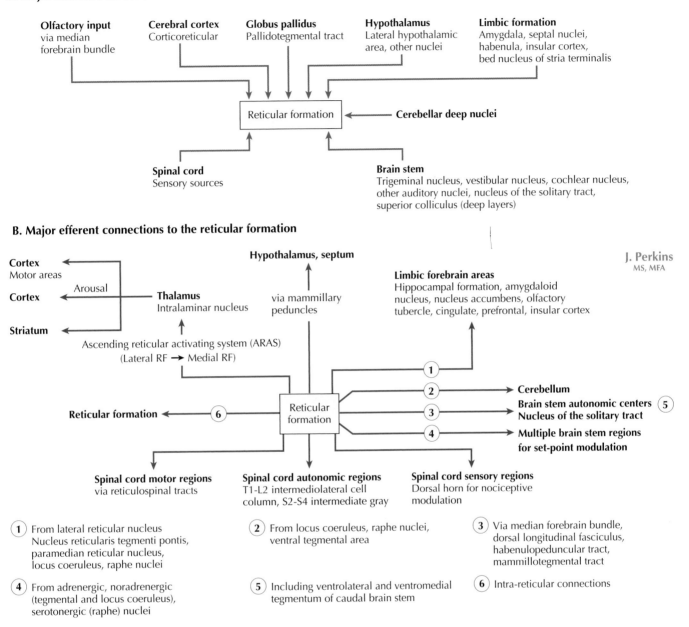

A. Major afferent connections to the reticular formation

Olfactory input
via median
forebrain bundle

Cerebral cortex
Corticoreticular

Globus pallidus
Pallidotegmental tract

Hypothalamus
Lateral hypothalamic
area, other nuclei

Limbic formation
Amygdala, septal nuclei,
habenula, insular cortex,
bed nucleus of stria terminalis

Reticular formation ◄— **Cerebellar deep nuclei**

Spinal cord
Sensory sources

Brain stem
Trigeminal nucleus, vestibular nucleus, cochlear nucleus,
other auditory nuclei, nucleus of the solitary tract,
superior colliculus (deep layers)

B. Major efferent connections to the reticular formation

J. Perkins
MS, MFA

Cortex
Motor areas

Arousal

Cortex

Striatum

Thalamus
Intralaminar nucleus

Hypothalamus, septum

via mammillary
peduncles

Limbic forebrain areas
Hippocampal formation, amygdaloid
nucleus, nucleus accumbens, olfactory
tubercle, cingulate, prefrontal, insular cortex

Ascending reticular activating system (ARAS)
(Lateral RF ➝ Medial RF)

Reticular formation ◄— ⑥

Reticular
formation

① **Cerebellum**

②

③ **Brain stem autonomic centers** ⑤
Nucleus of the solitary tract

④ **Multiple brain stem regions**
for set-point modulation

Spinal cord motor regions
via reticulospinal tracts

Spinal cord autonomic regions
T1-L2 intermediolateral cell
column, S2-S4 intermediate gray

Spinal cord sensory regions
Dorsal horn for nociceptive
modulation

① From lateral reticular nucleus
Nucleus reticularis tegmenti pontis,
paramedian reticular nucleus,
locus coeruleus, raphe nuclei

② From locus coeruleus, raphe nuclei,
ventral tegmental area

③ Via median forebrain bundle,
dorsal longitudinal fasciculus,
habenulopeduncular tract,
mammillotegmental tract

④ From adrenergic, noradrenergic
(tegmental and locus coeruleus),
serotonergic (raphe) nuclei

⑤ Including ventrolateral and ventromedial
tegmentum of caudal brain stem

⑥ Intra-reticular connections

11.32 MAJOR AFFERENT AND EFFERENT CONNECTIONS TO THE RETICULAR FORMATION

A, Extensive sensory information from spinal cord somatosensory sources (particularly nociceptive information) and from virtually all brain stem sensory modalities is sent to the lateral regions of the RF. Olfactory input arrives through olfactory tract projections into forebrain regions. Many limbic and hypothalamic structures provide input into the RF, particularly for visceral and autonomic regulatory functions. The cerebral cortex, the globus pallidus, and the cerebellum also provide input into the RF medial zones involved in motor regulation. **B,** The ascending reticular activating system (ARAS) of the RF is responsible for consciousness and arousal. It projects through nonspecific nuclei of the thalamus to the cerebral cortex; lesions in this area lead to coma. The RF sends extensive axonal projections to sensory, motor, and autonomic regions of the spinal cord, modulating nociceptive input, preganglionic autonomic outflow, and LMN outflow, respectively. The RF sends extensive connections to brain stem nuclei (such as nucleus tractus solitarius) and to autonomic regulatory centers and nuclei for modulation of visceral functions. Efferent RF projections to the hypothalamus, septal nuclei, and limbic forebrain areas help to modulate visceral autonomic functions, neuroendocrine outflow, and emotional responsiveness and behavior. Efferent RF projections to the cerebellum and basal ganglia participate in modulating UMN control of LMNs.

Nucleus basalis (cholinergics)

From retina

Preoptic hypothalamic area

Supra-chiasmatic nucleus

Interleukins; other blood-borne substances

Thalamus

Reticular formation

Sensory input

Locus coeruleus

To pineal (melatonin)

Area postrema

Nucleus tractus solitarius

Raphe nuclei

Sensory input

Spinal cord

Sympathetic chain ganglia

Areas associated with arousal

Areas associated with the induction of sleep

11.33 SLEEP-WAKEFULNESS CONTROL

Sleep is a normal physiological state involving a cyclic temporary loss of consciousness; it is readily reversed by appropriate sensory stimuli. Sleep is an active process initiated by brain activity in several chemical-specific collections of neurons of the brain: (1) the locus coeruleus of the pons (noradrenergic); (2) the raphe nuclei of the medulla and pons (serotonergic); (3) the nucleus solitarius of the medulla; (4) the cholinergic neurons of the brain stem tegmentum; (5) the lateral RF, particularly in the pons; (6) several regions of the hypothalamus (anterior region, posterior region, preoptic area); and (7) the reticular nucleus of the thalamus. Many of these regions actively inhibit the lateral (sensory) portion of the RF that is responsible for maintaining

a waking state and consciousness. Circulating substances such as interleukin-1 beta can act on key sites in the hypothalamus and brain stem to influence components of sleep. Illness behavior involves enhanced slow-wave sleep induced by interleukin-1 beta and other inflammatory mediators. Sleep that does not involve rapid eye movement (REM), or slow-wave sleep, is initiated by hypothalamic neurons and other regions and is accompanied by decreased activity in the locus coeruleus and the cholinergic tegmental neurons. During REM sleep, activity in noradrenergic locus coeruleus neurons and serotonergic raphe neurons greatly diminishes, which prevents the cerebral cortex from attending to external stimuli. Dreams probably occur because the cortex is attending to internal stimuli provided by stored memories.

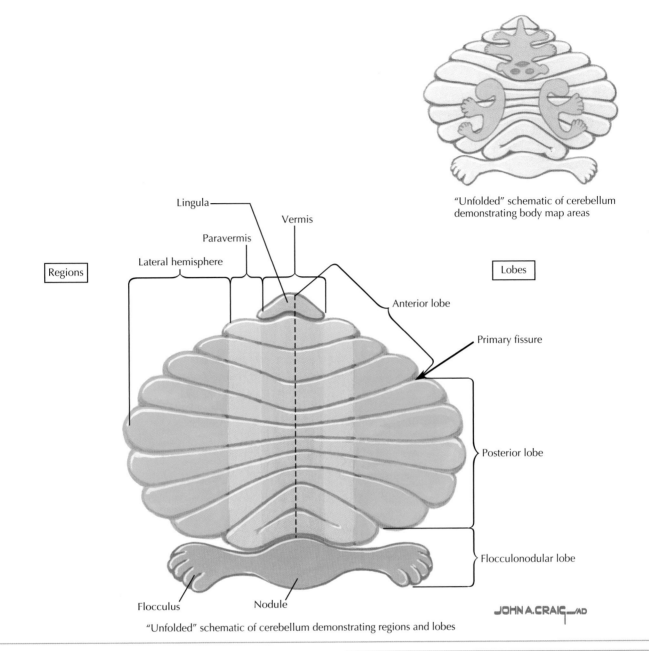

"Unfolded" schematic of cerebellum demonstrating body map areas

"Unfolded" schematic of cerebellum demonstrating regions and lobes

JOHN A.CRAIG—AD

CEREBELLUM

11.34 CEREBELLAR ORGANIZATION: LOBES AND REGIONS

The cerebellum is organized anatomically into three major lobes: (1) anterior, (2) posterior, and (3) flocculonodular. Distinct syndromes are associated with damage to each lobe. The functional organization of the cerebellar hemisphere follows a vertical organization: (1) vermis (midline); (2) paravermis; and (3) lateral hemispheres. Each of these functional regions is associated with specific deep nuclei (fastigial, globose and emboliform, and dentate, respectively) that help to regulate the activity of reticulospinal and vestibulospinal tracts, the rubrospinal tract, and the corticospinal tract, respectively. At least three representations of the body are mapped onto the cerebellar cortex. The cerebellar cortex has multiple, orderly, small infoldings, or convolutions, called folia.

CLINICAL POINT

The cerebellum demonstrates both a lobular organization (anterior lobe, posterior lobe, and flocculonodular lobe), commonly associated with cerebellar syndromes; and a longitudinal organization (vermis, paravermis, lateral hemispheres), commonly associated with regulatory control over specific groups of UMNs. The vascular supply to the cerebellum comes mainly from the superior, anterior inferior, and posterior inferior cerebellar arteries. The cerebellum is quite prone to intracerebellar bleeds and hematomas. The superior cerebellar artery has fine branches that can rupture in hypertensive conditions and damage the rostral cerebellum and deep nuclei such as the dentate nucleus. A cerebellar hematoma acts as a space-occupying lesion and also may induce further edema. As a result, increased intracranial pressure can occur, and the flow of cerebrospinal fluid can be disrupted, secondarily bringing about supratentorial increased intracranial pressure. The patient experiences headache, nausea and vomiting, and vertigo and then may lapse into a coma. Decerebrate posturing, blood pressure dysregulation, and respiratory failure may ensue. Without rapid drainage, such a hematoma is commonly fatal. Smaller intracerebellar bleeds result in ipsilateral symptoms that are characteristic of the affected region of cerebellum.

A. Posterior view

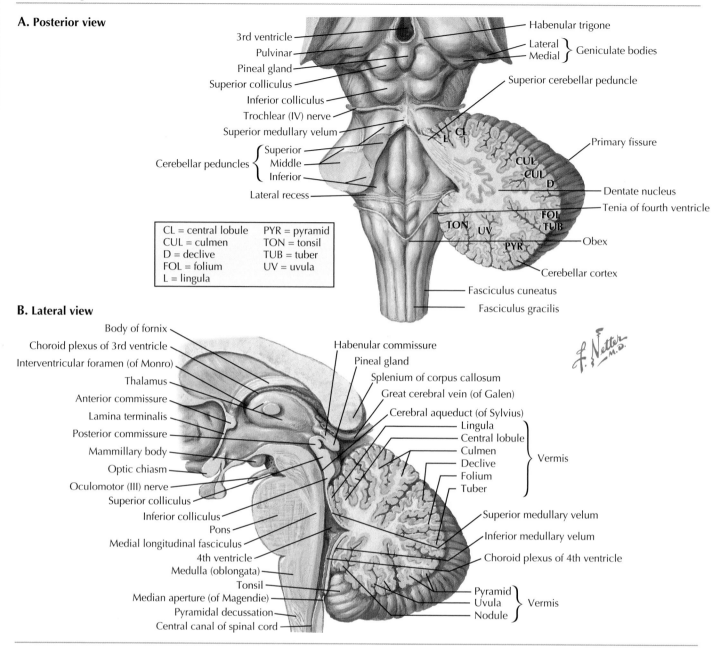

3rd ventricle
Pulvinar
Pineal gland
Superior colliculus
Inferior colliculus
Trochlear (IV) nerve
Superior medullary velum

Cerebellar peduncles { Superior / Middle / Inferior

Lateral recess

CL = central lobule   PYR = pyramid
CUL = culmen   TON = tonsil
D = declive   TUB = tuber
FOL = folium   UV = uvula
L = lingula

Habenular trigone
Lateral / Medial } Geniculate bodies
Superior cerebellar peduncle
Primary fissure
Dentate nucleus
Tenia of fourth ventricle
Obex
Cerebellar cortex
Fasciculus cuneatus
Fasciculus gracilis

L CL
CUL
CUL D
FOL TUB
TON UV
PYR

B. Lateral view

Body of fornix
Choroid plexus of 3rd ventricle
Interventricular foramen (of Monro)
Thalamus
Anterior commissure
Lamina terminalis
Posterior commissure
Mammillary body
Optic chiasm
Oculomotor (III) nerve
Superior colliculus
Inferior colliculus
Pons
Medial longitudinal fasciculus
4th ventricle
Medulla (oblongata)
Tonsil
Median aperture (of Magendie)
Pyramidal decussation
Central canal of spinal cord

Habenular commissure
Pineal gland
Splenium of corpus callosum
Great cerebral vein (of Galen)
Cerebral aqueduct (of Sylvius)
Lingula
Central lobule
Culmen
Declive
Folium
Tuber
} Vermis
Superior medullary velum
Inferior medullary velum
Choroid plexus of 4th ventricle
Pyramid
Uvula
Nodule
} Vermis

11.35 CEREBELLAR ANATOMY: LOBULES

A, Posterior view. In this horizontal (axial) section through the right cerebellar hemisphere, the left hemisphere has been removed, the cerebellar peduncles cut, and the fourth ventricle opened to show the dorsal surface of the brain stem below. The cerebellar cortex is organized into 10 lobules. The cerebellar peduncles provide the large regions through which afferents and efferents pass, connecting the cerebellum with the brain stem and diencephalon. **B,** Lateral view. The lobules of the cerebellum are shown in midsagittal section. Inputs into the cerebellar hemispheres show a similar general organization, with variation from lobule to lobule, particularly for noradrenergic inputs from the locus coeruleus. Inputs from a vast majority of nuclei projecting to the cerebellar hemispheres arrive as mossy fibers; the inferior olivary nucleus sends climbing fibers to end on Purkinje cell dendrites in the cerebellar hemispheres, and the locus coeruleus sends diffuse varicose inputs into all three layers of many regions of the cerebellar cortex. The deep nuclei provide the "coarse adjustment" upon which is superimposed the "fine adjustment" by the cerebellar cortex. The cerebellar cortex sends its output via Purkinje cell projections, using gamma-aminobutyric acid (GABA) as the principal neurotransmitter, to deep nuclei, which in turn project to UMNs.

CLINICAL POINT

Cerebellar tumors commonly start in a specific region of the cerebellum. Cerebellar medulloblastomas are childhood malignant tumors that often begin in the flocculonodular lobe and are detected initially because of truncal ataxia and a broad-based uncoordinated gait. However, as the tumor slowly grows, it involves additional areas of the cerebellum by means of pressure or by invading neighboring areas. Then, in addition to the truncal ataxia, additional limb ataxia, dysmetria, dysdiadochokinesia, intention tremor, hypotonia, and other characteristics of lateral cerebellar damage are seen. Because the posterior fossa is involved, and not supratentorial regions, papilledema does not occur and does not provide a clue for diagnosis; rather, the increased posterior fossa pressure results in occipital headaches with nausea, vomiting, and nystagmus. The two most common cerebellar tumors of childhood are medulloblastomas, which can spread to adjacent portions of the CNS; and astrocytomas, which commonly are not highly invasive in the cerebellum but do grow as space-occupying masses.

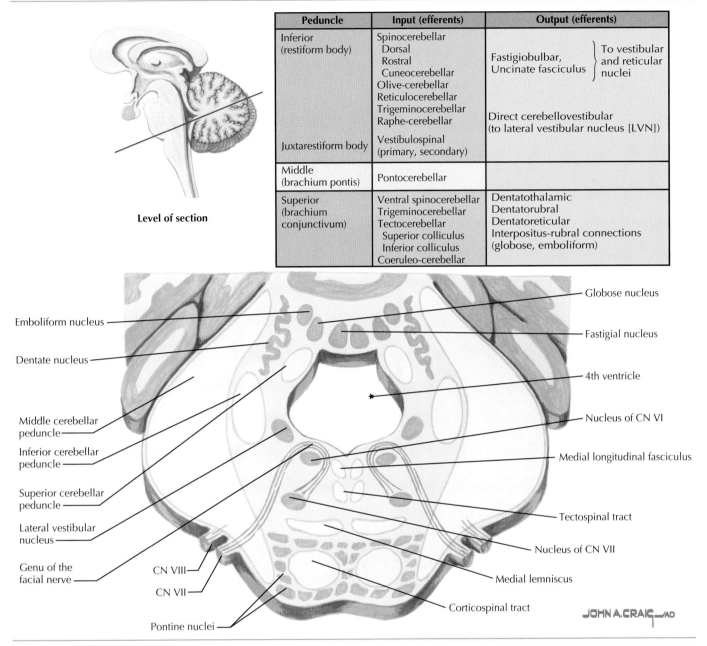

Peduncle	Input (efferents)	Output (efferents)

Inferior (restiform body)	Spinocerebellar
	  Dorsal
	  Rostral
	  Cuneocerebellar
	Olive-cerebellar
	Reticulocerebellar
	Trigeminocerebellar
	Raphe-cerebellar
		Fastigiobulbar, Uncinate fasciculus } To vestibular and reticular nuclei
		
		Direct cerebellovestibular (to lateral vestibular nucleus [LVN])

Juxtarestiform body	Vestibulospinal (primary, secondary)	
Middle (brachium pontis)	Pontocerebellar	

Superior (brachium conjunctivum)	Ventral spinocerebellar
	Trigeminocerebellar
	Tectocerebellar
	  Superior colliculus
	  Inferior colliculus
	Coeruleo-cerebellar
		Dentatothalamic
		Dentatorubral
		Dentatoreticular
		Interpositus-rubral connections (globose, emboliform)

Level of section

Emboliform nucleus

Dentate nucleus

Middle cerebellar peduncle

Inferior cerebellar peduncle

Superior cerebellar peduncle

Lateral vestibular nucleus

Genu of the facial nerve

CN VIII

CN VII

Pontine nuclei

Globose nucleus

Fastigial nucleus

4th ventricle

Nucleus of CN VI

Medial longitudinal fasciculus

Tectospinal tract

Nucleus of CN VII

Medial lemniscus

Corticospinal tract

JOHN A.CRAIG—AD

11.36 CEREBELLAR ANATOMY: DEEP NUCLEI AND CEREBELLAR PEDUNCLES

The deep cerebellar nuclei are found at the roof of the fourth ventricle in a cross-sectional view of the pons at the level of cranial motor nuclei for CNs VI and VII. The fastigial nucleus receives input from the vermis and sends projections to reticular and vestibular nuclei, the cells of origin of the reticulospinal and vestibulospinal tracts. Some vermal and flocculonodular Purkinje cells project directly to the lateral vestibular nuclei, which some authors consider to be a fifth deep cerebellar nucleus; this nucleus also is the UMN cell group for the vestibulospinal tract. The globose and emboliform nuclei receive input from the paravermis and project to the red nucleus, the cells of origin for the rubrospinal tract. The dentate nucleus receives input from the lateral hemispheres and projects to the ventrolateral and ventral anterior nuclei of the thalamus; these thalamic nuclei project to the cells of origin of the corticospinal and corticobulbar tracts. All three cerebellar peduncles can be seen in this cross-section. The table lists the major afferent and efferent projections through the three cerebellar peduncles.

CLINICAL POINT

The inferior cerebellar peduncle conveys many afferents to the cerebellum from the spinocerebellar system, reticular formation, vestibular system, and trigeminal system, and it conveys efferents from the fastigial nucleus and flocculonodular lobe to vestibulospinal and reticulospinal UMN systems. The middle cerebellar peduncle mainly conveys afferents to the cerebellum from the cortico-ponto-cerebellar system. The superior cerebellar peduncle conveys selective afferents to the cerebellum and carries extensive efferents from the globose, emboliform, and dentate nuclei to the red nucleus and ventrolateral thalamus for regulation of the rubrospinal and corticospinal UMN systems. An infarct in the superior cerebellar artery can damage the blood supply to the superior and middle peduncles and the deep nuclei on one side. Lesions in these structures commonly have longer lasting and more severe clinical effects than lesions that affect only the cerebellar cortex. A superior cerebellar artery infarct can result in ipsilateral limb ataxia, dysmetria, dysdiadochokinesia, intention tremor, hypotonus, and other characteristics of lateral cerebellar damage. In addition, some midbrain structures are supplied by this artery; an infarct causes added brain stem problems, such as nystagmus and eye movement problems.

12

DIENCEPHALON

Thalamocortical radiations

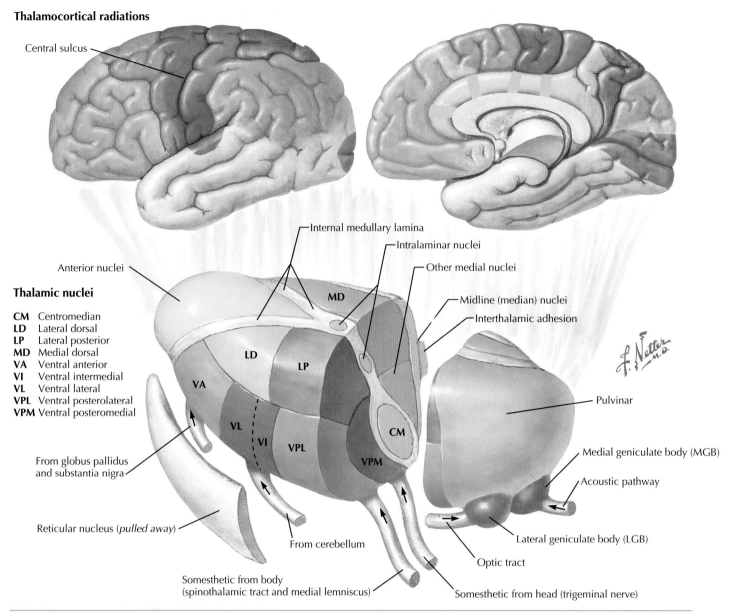

Central sulcus

Internal medullary lamina

Intralaminar nuclei

Other medial nuclei

Anterior nuclei

MD

Midline (median) nuclei

Interthalamic adhesion

Thalamic nuclei

CM Centromedian
LD Lateral dorsal
LP Lateral posterior
MD Medial dorsal
VA Ventral anterior
VI Ventral intermedial
VL Ventral lateral
VPL Ventral posterolateral
VPM Ventral posteromedial

LD

LP

VA

Pulvinar

VL

VI

VPL

CM

VPM

Medial geniculate body (MGB)

Acoustic pathway

From globus pallidus and substantia nigra

Reticular nucleus (*pulled away*)

From cerebellum

Lateral geniculate body (LGB)

Optic tract

Somesthetic from body (spinothalamic tract and medial lemniscus)

Somesthetic from head (trigeminal nerve)

12.1 THALAMIC ANATOMY AND INTERCONNECTIONS WITH THE CEREBRAL CORTEX

The thalamus, the gateway to the cerebral cortex, conveys extensive sensory, motor, and autonomic information from the brain stem and spinal cord to the cortex. All sensory projections to the cortex except olfaction are processed through thalamic nuclei. Thalamic nuclei are reciprocally interconnected with regions of cortex. Specific thalamic nuclei project to circumscribed regions of cortex. These nuclei include (1) sensory projection nuclei (VPL: somatosensory; VPM: trigeminal; LGB: visual; MGB: auditory; pulvinar: sensory); (2) motor-related nuclei (VL and VI: cerebellum; VA and VL: basal ganglia); (3) autonomic- and limbic-related nuclei (anterior and LD: cingulate cortex; MD: frontal and cingulate cortex); and (4) nuclei related to association areas (pulvinar and LP: parietal cortex). Nonspecific thalamic nuclei (intralaminar nuclei, such as CM, parafascicular, and medial VA) send diffuse connections to widespread regions of cerebral cortex and to other thalamic nuclei. The reticular nucleus of the thalamus helps to regulate the

excitability of thalamic projection nuclei. Specific lesions of the thalamus can result in diminished sensory, motor, or autonomic activity related to loss of the specific modalities processed. Some thalamic lesions can lead to excruciating paroxysms of neuropathic pain, which is referred to as thalamic syndrome.

CLINICAL POINT

The thalamus has a complex blood supply that is derived extensively from the penetrating posterior cerebral, posterior communicating, and other nearby arteries. Thalamic nuclei are seldom individually affected by infarcts and lesions but are damaged along with nearby regions. Lesions that affect one side of the thalamus seldom produce permanent deficits unless sensory nuclei are involved. Thalamic lesions can result in changes in consciousness and alertness (intralaminar, reticular nuclei); affective behavior (medial dorsal, ventral anterior, intralaminar nuclei); memory functions (midline, medial, mammillary, and possibly anterior nuclei); motor activity (ventrolateral, ventral anterior, posterior, other nuclei); somatic sensation (ventral posterolateral and posteromedial nuclei); vision (lateral geniculate nuclei); and perceptions and hallucinations (dorsomedial, intralaminar nuclei). Medial dorsal lesions may produce a reciprocal disconnect with the prefrontal cortex and bring about a deficit in frontal functions.

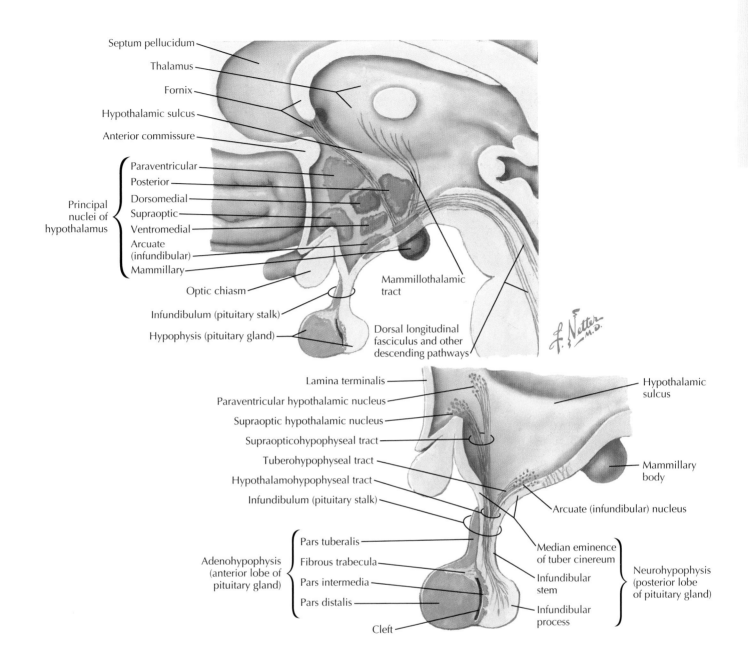

Septum pellucidum
Thalamus
Fornix
Hypothalamic sulcus
Anterior commissure

Principal nuclei of hypothalamus
- Paraventricular
- Posterior
- Dorsomedial
- Supraoptic
- Ventromedial
- Arcuate (infundibular)
- Mammillary

Optic chiasm
Infundibulum (pituitary stalk)
Hypophysis (pituitary gland)

Mammillothalamic tract

Dorsal longitudinal fasciculus and other descending pathways

Lamina terminalis
Paraventricular hypothalamic nucleus
Supraoptic hypothalamic nucleus
Supraopticohypophyseal tract
Tuberohypophyseal tract
Hypothalamohypophyseal tract
Infundibulum (pituitary stalk)

Hypothalamic sulcus

Mammillary body

Arcuate (infundibular) nucleus

Median eminence of tuber cinereum

Infundibular stem

Infundibular process

Neurohypophysis (posterior lobe of pituitary gland)

Adenohypophysis (anterior lobe of pituitary gland)
- Pars tuberalis
- Fibrous trabecula
- Pars intermedia
- Pars distalis

Cleft

12.2 HYPOTHALAMUS AND PITUITARY GLAND

The hypothalamus is the major region of the central nervous system involved in neuroendocrine regulation and control of visceral functions, such as temperature regulation, food and appetite regulation, thirst and water balance, reproduction and sexual behavior, parturition and control of lactation, respiratory and cardiovascular regulation, gastrointestinal regulation, stress responses, and reparative states. The hypothalamus is located between the rostral midbrain and the lamina terminalis, ventral to the thalamus; it surrounds the third ventricle. The hypothalamus is subdivided in rostral-to-caudal zones (preoptic, anterior or supraoptic, tuberal, and mammillary or posterior) as well as medial-to-lateral zones (periventricular, medial, lateral). These zones contain some discrete nuclei and even discrete chemical-specific subnuclei, such as the paraventricular nucleus (PVN) and more diffuse centers, regions, or areas (such as anterior, posterior, and lateral regions). The neuroendocrine portion of the hypothalamus consists of (1) magnocellular portions of the PVN and the supraoptic nucleus, which send axons directly to the posterior pituitary and release vasopressin and oxytocin into the general circulation; (2) releasing-factor and inhibitory-factor neurons, which project axons to the hypophyseal-portal vasculature in the contact zone of the median eminence, through which very high concentrations of these factors (hormones) induce the release of anterior pituitary hormones into the general circulation; and (3) the tuberoinfundibular system and ascending systems (monoamine and other chemical-specific neurons) that modulate the release of releasing and inhibitory factors into the hypophyseal-portal vasculature.

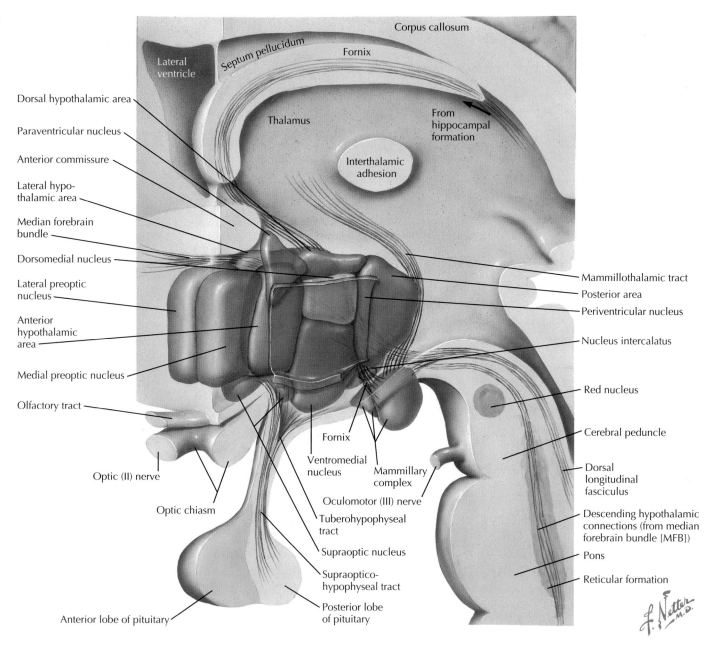

Illustration of Hypothalamic Nuclei

12.3 ILLUSTRATION OF HYPOTHALAMIC NUCLEI

Hypothalamic nuclei and areas are associated with many visceral and neuroendocrine functions. The magnocellular neurons of the PVN and supraoptic nucleus release oxytocin and vasopressin into the posterior pituitary general circulation. PVN parvocellular neurons containing corticotrophin-releasing hormone project to the hypophyseal portal system in the contact zone of the median eminence and induce the release of adrenocorticotropic hormone (which stimulates the release of cortisol from the adrenal cortex). Descending axons of the PVN also project to the dorsal (motor) nucleus of CN X, the nucleus solitarius, and the intermediolateral cell column preganglionic sympathetic neurons, and they regulate preganglionic outflow from the autonomic nervous system. The anterior and posterior areas coordinate parasympathetic and sympathetic outflow, respectively. The dorsomedial (DM) and ventromedial (VM) nuclei and the lateral hypothalamic area regulate appetite, drinking, and reproductive behavior. The preoptic area regulates cyclic neuroendocrine behavior and thermoregulation. The suprachiasmatic nucleus receives visual inputs from the optic tract and regulates circadian rhythms. Several hypothalamic regions are involved in the regulation of sleep.

CLINICAL POINT

Hypothalamic nuclei often appear as discrete nuclei and regions that may subserve discrete functions. Early studies of lesions in the hypothalamus led to this impression, resulting in a description of centers, such as the ventromedial nucleus satiety center (lesions led to hyperphagia and obesity) and a lateral appetitive stimulatory center (lesions led to aphagia and cachexia). However, such lesions often damaged passing fiber tracts (e.g., passing axons of the monoaminergic systems) and connections, sometimes even those not associated with the primary functions studied. We now know that many hormones are involved in the control of appetite and food intake. When food is ingested, cholecyctokinin and glucagon-like peptide-1 are released by neuroendocrine cells in the intestine, and they act in the brain to suppress appetite and give the sensation of satiety. In the absence of food, these hormone levels are low, permitting appetite and food-seeking behavior. Long-term regulation of food intake also involves the hormone leptin, produced by fat cells. When fat stores are high, leptin is released and acts on the hypothalamus to suppress appetite. When body nutrient stores are depleted, leptin levels are lowered. Other hormones, such as ghrelins, also regulate appetite and eating behavior. Hypothalamic physiology awaits further studies to fully integrate the complex hypothalamic circuitry with the complex hormonal regulation, over which volitional and affective control from higher brain regions is further superimposed. Given the epidemic of obesity in the United States and other "fast-food countries," a better understanding of the physiology of eating and appetite is urgently needed.

CLINICAL POINT

The hypothalamus is a small but complex region of the central nervous system that interconnects the limbic forebrain and the brain stem. The principal functions of the hypothalamus are neuroendocrine regulation, especially through the pituitary gland, and regulation of autonomic function. Thermoregulation is one example of the latter. Several hypothalamic sites, including the anterior and posterior hypothalamic areas, regulate the set point for body temperature within relatively tight parameters. Damage to these mechanisms by head trauma, tumor, surgery, increased intracranial pressure, or vascular problems can induce a change in thermoregulation. Posterior hypothalamic damage is often accompanied by hypothermia, whereas anterior hypothalamic damage is often accompanied by hyperthermia. In addition, inflammatory mediators such as interleukin-1 beta and interleukin-6, whether derived from an infectious process (endotoxin or pyrogen) or from other sources of inflammation, can activate some of the anterior regions of the hypothalamus such as the preoptic area and can induce fever. These inflammatory mediators also can produce classic illness behavior and can powerfully activate both the hypothalamo-pituitary-adrenal axis and the hypothalamo-sympathetic axis, driving a classic stress response. Altered internal body temperature also can be affected by intracranial surgery, susceptibility to some anesthetic agents (malignant hyperthermia), and susceptibility to some neuroleptic drugs.

A major role of the hypothalamus is neuroendocrine regulation of the anterior and posterior pituitary. Neurons in the supraoptic and paraventricular nuclei send axonal connections directly to the posterior pituitary to release oxytocin and vasopressin into the general circulation. Many other collections of neurons, in the hypothalamus and elsewhere, send axonal connections to the hypophyseal-portal vascular system in the contact zone of the median eminence and release releasing factors (hormones) and inhibitory factors (hormones) that regulate the secretion of a variety of hormones from pituicytes in the anterior pituitary. These releasing-factor neurons and inhibitory-factor neurons receive extensive input from brain stem, hypothalamic, and limbic forebrain sources. Some of these neurons (such as the corticotrophin-releasing factor neurons in the PVN) also receive input from chemical sources, such as interleukin-1 beta, prostaglandin E2, and nitric oxide. Interleukin-1 beta, both directly and indirectly, can drive the response of corticotrophin-releasing factor, thereby activating the hypothalamo-pituitary-adrenal system to stimulate cortisol production and drive the hypothalamo-sympathetic system to stimulate the release of catecholamines. Some neurotransmitters in these releasing-factor neurons and inhibitory-factor neurons can be influenced pharmacologically. Dopamine in the arcuate nucleus acts as a prolactin-inhibitory factor. A dopamine agonist can suppress prolactin output by a prolactin-secreting pituitary tumor (chromophobe adenoma).

13

TELENCEPHALON

Level 1: Mid Pons

Level of section
(mid pons)

CN V
Uncus
Basis pontis
Corticospinal tract fibers
Basilar artery
Temporal lobe
*
Lateral cerebellar hemisphere
Superior cerebellar peduncle
Medial lemniscus
Pontine tegmentum
Cerebellar vermis
Fourth ventricle

JOHN A.CRAIG—AD

13.1A AXIAL (HORIZONTAL) SECTIONS THROUGH THE FOREBRAIN: LEVEL 1—MID PONS

These axial (horizontal) sections compare anatomical sections and high-resolution magnetic resonance (MR) images. They are cut in the true horizontal (axial) plane, not in the older 25-degree tilt. The most important anatomical relationships in these sections center on the internal capsule (IC). The head of the caudate nucleus is medial to the anterior limb of the IC and forms the lateral margin of the frontal pole of the lateral ventricle. The thalamus is medial to the posterior limb of the IC. The globus pallidus and putamen are lateral to the wedge-shaped IC. The posterior limb of the IC carries the major descending corticospinal, corticorubral, and corticoreticular fibers and the ascending sensory fibers of the somatosensory and trigeminal systems. The most posterior portions of the posterior limb also carry the auditory and visual projections to their respective cortices. The genu of the IC carries the corticobulbar fibers. The anterior limb of the IC carries cortical projections to the striatum and the pontine nuclei (pontocerebellar system). The full-plate MR images are T1-weighted; the ventricles appear dark. The scout MRI images that accompany the drawings are T2-weighted MR images, in which the CSF appears white.

Basilar artery

Basis pontis (with corticospinal system)

Medial longitudinal fasciculus

Fourth ventricle

Lateral cerebellar hemisphere

Temporal lobe

Pontine tegmentum

Middle cerebellar peduncle

Superior cerebellar peduncle

13.1B AXIAL (HORIZONTAL) SECTIONS THROUGH THE FOREBRAIN: LEVEL 1—MID PONS

Level 2: Rostral Pons

Level of section
(rostral pons)

Amygdala

Temporal lobe

Basis pontis

Corticospinal tract fibers

Basilar artery

Superior
cerebellar
peduncle

Fourth
ventricle

Lateral cerebellar
hemisphere

Vermis of cerebellum

Medial
lemniscus

Pontine
tegmentum

JOHN A. CRAIG—AD

13.2A AXIAL (HORIZONTAL) SECTIONS THROUGH THE FOREBRAIN: LEVEL 2—ROSTRAL PONS

Temporal lobe

Basis pontis (with
corticospinal system)

Pontine tegmentum

Fourth ventricle

Superior cerebellar
peduncle

Lateral hemisphere
of cerebellum

Cerebellar vermis

**13.2B AXIAL (HORIZONTAL) SECTIONS THROUGH THE FOREBRAIN: LEVEL 2—ROSTRAL PONS
(CONTINUED)**

Level 3: Midbrain

Level of section
(midbrain)

Posterior cerebral arteries

CN III (oculomotor)

CN II (optic)

Temporal lobe

Substantia nigra

Cerebral peduncle

Amygdala

Tail of caudate nucleus

Hippocampal formation

Inferior horn of lateral ventricle

Entorhinal cortex

Cerebral aqueduct

Occipital lobe

Decussation of superior cerebellar peduncle

Cerebellar vermis

JOHN A. CRAIG—AD

13.3A AXIAL (HORIZONTAL) SECTIONS THROUGH THE FOREBRAIN: LEVEL 3—MIDBRAIN

CLINICAL POINT

The temporal lobe includes the amygdaloid nuclei, the hippocampal formation and associated cortex, the transverse gyrus of Heschl, some language-associated cortical regions (Wernicke's area in the dominant hemisphere), Meyer's loop of geniculocalcarine axons, the inferior horn of the lateral ventricle, and extensive cortical areas (superior, middle, and inferior temporal gyri). The temporal lobe can be damaged by trauma, infarcts, tumors, abscesses, and other pathological conditions. Such damage can result in auditory hallucinations, delirium and psychotic behavior, sometimes a contralateral upper quadrantanopia (if Meyer's loop is damaged), and receptive aphasia (Wernicke's aphasia) that involves a lack of understanding of verbal information (in a lesion of the dominant hemisphere). Some very specific lesions in the temporal lobe result in an agnosia for recognition of faces (prosopagnosia).

Amygdala

Inferior horn of
lateral ventricle

Hippocampal formation

Orbitofrontal cortex

Temporal lobe

Cerebral peduncle

Aqueduct

Superior colliculus

Cerebellar vermis

Occipital lobe

13.3B AXIAL (HORIZONTAL) SECTIONS THROUGH THE FOREBRAIN: LEVEL 3—MIDBRAIN (CONTINUED)

Level 4: Rostral Midbrain and Hypothalamus

**Level of section
(rostral midbrain
and hypothalamus)**

Substantia nigra

Cerebral peduncle

Red nucleus

Medial geniculate
nucleus

Orbitofrontal cortex

Amygdala

Mammillary bodies

Lateral geniculate
nucleus

Anterior cerebral
artery

Hippocampal
formation

Temporal lobe

Tail of caudate
nucleus

Temporal horn of
lateral ventricle

Entorhinal
cortex

Periaqueductal
gray matter

Superior
colliculus

Occipital lobe

Cerebral
aqueduct

Cerebellar
vermis

Optic tract

Posterior
cerebral
artery

JOHN A. CRAIG—AD

**13.4A   AXIAL (HORIZONTAL) SECTIONS THROUGH THE FOREBRAIN: LEVEL 4—ROSTRAL MIDBRAIN
AND HYPOTHALAMUS**

Orbitofrontal cortex

Cerebellar peduncle

Lateral geniculate nucleus

Temporal lobe

Medial geniculate nucleus

Hippocampal formation

Temporal horn of
lateral ventricle

Superior colliculus

Cerebellar vermis

Occipital lobe

13.4B AXIAL (HORIZONTAL) SECTIONS THROUGH THE FOREBRAIN: LEVEL 4—ROSTRAL MIDBRAIN AND HYPOTHALAMUS (CONTINUED)

Level 5: Anterior Commissure and Caudal Thalamus

Level of section (anterior commissure and caudal thalamus)

Orbitofrontal cortex

Putamen

Claustrum

Insular cortex

Posterior limb of internal capsule

Thalamus

Temporal lobe

Choroid plexus

Tail of caudate nucleus

Atrium of lateral ventricle

Anterior limb of internal capsule

Globus pallidus (internal and external segments)

Head of caudate nucleus

Anterior commissure

Columns of fornix

Extreme capsule

External capsule

Third ventricle

Habenular commissure

Hippocampal formation

Pulvinar

Occipital lobe

JOHN A. CRAIG—AD

13.5A AXIAL (HORIZONTAL) SECTIONS THROUGH THE FOREBRAIN: LEVEL 5—ANTERIOR COMMISSURE AND CAUDAL THALAMUS

CLINICAL POINT

The basal ganglia assist the cerebral cortex in planning and generating desired programs of activity and suppressing undesired programs of activity. The most conspicuous arena in which these functions are observed is motor activity. Basal ganglia disorders produce movement problems that are often involuntary in nature and are commonly accompanied by cognitive and affective symptoms (e.g., Huntington's disease). The principal route of information flow from the basal ganglia is from the thalamus and cerebral cortex to the striatum (caudate nucleus and putamen), then to the globus pallidus, then back to the thalamus and cortex, completing the loop. Disruption of this loop can produce excessive movements (e.g., choreiform and athetoid movements, tremor) or diminished movements (bradykinesia). In some instances, specific nuclei are known to be associated with such changes. A small lacunar infarct in the subthalamic nucleus results in wild, flinging (ballistic) movements in the contralateral limbs. However, a surgical lesion in the subthalamic nucleus may ameliorate some of the movement problems seen in Parkinson's disease. The subthalamus most likely drives activity in the internal segment of the globus pallidus, which in turn can be modified by the external segment. A pathological lesion in the globus pallidus can produce rigidity and akinesia; a surgical pallidal lesion may reduce excessive movements in other basal ganglia disorders.

Anterior commissure

Temporal lobe

Columns of fornix

Third ventricle

Habenula

Hippocampal formation

Orbitofrontal cortex

Head of caudate nucleus

Putamen

Thalamus

Pulvinar

Tail of caudate nucleus

Atrium of lateral ventricle

Occipital lobe

13.5B AXIAL (HORIZONTAL) SECTIONS THROUGH THE FOREBRAIN: LEVEL 5—ANTERIOR COMMISSURE AND CAUDAL THALAMUS (CONTINUED)

Level 6: Head of Caudate and Mid Thalamus

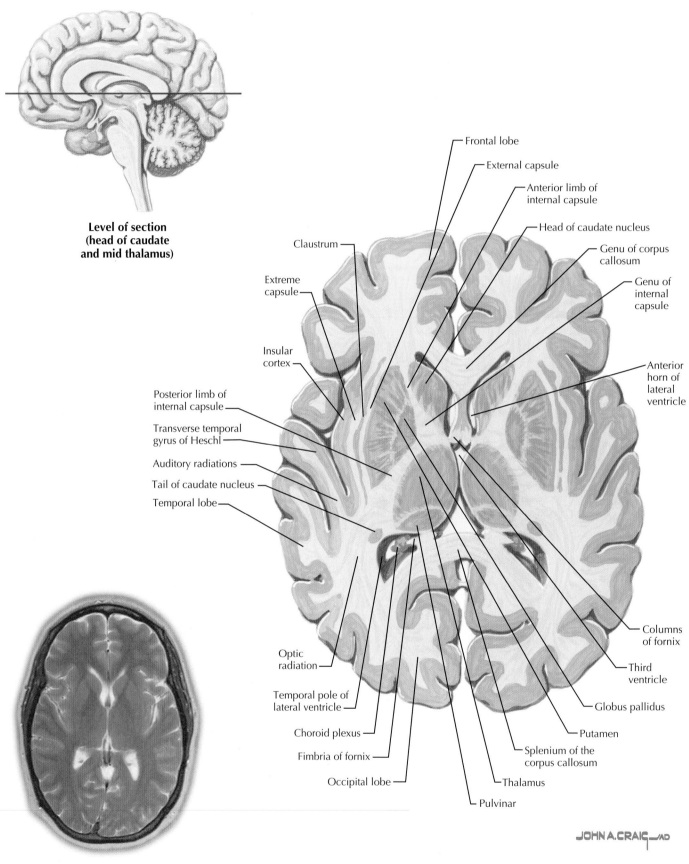

Level of section
(head of caudate
and mid thalamus)

Frontal lobe

External capsule

Anterior limb of
internal capsule

Head of caudate nucleus

Genu of corpus
callosum

Genu of
internal
capsule

Anterior
horn of
lateral
ventricle

Claustrum

Extreme
capsule

Insular
cortex

Posterior limb of
internal capsule

Transverse temporal
gyrus of Heschl

Auditory radiations

Tail of caudate nucleus

Temporal lobe

Optic
radiation

Temporal pole of
lateral ventricle

Choroid plexus

Fimbria of fornix

Occipital lobe

Columns
of fornix

Third
ventricle

Globus pallidus

Putamen

Splenium of the
corpus callosum

Thalamus

Pulvinar

JOHN A. CRAIG—AD

**13.6A AXIAL (HORIZONTAL) SECTIONS THROUGH THE FOREBRAIN: LEVEL 6—HEAD OF CAUDATE
AND MID THALAMUS**

Frontal cortex

Genu of corpus callosum

Head of caudate nucleus

Anterior horn of
lateral ventricle

Globus pallidus

Insular cortex

Putamen

Temporal pole of
lateral ventricle

Optic radiations

Anterior limb
of internal capsule

Columns of fornix

Genu of internal capsule

Posterior limb
of internal capsule

Lateral fissure

Thalamus

Tail of caudate nucleus

Splenium of
corpus callosum

13.6B AXIAL (HORIZONTAL) SECTIONS THROUGH THE FOREBRAIN: LEVEL 6—HEAD OF CAUDATE AND MID THALAMUS (CONTINUED)

Level 7: Basal Ganglia and Internal Capsule

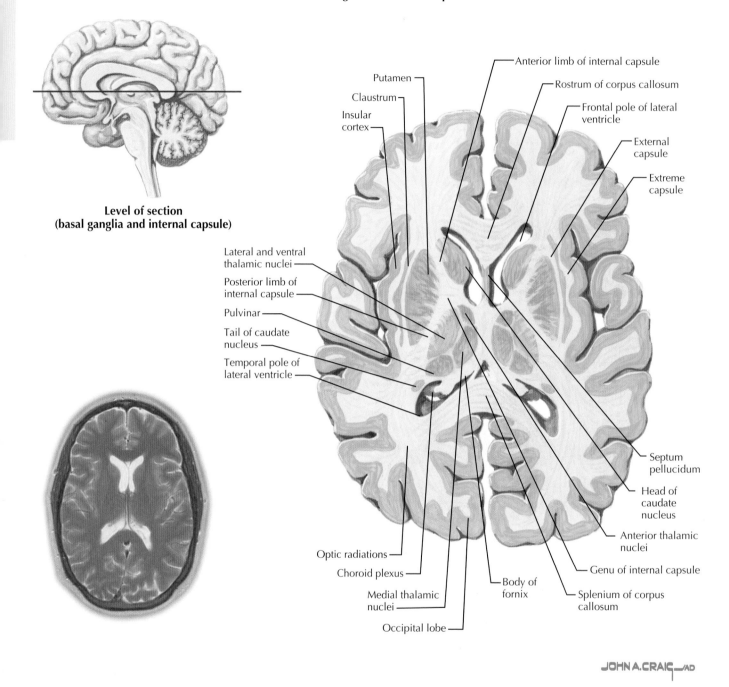

**Level of section
(basal ganglia and internal capsule)**

Putamen

Claustrum

Insular cortex

Lateral and ventral thalamic nuclei

Posterior limb of internal capsule

Pulvinar

Tail of caudate nucleus

Temporal pole of lateral ventricle

Anterior limb of internal capsule

Rostrum of corpus callosum

Frontal pole of lateral ventricle

External capsule

Extreme capsule

Septum pellucidum

Head of caudate nucleus

Anterior thalamic nuclei

Genu of internal capsule

Splenium of corpus callosum

Optic radiations

Choroid plexus

Medial thalamic nuclei

Body of fornix

Occipital lobe

JOHN A. CRAIG—AD

13.7A AXIAL (HORIZONTAL) SECTIONS THROUGH THE FOREBRAIN: LEVEL 7—BASAL GANGLIA AND INTERNAL CAPSULE

CLINICAL POINT

Huntington's disease is an autosomal dominant disorder caused by a trinucleotide repeat (CAG) on the short arm of chromosome 4. It results in a progressive, untreatable disease that includes a movement disorder (choreiform movements: brisk, jerky, forcible, arrhythmic movements), progressive cognitive impairment, and affective disorders (such as depression, psychotic behavior). This disease progresses from a state of minor impairment (clumsiness) with minor behavioral problems (irritability and depression) to major impairment, dementia, and a decline that leads to incapacitation and ultimately to an early death. The anatomical hallmark of this disease is marked degeneration of the caudate nucleus (also the putamen). The characteristic bulge of the head of the caudate into the frontal pole of the lateral ventricle is lost. Most of the medium spiny caudate neurons that project to the globus pallidus degenerate as the result of damage from excess Ca^{++} influx caused by glutamate excitotoxic damage via activation of receptors of N-methyl-D-aspartate (NMDA). The intrinsic cholinergic interneurons of the striatum also degenerate in Huntington's disease.

Frontal cortex

Head of
caudate nucleus

Putamen

Insular cortex

Temporal pole
of lateral ventricle

Occipital lobe

Genu of corpus callosum

Septum pellucidum

Anterior limb
of internal capsule

Columns of fornix

Posterior limb
of internal capsule

Lateral fissure

Thalamus

Body of fornix

Splenium of
corpus callosum

Optic radiations

13.7B AXIAL (HORIZONTAL) SECTIONS THROUGH THE FOREBRAIN: LEVEL 7—BASAL GANGLIA AND INTERNAL CAPSULE (CONTINUED)

Level 8: Dorsal Caudate, Splenium, and Genu of Corpus Callosum

Level of section
(dorsal caudate, splenium, and genu
of corpus callosum)

Cingulate cortex

Genu of corpus callosum

Frontal lobe

Body of lateral ventricle

Body of caudate nucleus

Insular cortex

Parietal lobe

Frontal pole of lateral ventricle

Septum pellucidum

Occipital lobe

Splenium of corpus callosum

JOHN A.CRAIG—AD

13.8A AXIAL (HORIZONTAL) SECTIONS THROUGH THE FOREBRAIN: LEVEL 8—DORSAL CAUDATE, SPLENIUM, AND GENU OF CORPUS CALLOSUM

Frontal lobe

Body of caudate nucleus

Septum pellucidum

Cingulate cortex

Frontal pole of lateral ventricle

Body of lateral ventricle

Parietal lobe

Splenium of corpus callosum

Occipital lobe

13.8B AXIAL (HORIZONTAL) SECTIONS THROUGH THE FOREBRAIN: LEVEL 8—DORSAL CAUDATE, SPLENIUM, AND GENU OF CORPUS CALLOSUM (CONTINUED)

Level 9: Body of Corpus Callosum

Level of section
(body of corpus callosum)

Anterior cingulate cortex

Frontal lobe

Centrum semiovale

Body of caudate nucleus

Parietal lobe

Occipital lobe

Visual cortex

Body of lateral ventricle

Body of corpus callosum

JOHN A.CRAIG—AD

13.9A AXIAL (HORIZONTAL) SECTIONS THROUGH THE FOREBRAIN: LEVEL 9—BODY OF CORPUS CALLOSUM

Anterior cingulate cortex

Body of caudate nucleus

Body of corpus callosum

Parietal lobe

Visual cortex

Body of lateral ventricle

Centrum semiovale

Occipital lobe

13.9B AXIAL (HORIZONTAL) SECTIONS THROUGH THE FOREBRAIN: LEVEL 9—BODY OF CORPUS CALLOSUM (CONTINUED)

Level 10: Centrum Semiovale

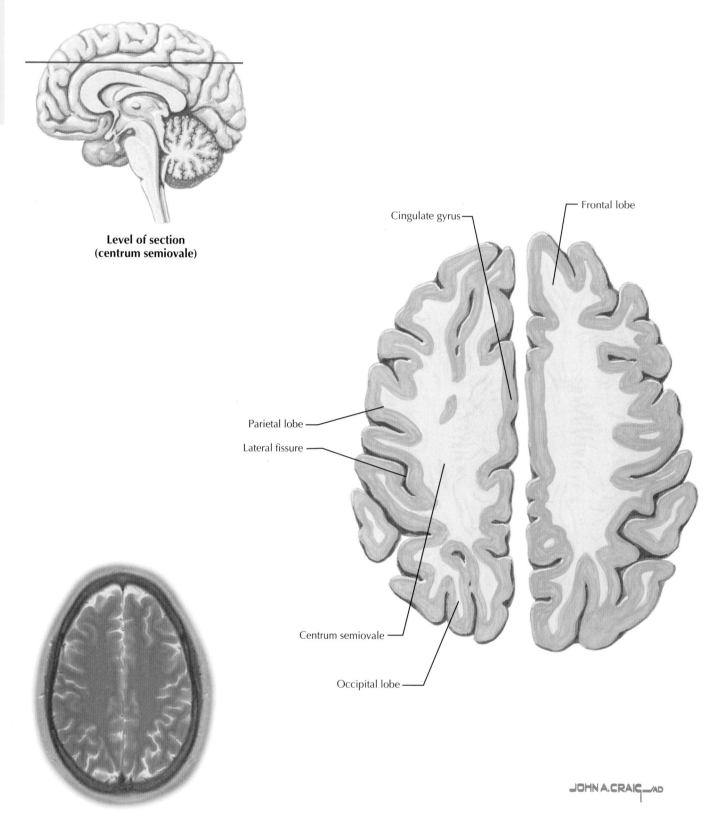

Level of section
(centrum semiovale)

Cingulate gyrus

Frontal lobe

Parietal lobe

Lateral fissure

Centrum semiovale

Occipital lobe

JOHN A. CRAIG⌐AD

13.10A AXIAL (HORIZONTAL) SECTIONS THROUGH THE FOREBRAIN: LEVEL 10—CENTRUM SEMIOVALE

Frontal lobe

Cingulate gyrus

Parietal lobe

Centrum semiovale

Lateral fissure

Occipital lobe

13.10B AXIAL (HORIZONTAL) SECTIONS THROUGH THE FOREBRAIN: LEVEL 10—CENTRUM SEMIOVALE (CONTINUED)

Level 1: Genu of Corpus Callosum

**Level of section
(genu of corpus callosum)**

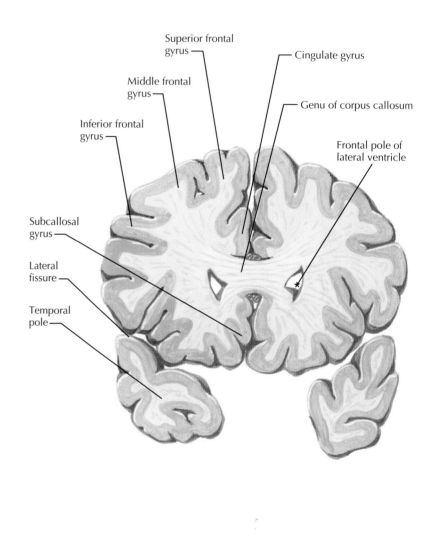

Superior frontal gyrus

Middle frontal gyrus

Inferior frontal gyrus

Cingulate gyrus

Genu of corpus callosum

Frontal pole of lateral ventricle

Subcallosal gyrus

Lateral fissure

Temporal pole

JOHN A. CRAIG—AD

13.11A CORONAL SECTIONS THROUGH THE FOREBRAIN: LEVEL 1—GENU OF CORPUS CALLOSUM

These coronal sections compare anatomical sections and high-resolution MR images. They show important relationships among the internal capsule, basal ganglia, and thalamus. These sections show basal forebrain structures, such as nucleus accumbens, substantia innominata, and nucleus basalis (cholinergic forebrain nucleus), some individual thalamic nuclei, and the important temporal lobe structures (amygdaloid nuclei, hippocampal formation) and pathways (fornix, stria terminalis). The full-page MR images are T1-weighted; the ventricles appear dark. The scout MR images that accompany the drawings are T2-weighted MR images in which the CSF appears white.

Superior frontal gyrus

Middle frontal gyrus

Inferior frontal gyrus

Cingulate gyrus

Genu of corpus callosum

Frontal pole of lateral ventricle

Subcallosal gyrus

Lateral fissure

Temporal pole

13.11B   CORONAL SECTIONS THROUGH THE FOREBRAIN: LEVEL 1—GENU OF CORPUS CALLOSUM (CONTINUED)

Level 2: Head of Caudate Nucleus/Nucleus Accumbens

**Level of section
(head of caudate nucleus/
nucleus accumbens)**

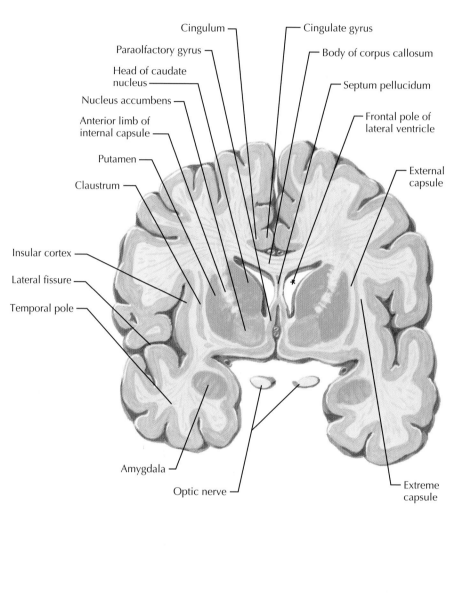

Cingulum

Cingulate gyrus

Paraolfactory gyrus

Body of corpus callosum

Head of caudate nucleus

Septum pellucidum

Nucleus accumbens

Anterior limb of internal capsule

Frontal pole of lateral ventricle

Putamen

External capsule

Claustrum

Insular cortex

Lateral fissure

Temporal pole

Amygdala

Optic nerve

Extreme capsule

JOHN A.CRAIG—AD

13.12A CORONAL SECTIONS THROUGH THE FOREBRAIN: LEVEL 2—HEAD OF CAUDATE NUCLEUS/NUCLEUS ACCUMBENS

CLINICAL POINT

The nucleus accumbens is located at the anterior end of the striatum in the ventral part of the forebrain. It receives a variety of inputs from limbic structures, such as the amygdala, hypocampal formation, and bed nucleus of the stria terminalis. A major dopaminergic (DA) input innervates the nucleus accumbens via the mesolimbic DA pathway, which derives from the ventral tegmental area in the ventral midbrain. The nucleus accumbens is central to motivational states and addictive behavior, driven by DA neurotransmission. The nucleus accumbens is also a principal region of brain circuitry associated with reward, such as joy, pleasure, and gratification. This nucleus has a looped circuitry through the thalamus and cortex that helps to provide motor expression of emotional responses and accompanying gestures and behaviors.

Cingulate gyrus

Body of corpus callosum

Septum pellucidum

Claustrum

Insular cortex

Lateral fissure

Temporal lobe

Amygdala

Frontal pole of lateral ventricle

Head of caudate nucleus

Anterior limb of internal capsule

Putamen

Nucleus accumbens

Optic chiasm

13.12B CORONAL SECTIONS THROUGH THE FOREBRAIN: LEVEL 2 — HEAD OF CAUDATE NUCLEUS/ NUCLEUS ACCUMBENS (CONTINUED)

Level 3: Anterior Commissure/Columns of Fornix

**Level of section
(anterior commissure/
columns of fornix)**

Columns of fornix

Cingulum

Head of caudate nucleus

Anterior commissure

Anterior limb of internal capsule

Globus pallidus

Claustrum

Insular cortex

Putamen

Lateral fissure

Nucleus basalis

Temporal lobe

Amygdala

Third ventricle

Supraoptic recess

Optic chiasm

Cingulate gyrus

Body of corpus callosum

Septum pellucidum

Frontal pole of lateral ventricle

Extreme capsule

External capsule

JOHN A. CRAIG—AD

**13.13A CORONAL SECTIONS THROUGH THE FOREBRAIN: LEVEL 3—ANTERIOR COMMISSURE/
COLUMNS OF FORNIX**

Frontal pole of lateral ventricle

Head of caudate nucleus

Anterior limb of internal capsule

Putamen

Globus pallidus

Temporal lobe

Anterior commissure

Nucleus basalis

Amygdala

Cingulate cortex

Cingulum

Body of corpus callosum

Septum pellucidum

External capsule

Insular cortex

Lateral fissure

Third ventricle

Optic tract

13.13B CORONAL SECTIONS THROUGH THE FOREBRAIN: LEVEL 3—ANTERIOR COMMISSURE/ COLUMNS OF FORNIX (CONTINUED)

Level 4: Amygdala, Anterior Limb of Internal Capsule

**Level of section
(amygdala, anterior limb
of internal capsule)**

Cingulum

Stria terminalis
and terminal vein

Cingulate gyrus

Body of caudate
nucleus

Body of corpus callosum

Anterior limb of
internal capsule

Body of lateral
ventricle

Claustrum

Putamen

Insular cortex

Globus pallidus
external segment

Temporal cortex

Amygdala

Columns of fornix

Globus pallidus
internal segment

Third ventricle

Optic tract

Hypothalamus

JOHN A.CRAIG—AD

13.14A CORONAL SECTIONS THROUGH THE FOREBRAIN: LEVEL 4—AMYGDALA, ANTERIOR LIMB OF INTERNAL CAPSULE

CLINICAL POINT

The corpus callosum is the principal interhemispheric or commissural pathway in the brain. It interconnects one hemisphere with its counterpart on the other side, with the exception of part of the temporal lobe that is interconnected by the anterior commissure. Some large lesions resulting from trauma or tumor can damage the corpus callosum, but this is usually accompanied by a large amount of additional forebrain damage. However, specific surgical sectioning of the corpus callosum has been performed in an attempt to alleviate the spread of seizure activity from one side of the brain to the other. This "split-brain" surgery causes each hemisphere to be unaware of specific activity occurring in the other hemisphere. Thus, the left brain cannot identify a visual or somatosensory stimulus presented to the right hemisphere and does not know where the left hand and arm are located if they are kept from the left hemisphere's view. Sometimes, the left hand may act independently of the conscious intent of the left hemisphere. Some emotional information appears to transfer through brain stem regions between the two parts of the split brain, providing a limbic context that may be perceived to some extent by both hemispheres.

Body of corpus callosum

Septum pellucidum

Lateral fissure

Insular cortex

Columns of fornix

Inferior horn of lateral ventricle

Amygdala

Hypothalamus

Cingulate cortex

Cingulum

Body of lateral ventricle

Body of caudate nucleus

Genu/anterior limb of internal capsule

Putamen

Temporal lobe

Globus pallidus

Optic tract

Third ventricle

13.14B CORONAL SECTIONS THROUGH THE FOREBRAIN: LEVEL 4—AMYGDALA, ANTERIOR LIMB OF INTERNAL CAPSULE (CONTINUED)

Level 5: Mammillary Bodies

**Level of section
(mammillary bodies)**

Third ventricle

Rostral thalamus

Hypothalamus

Posterior limb of
internal capsule

Globus pallidus
internal segment

Putamen

Globus pallidus
external segment

Insular cortex

Lateral fissure

Claustrum

Inferior horn of
lateral ventricle

Temporal lobe

Amygdala

Optic tract

Hippocampal
formation

Interpeduncular fossa

Mammillary body

Cerebral peduncle

Cingulate gyrus

Body of corpus callosum

Cingulum

Columns of fornix

Body of lateral
ventricle

Body of caudate
nucleus

Extreme capsule

External capsule

Middle cerebral artery

Basis pontis

Corticospinal tract
in basis pontis

JOHN A.CRAIG—AD

13.15A CORONAL SECTIONS THROUGH THE FOREBRAIN: LEVEL 5—MAMMILLARY BODY

Cingulate cortex
Cingulum
Body of caudate nucleus
Putamen
Insular cortex
Lateral fissure
Third ventricle
Hypothalamus

Body of lateral ventricle
Columns of fornix
Rostral thalamus
Posterior limb of internal capsule
Claustrum
Temporal lobe
Amygdala
Inferior horn of lateral ventricle
Hippocampal formation
Corticospinal tract in basis pontis
Basis pontis

13.15B CORONAL SECTIONS THROUGH THE FOREBRAIN: LEVEL 5—MAMMILLARY BODY (CONTINUED)

Level 6: Mammillothalamic Tract/Substantia Nigra, Rostral Hippocampus

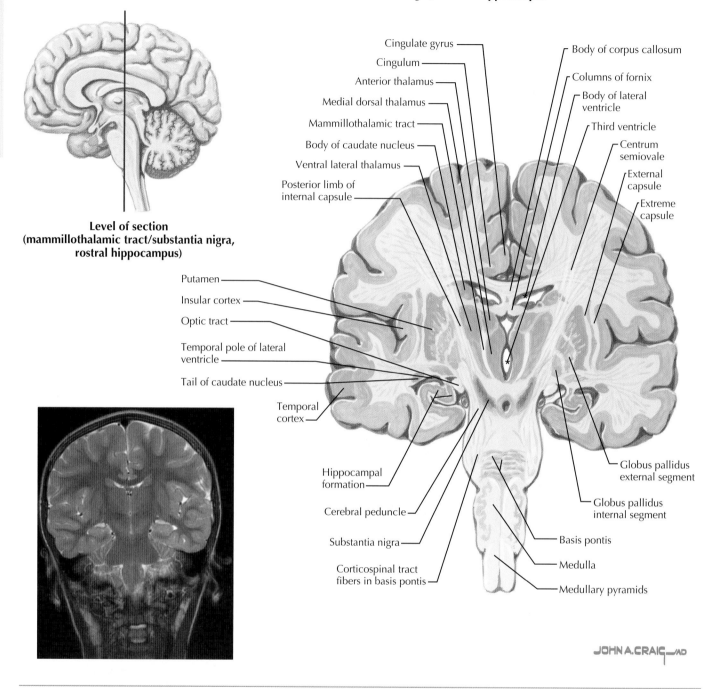

Level of section
(mammillothalamic tract/substantia nigra,
rostral hippocampus)

Cingulate gyrus

Cingulum

Anterior thalamus

Medial dorsal thalamus

Mammillothalamic tract

Body of caudate nucleus

Ventral lateral thalamus

Posterior limb of internal capsule

Body of corpus callosum

Columns of fornix

Body of lateral ventricle

Third ventricle

Centrum semiovale

External capsule

Extreme capsule

Putamen

Insular cortex

Optic tract

Temporal pole of lateral ventricle

Tail of caudate nucleus

Temporal cortex

Hippocampal formation

Cerebral peduncle

Substantia nigra

Corticospinal tract fibers in basis pontis

Globus pallidus external segment

Globus pallidus internal segment

Basis pontis

Medulla

Medullary pyramids

JOHN A. CRAIG—AD

13.16A CORONAL SECTIONS THROUGH THE FOREBRAIN: LEVEL 6—MAMMILLO-THALAMIC TRACT/SUBSTANTIA NIGRA, ROSTRAL HIPPOCAMPUS

CLINICAL POINT

The posterior limb of the IC is the major afferent and efferent route through which the cerebral cortex is connected with the rest of the brain. The cerebral cortex sends descending fibers through the IC that are destined for the spinal cord, brain stem, cerebellum (via pontine nuclei), striatum and related nuclei, thalamus, and limbic structures. Of particular importance for movement are the corticospinal system and cortical connections to other upper motor neuron regions (such as the red nucleus) arising from the motor and premotor/supplemental motor cortices, which help to control skilled movements of the contralateral limbs; and the corticobulbar tract, which supplies motor cranial nerve nuclei with descending control, all bilaterally except for the lower facial nucleus, which receives exclusively contralateral input. The corticospinal tract travels in the posterior limb of the IC, and the corticobulbar tract travels in the genu of the IC. The posterior limb of the IC also conveys the ascending somatosensory and trigeminal sensory axons from the ventral posterolateral and posteromedial thalamus, which are susceptible to vascular infarcts in the middle cerebral artery and fine penetrating lenticulostriate arteries. Such an infarct acutely produces contralateral hemiplegia and a drooping lower face, with loss of somatic sensation. With time, the hemiplegia becomes spastic, with hyperreflexia, hypertonus, and pathological reflexes (Babinski's reflex, or plantar extensory response).

Cingulum

Body of lateral ventricle

Insular cortex

Lateral fissure

Thalamus

Tail of caudate nucleus

Substantia nigra

Cerebral peduncle

Cingulate cortex

Body of corpus callosum

Body of caudate nucleus

Columns of fornix

Putamen

Posterior limb of internal capsule

Third ventricle

Inferior horn of lateral ventricle

Hippocampal formation

Corticospinal tract in basis pontis

Basis pontis

13.16B CORONAL SECTIONS THROUGH THE FOREBRAIN: LEVEL 6—MAMMILLOTHALAMIC TRACT/ SUBSTANTIA NIGRA, ROSTRAL HIPPOCAMPUS (CONTINUED)

Level 7: Midthalamus

Level of section
(midthalamus)

Body of corpus callosum

Cingulate cortex

Interventricular
foramen of Munro

Cingulum

Stria terminalis

Body of caudate
nucleus

Columns of fornix

Third ventricle

Body of lateral
ventricle

Medial dorsal thalamus

Insular cortex

Lateral thalamus

Lateral geniculate nucleus

Centromedian thalamus

Tail of the caudate nucleus

Hippocampal
formation

Medial
geniculate
nucleus

Cortex of
cerebellum

Entorhinal
cortex

Superior
cerebellar peduncle

Pons (floor of
fourth ventricle)

Inferior cerebellar
peduncle

Medulla

JOHN A. CRAIG—AD

13.17A CORONAL SECTIONS THROUGH THE FOREBRAIN: LEVEL 7—MIDTHALAMUS

Cingulum

Body of lateral ventricle

Columns of fornix

Thalamus

Lateral geniculate nucleus

Temporal lobe

Medial geniculate nucleus

Superior cerebellar peduncle

Cingulate cortex

Body of corpus callosum

Body of caudate nucleus

Stria terminalis

Third ventricle

Hippocampal formation

Middle cerebellar peduncle

Inferior cerebellar peduncle

13.17B CORONAL SECTIONS THROUGH THE FOREBRAIN: LEVEL 7—MIDTHALAMUS (CONTINUED)

Level 8: Geniculate Nuclei

Level of section
(geniculate nuclei)

Labels (clockwise/around figure):
Cingulate gyrus
Cingulum
Body of caudate nucleus
Pulvinar
Body of corpus callosum
Body of fornix
Third ventricle
Body of lateral ventricle
Medial geniculate nucleus
Lateral geniculate nucleus
Tail of caudate nucleus
Inferior pole of lateral ventricle
Hippocampal formation
Pretectum
Cerebellar cortex
Middle cerebellar peduncle
Decussation of superior cerebellar peduncle
Pons
Medulla
Cerebral aqueduct
Periaqueducial gray matter
Posterior commissure

JOHN A. CRAIG _AD

13.18A CORONAL SECTIONS THROUGH THE FOREBRAIN: LEVEL 8—GENICULATE NUCLEI

CLINICAL POINT

Several thalamic nuclei in the posterior thalamus are important for conveying visual and auditory information to the cerebral cortex. The lateral geniculate nucleus receives segregated input from the temporal hemiretina of the ipsilateral eye and from the nasal hemiretina of the contralateral eye, and it conveys this topographical information to area 17, the primary visual cortex, located on the banks of the calcarine fissure. A lesion in the lateral geniculate nucleus results in contralateral hemianopia. The pulvinar receives visual input from the superior colliculus and also conveys visual information to the visual cortex, to areas 18 and 19 (associative visual cortex). A lesion in the pulvinar can lead to contralateral visual neglect. The medial geniculate nucleus receives input from the inferior colliculus through the brachium of the inferior colliculus. However, because the auditory system is bilaterally represented at this level, a lesion in the medial geniculate nucleus on one side does not result in contralateral deafness. There may be some diminution of hearing contralateral to the lesion, but it is not a profound deficit. Visual areas 17, 18, and 19 correspond to visual cortices 1, 11, and 111, as illustrated in Figure 13.26.

Cingulate cortex

Cingulum

Columns of fornix

Tail of caudate nucleus

Middle cerebellar peduncle

Lateral cerebellar hemisphere

Body of corpus callosum

Body of lateral ventricle

Body of caudate nucleus

Pulvinar

Inferior horn of lateral ventricle

Hippocampal formation

Superior cerebellar peduncle

Pons

Medulla

Cervical spinal cord

13.18B CORONAL SECTIONS THROUGH THE FOREBRAIN: LEVEL 8—GENICULATE NUCLEI (CONTINUED)

Level 9: Caudal Pulvinar and Superior Colliculus

Level of section
(caudal pulvinar and superior colliculus)

Cingulate gyrus

Cingulum

Superior colliculus

Pulvinar

Body of caudate nucleus

Body of corpus callosum

Crus of fornix

Habenula

Third ventricle

Body of lateral ventricle

Tail of caudate nucleus

Fimbria of hippocampal formation

Inferior pole of lateral ventricle

Hippocampal formation

Lateral cerebellar hemisphere

Entorhinal cortex

Middle cerebellar peduncle

Superior cerebellar peduncle

Inferior colliculus

Cerebellar vermis

Fourth ventricle

JOHN A. CRAIG AD

13.19A CORONAL SECTIONS THROUGH THE FOREBRAIN: LEVEL 9—CAUDAL PULVINAR AND SUPERIOR COLLICULUS

Cingulate cortex

Cingulum

Parietal lobe

Body of corpus callosum

Body of lateral ventricle

Columns of fornix at transition to body

Superior colliculus

Confluence of inferior horn
and body of lateral ventricle

Hippocampal formation

Pulvinar

Inferior colliculus

Superior cerebellar peduncle

Fourth ventricle

Lateral cerebellar hemisphere

Medulla

Middle cerebellar peduncle

**13.19B CORONAL SECTIONS THROUGH THE FOREBRAIN: LEVEL 9—CAUDAL PULVINAR
AND SUPERIOR COLLICULUS (CONTINUED)**

Level 10: Splenium of Corpus Callosum

Level of section
(splenium of corpus callosum)

Cingulate gyrus

Cingulum

Crus of fornix

Pulvinar

Splenium of corpus callosum

Pineal

Trigone of lateral ventricle

Choroid plexus

Inferior pole of lateral ventricle

Tail of caudate nucleus

Optic radiations

Hippocampal formation

Temporal lobe

Lateral cerebellar hemisphere

Dentate nucleus

Cerebellar vermis

Fourth ventricle

JOHN A.CRAIG—AD

13.20A CORONAL SECTIONS THROUGH THE FOREBRAIN: LEVEL 10—SPLENIUM OF CORPUS CALLOSUM

Splenium of corpus callosum

Pineal

Crus of fornix

Choroid plexus in ventricle

Optic radiations

Temporal lobe

Fourth ventricle

Cingulate cortex

Cingulum

Parietal lobe

Trigone of lateral ventricle

Hippocampal formation

Deep cerebellar nuclei

Lateral cerebellar hemisphere

Cerebellar vermis

13.20B CORONAL SECTIONS THROUGH THE FOREBRAIN: LEVEL 10—SPLENIUM OF CORPUS CALLOSUM (CONTINUED)

Noradrenergic axon from locus coeruleus

Serotonergic axon from rostral raphe nuclei

Specific afferents

From other parts of cortex

Association fibers

To other parts of cortex

Motor fibers

13.21 LAYERS OF THE CEREBRAL CORTEX

Regions of cerebral cortex with specific functional roles, such as the somatosensory cortex and the motor cortex, demonstrate histological characteristics that reflect that function. The sensory cortex has large granule cell layers (granular cortex) for receiving extensive input, whereas the motor cortex has sparse granule cell layers and extensive pyramidal cell layers, reflecting extensive output. Specific and nonspecific afferents terminate differentially in these structurally unique regions of the cortex. Monoamine inputs terminate more diffusely than do the specific inputs, reflecting the role of monoamines as modulators and enhancers of the activity of other neuronal systems.

Key for Abbreviations
a Horizontal cell
b Cell of Martinotti
c Chandelier cell
d Aspiny granule cell
e Spiny granule cell
f Stellate (granule) cell
g Small pyramidal cell of layers II, III
h Small pyramidal association cell
i Small pyramidal association and projection cells of layer V
j Large pyramidal projection cell (Betz cell)

Cortical interneurons

Cortical association neurons

Efferent neuron

Black—cell bodies and dendrites   **Brown—axons of interneurons and association neurons**   **Red—axon of efferent neurons**

13.22 **CORTICAL NEURONAL CELL TYPES**

The cerebral cortex has many anatomically unique cell types that have characteristic cell bodies, dendritic arborizations, and axonal distributions. Granule cells are local circuit neurons with small cell bodies, localized dendritic trees, and axons that distribute locally. Granule cells function as receiving neurons for thalamic and other inputs, and they modulate the excitability of other cortical neurons. Pyramidal cells possess more varied cell bodies (some large, some small) that have large basolateral dendritic branching patterns and apical dendritic arborizations that run perpendicular to the cortical surface and arborize in upper layers. The axons of pyramidal cells, which function as projection neurons (e.g., corticospinal tract neurons), leave the cortex and may extend for as long as a meter before synapsing on target neurons. These unique anatomical characteristics give rise to the concept that neuronal structure explains neuronal function.

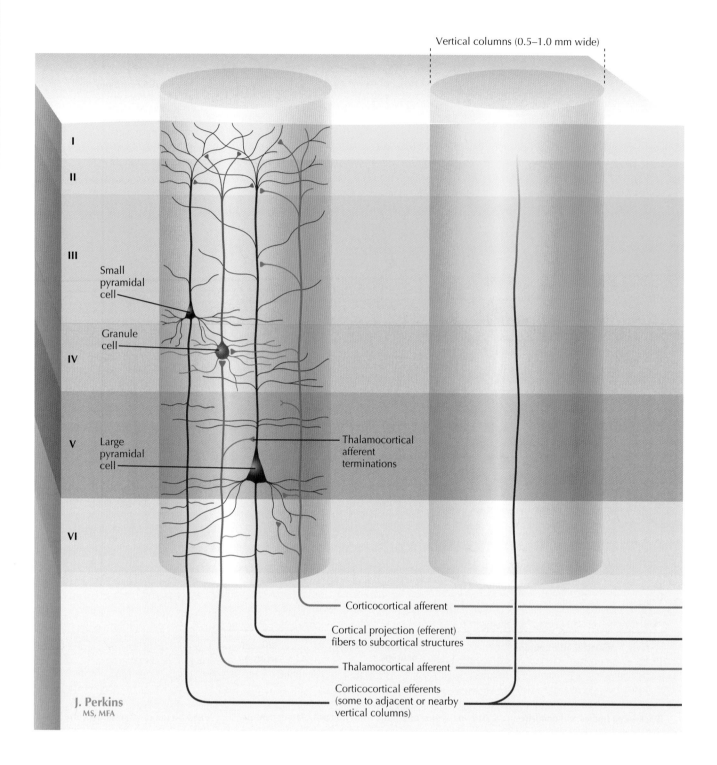

Vertical columns (0.5–1.0 mm wide)

I

II

III

Small pyramidal cell

Granule cell

IV

V

Large pyramidal cell

Thalamocortical afferent terminations

VI

Corticocortical afferent

Cortical projection (efferent) fibers to subcortical structures

Thalamocortical afferent

Corticocortical efferents (some to adjacent or nearby vertical columns)

J. Perkins
MS, MFA

13.23 VERTICAL COLUMNS: FUNCTIONAL UNITS OF THE CEREBRAL CORTEX

Experimental studies of sensory regions of the cerebral cortex provided anatomical and physiological evidence that discrete information that comes from a specific region or that conveys specific functional characteristics is processed in a cylindrical vertical zone of neurons in the cortex that spans all six layers of the neocortex. These vertical units vary from 0.5 to 1.0 mm in diameter. The diameter corresponds to the major horizontal expanse of a larger pyramidal cell in that unit. Both thalamic and cortical afferents arborize in the vertical column and synapse on both stellate (granule) cells and pyramidal neuron dendrites. Information from a vertical column can be sent to an adjacent or nearby column via corticocortical efferents or can be sent to distant structures by commissural fibers (cortex on the other side) or by projection fibers (subcortical structures). The minimal elements of the vertical unit are shown.

Association Fibers
 Long - to distant regions of
   ipsilateral hemisphere
 Short - to nearby regions of
   ipsilateral hemisphere

Commissural Fibers
 To cortical regions of
 contralateral hemisphere

Projection Fibers
 Corticospinal tract
 Corticobulbar tract
 Corticorubrospinal system
 Corticoreticulospinal system
 Corticobulbospinal system
   (polysynaptic)
 Corticotectal fibers
 Corticopontine fibers
   (to cerebellum)
 Corticostriate fibers
   (to basal ganglia)
 Corticonigral and
   corticosubthalamic fibers
 Corticonuclear fibers (to secondary
   sensory nuclei)
 Corticothalamic projections
 Corticohypothalamic and corticoautonomic fibers
 Cortico-olivary fibers
 Corticolimbic fibers (in subcortical forebrain)

Caudate
nucleus

Thalamus

Putamen

Globus
pallidus

Third ventricle

Hypothalamus

Hippocampus

Lateral
fissure

Lateral ventricle
(lateral pole)

J. Perkins
MS, MFA

13.24 EFFERENT CONNECTIONS OF THE CEREBRAL CORTEX

Neurons of the cerebral cortex send efferent connections to three major regions: (1) association fibers are sent to other cortical regions of the same hemisphere, either nearby (short-association fibers) or at a distance (long-association fibers); (2) commissural fibers are sent to cortical regions of the other hemisphere through the corpus callosum or the anterior commissure; and (3) projection fibers are sent to numerous subcortical structures in the telencephalon, diencephalon, brain stem, and spinal cord. The major sites of termination of these connections are listed in the diagram.

accomplishment. The cortex does this through three types of efferent pathways: (1) association fibers; (2) commissural fibers; and (3) projection fibers. Association fibers interconnect with either nearby (short) or distant (long) regions of cortex. Damage to long-association fibers can disconnect regions of cortex that normally need to communicate; this can result in altered language function, altered behavior, and other cortex-related problems. Damage to commissural fibers, especially the corpus callosum and anterior commissure, sometimes done deliberately to alleviate the spread of seizure activity, can result in a disconnection between the left and right hemispheres, with each hemisphere not being fully aware of what the other is doing because it does not have separate input. Damage to the projection fibers, which commonly accompanies infarcts or lesions in the internal capsule, can disrupt cortical outflow to the spinal cord, brain stem, cerebellum, thalamus and hypothalamus, basal ganglia, and limbic forebrain structures. As a consequence, major sensory deficits (especially in the opposite side for somatic sensation and vision), contralateral spastic hemiplegia with central facial involvement, hemianopia, and other motor, sensory, and behavioral deficits may occur.

CLINICAL POINT

The cerebral cortex provides the highest level of regulation over motor and sensory systems, behavior, cognition, and the functional capacities of the brain that are most characteristic of human

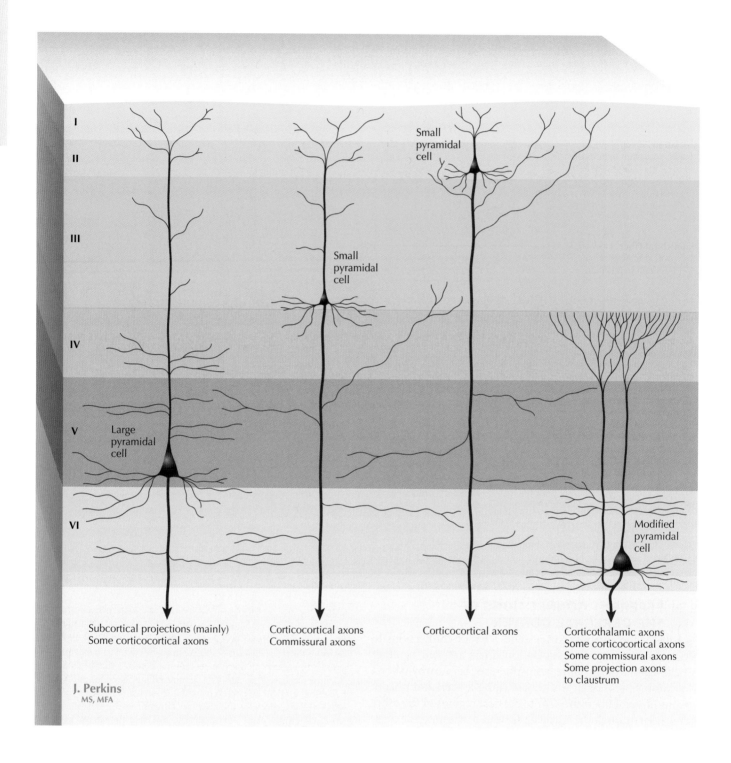

I

II

III

Small
pyramidal
cell

Small
pyramidal
cell

IV

V   Large
pyramidal
cell

Modified
pyramidal
cell

VI

Subcortical projections (mainly)
Some corticocortical axons

Corticocortical axons
Commissural axons

Corticocortical axons

Corticothalamic axons
Some corticocortical axons
Some commissural axons
Some projection axons
to claustrum

J. Perkins
MS, MFA

13.25 NEURONAL ORIGINS OF EFFERENT CONNECTIONS OF THE CEREBRAL CORTEX

Association fibers destined for cortical regions of the same hemisphere arise mainly from smaller pyramidal cells in cortical layers II and III and from modified pyramidal cells in layer VI. Commissural fibers destined for cortical regions of the opposite hemisphere arise mainly from small pyramidal cells in cortical layer III and from some modified pyramidal cells in layer VI. Projection fibers arise from larger pyramidal cells in layer V and also from smaller pyramidal cells in layers V and VI. Only a small number of projection fibers arise from the giant Betz cells in layer V.

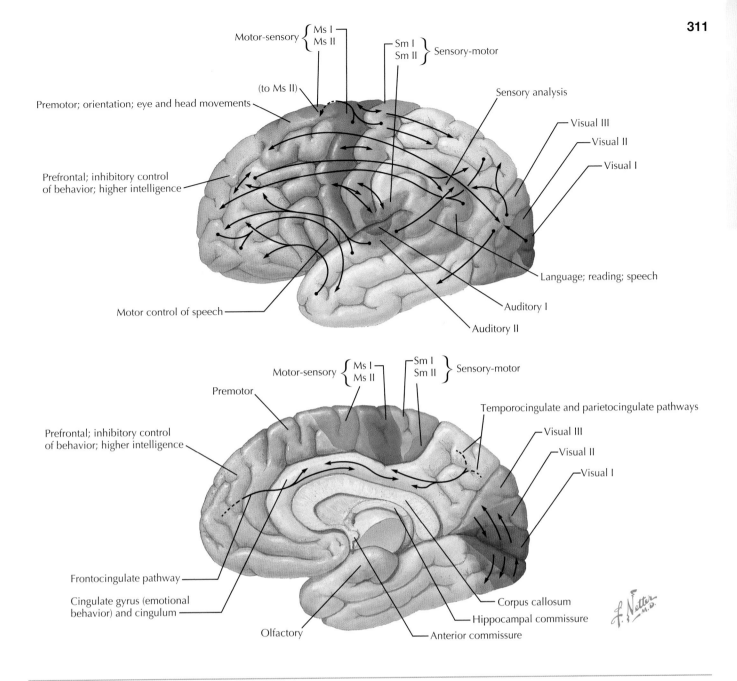

Motor-sensory { Ms I / Ms II

(to Ms II)

Sm I / Sm II } Sensory-motor

Premotor; orientation; eye and head movements

Sensory analysis

Visual III

Visual II

Visual I

Prefrontal; inhibitory control of behavior; higher intelligence

Language; reading; speech

Motor control of speech

Auditory I

Auditory II

Motor-sensory { Ms I / Ms II

Premotor

Sm I / Sm II } Sensory-motor

Temporocingulate and parietocingulate pathways

Visual III

Visual II

Visual I

Prefrontal; inhibitory control of behavior; higher intelligence

Frontocingulate pathway

Cingulate gyrus (emotional behavior) and cingulum

Olfactory

Anterior commissure

Hippocampal commissure

Corpus callosum

13.26 CORTICAL ASSOCIATION PATHWAYS

Neurons of the cerebral cortex have extensive connections with other regions of the brain (projection neurons); with the opposite hemisphere (commissural neurons); and with other regions of the ipsilateral hemisphere (association fibers). The cortical association fibers may connect a primary sensory cortex with adjacent association areas (e.g., visual cortex, somatosensory cortex) or may link multiple regions of cortex into complex association areas (e.g., polysensory analysis regions) or interlink important areas involved in language function, cognitive function, and emotional behavior and analysis. Damage to these pathways and associated cortical regions can result in loss of specific sensory and motor capabilities, aphasias (language disorders), agnosias (failures of recognition), and apraxias (performance deficits).

CLINICAL POINT

Long cortical association pathways link regions of cortex with each other. Some pathways link multiple sensory areas with multimodal cortical association cortex, providing the substrate for integrated interpretation of the outside world. Some association pathways connect language areas

in the dominant hemisphere with each other. Broca's area of the frontal cortex and Wernicke's area in the parietotemporal region are interconnected by long-association fibers of the arcuate fasciculus or superior longitudinal fasciculus. When these association fibers are damaged, Broca's area and Wernicke's area are disconnected. The patient does not demonstrate a classic expressive or receptive aphasia but demonstrates the inability to repeat complex words or sentences. This is called conduction aphasia.

Subcortical white matter plays an important role in human behavior. Many types of pathology can affect subcortical white matter such as multi-infarct damage or demyelination. These conditions cause a disconnection between regions of cerebral cortex or between subcortical regions and cortex. With multiple regions of white matter damage, dementia can occur, including inattention, emotional changes, and memory problems; such changes generally occur in the absence of movement disorders or aphasias. Multi-infarct damage to the ascending catecholamine and serotonin pathways from the brain stem can occur with destruction of the axons in the cingulum, resulting in depression and bipolar disorder, as well as attention deficits, especially with lesions involving ascending noradrenergic and reticular activating circuitry. Bilateral damage to white matter of the frontal lobe may result in euphoria and inappropriate affect, whereas damage to the long-association fibers interconnecting the frontal lobes with limbic forebrain structures may result in psychotic behavior.

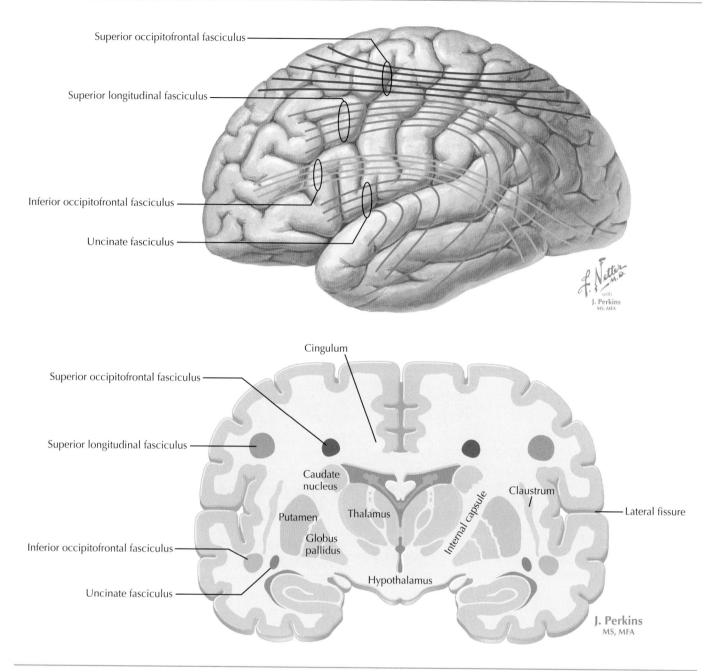

13.27 MAJOR CORTICAL ASSOCIATION BUNDLES

Association fibers interconnecting cortical regions in one hemisphere with adjacent or distant regions of the same hemisphere are categorized as short-association fibers (arcuate fibers) or long-association fibers. The long-association fibers often are recognized anatomically as specific association bundles and may have numerous fiber systems entering, exiting, and traversing them. Important named bundles include the uncinate fasciculus, the superior longitudinal fasciculus, the superior and inferior occipitofrontal fasciculi, and the cingulum. The cingulum is a bundle through which the major monoamines (dopamine, norepinephrine, serotonin) and part of the cholinergic projections travel to their widespread target sites.

CLINICAL POINT

Cortical association pathways, or bundles, can become demyelinated in multiple sclerosis and other demyelinating diseases, leading to cognitive and emotional problems in addition to the sensory, motor, and autonomic involvement that is well known in such disorders. Diminished attention and vigilance can occur with demyelination of association pathways, and that may contribute to some of the memory impairment seen in recall tasks. Inappropriate expression of emotion and euphoria or emotional disinhibition (sometimes called pseudobulbar affect) can occur with damage to frontal association pathways. Both depressive and bipolar disorders occur more commonly in patients with multiple sclerosis than in controls, and there is some correlation with the presence of demyelinating lesions in the temporal lobe, although monoaminergic pathways also may be involved. Although many clinicians view some of the demyelinating plaques that form in subcortical white matter to be "silent lesions" that produce no pathology, the end point for evaluation usually has been classic motor and sensory symptoms, not emotional and cognitive dysfunction. Although such deficits may be more common than previously supposed, the ability of the brain to repair demyelinated lesions often can ameliorate such deficits.

A. Axial view

Superior longitudinal fasciculus

Occipital-temporal association fibers

Cortical projection fibers

Superior longitudinal fasciculus

Splenium, corpus callosum

Arcuate fasciculus

Genu, corpus callosum

B. Sagittal view

13.28 COLOR IMAGING OF ASSOCIATION PATHWAYS

These diffusion tensor images show the association pathways of the forebrain in green (anterior-posterior direction) in an axial section and in a sagittal section. The most conspicuous association fibers in these images are the long-association pathways. Commissural fibers appear red/orange (left-right direction), and projection fibers appear blue (superior-inferior direction).

A. Sagittal view

Corona radiata coalescing into the internal capsule

Cingulum

Fibers of superior longitudinal fasciculus

Fornix

Fibers of inferior longitudinal fasciculus

Internal capsule

Superior cerebellar peduncle

Middle cerebellar peduncle

Pyramidal tract

Dorsal column system

Corona radiata

Corpus callosum

Fibers of uncinate fasciculus

Inferior longitudinal fasciculus

Motor fibers in basis pontis

Superior cerebellar peduncle

Pyramidal tract

Ascending sensory fibers from brain stem and spinal cord

B. Sagittal view

13.29 COLOR IMAGING OF PROJECTION PATHWAYS FROM THE CEREBRAL CORTEX

These diffusion tensor images show the projection pathways of the forebrain in blue in two sagittal sections. The widespread cortical projection bundles channel into a narrow zone of the internal capsule and then proceed to their sites of projection in the forebrain, brain stem, or spinal cord. The descending corticospinal/corticobulbar system is particularly prominent. Projection systems associated with the cerebellum also are present. In addition, green association fibers and red commissural fibers also can be seen.

A. Coronal section showing midline motor cortex response to alternating movement of the toes.

B. Coronal section showing contra-lateral convexity motor cortex response and ipsilateral cerebellar response to rapid alternating sequential tapping movement of the fingers bilaterally.

C. Coronal section showing Broca's area response to a language task in which subjects must silently discriminate word characteristics as abstract, concrete, single, double, upper case, or lower case over a 30-second time span.

D. Axial section showing occipital cortex response to a visual task of viewing flickering alternating bands on a screen.

13.30 FUNCTIONAL MAGNETIC RESONANCE IMAGING

Functional magnetic resonance imaging (fMRI) is a non-invasive method that uses no radioactive tracers; it takes advantage of the fact that there is a difference in magnetic states of arterial and venous blood, thus providing an intrinsic mechanism of contrast for brain activation studies. The origin of this dual state of blood is due to the fact that the magnetic state of hemoglobin (Hb) depends on its oxygentation; the oxyhemoglobin state (arterial blood) is diamagnetic, and the venous deoxyhemoglobin state (venous blood) is paramagnetic. The change in oxygen saturation of the hemoglobin produces a detectable small signal change; hence, it is called the blood oxygenation level-dependent (BOLD) effect.

During neural activity, the supposition behind BOLD-fMRI is that the involved neurons represent a region of relatively greater oxygenated hemoglobin compared with non-active regions in T2*-weighted images. However, there is a delay of several seconds between increased neural activity and increased oxygenated arterial blood flow to that region. BOLD-fMRI compares images during specific activity to images of the same region without such activity and can be used for processes that occur rapidly, such as language function, vision, audition, movement, cognitive tasks, and emotional responsiveness. The above images are taken from a sequence of coronal and axial sections showing regions of brain that are activated during A) movement of toes, B) sequential finger tapping, C) language task, and D) visual stimulation.

Temporal lobe

Locus coeruleus

A5, A7

A1, A2

13.31 NORADRENERGIC PATHWAYS

Noradrenergic neurons in the brain stem project to widespread areas of the central nervous system (CNS). The neurons are found in the locus coeruleus (group A6) and in several cell groups in the reticular formation (RF; tegmentum) of the medulla and pons (A1, A2, A5, and A7 groups). Axonal projections of the locus coeruleus branch to the cerebral cortex, hippocampus, hypothalamus, cerebellum, brain stem nuclei, and spinal cord. The locus coeruleus acts as a modulator of the excitability of other projection systems such as the glutamate system and helps to regulate attention and alertness, the sleep-wake cycle, and appropriate responses to stressors, including pain. The RF groups are interconnected extensively with the spinal cord, brain stem, hypothalamic, and limbic regions involved in neuroendocrine control, visceral functions (temperature regulation, feeding and drinking behavior, reproductive behavior, autonomic regulation) and with emotional behavior. Serotonergic neurons of the raphe system overlap with many of these noradrenergic connections, and comodulate related functional activities. A sparse set of epinephrine-containing neurons in the medullary RF are similarly interconnected. These RF noradrenergic neurons can work in concert with the locus coeruleus during challenge or in response to a stressor to coordinate alertness and appropriate neuroendocrine and autonomic responsiveness. The central noradrenergic and adrenergic neurons and their receptors are the targets of many pharmacological agents, including those that target depression, analgesia, hypertension, and many other conditions.

CLINICAL POINT

The axonal projections of the brain stem noradrenergic cell groups have incredibly widespread distribution to virtually all subdivisions of the CNS. The locus coeruleus acts as a modulator of the excitability of other axonal systems and can augment both glutamate excitability and gamma aminobutyric acid (GABA) inhibition within the same neurons (Purkinje cells). In keeping with such a modulatory role, the locus coeruleus system appears to help regulate attention, alertness, and sleep-wakefulness cycles. Similarly, the brain stem tegmental noradrenergic systems have projections to spinal cord, brain stem, hypothalamic, and limbic regions and help to regulate neuroendocrine outflow and visceral functions, such as feeding, drinking, reproductive behavior, and autonomic regulation. In the spinal cord, descending noradrenergic projections modulate the excitability of lower motor neurons in the ventral horn.

Central noradrenergic forebrain projections also influence emotional behavior and are integral to the catecholamine hypothesis of affective disorders, especially depression. Depression is hypothesized to be the result of diminished functioning of central noradrenergic connections (although serotonergic dysfunction is probably involved as well). All three major classes of drugs used for treating depression (monoamine oxidase inhibitors, tricyclic antidepressants, and psychomotor stimulants) enhance noradrenergic neurotransmission. MHPG (3-methoxy-4-hydroxyphenylglycol), the major metabolite of central norepinephrine, is diminished in many depressed individuals. As a phenomenon accompanying depression, the altered noradrenergic activity in the brain of depressed patients may exert a regulatory impact on the ability of the paraventricular nucleus of the hypothalamus to activate the stress axes, accounting for the increased cortisol and peripheral catecholamine secretion seen in many depressed individuals.

Basal ganglia

Thalamus

Temporal lobe

Raphe dorsalis

Raphe pontis centralis superior

Raphe pontis

Raphe magnus

Raphe pallidus and obscurus

13.32 SEROTONERGIC PATHWAYS

Serotonergic neurons (5-hydroxytryptamine; 5-HT), found in the raphe nuclei of the brain stem and adjacent wings of cells in the RF, have widespread projections that innervate every major subdivision in the CNS. The rostral serotonergic neurons in nucleus raphe dorsalis and centralis superior project rostrally to innervate the cerebral cortex, many limbic forebrain structures (hippocampus, amygdala), the basal ganglia, many hypothalamic nuclei and areas, and some thalamic regions. The caudal serotonergic neurons in the nuclei raphe magnus, pontis, pallidus, and obscurus project more caudally to innervate many brain stem regions, the cerebellum, and the spinal cord. Of particular importance are the projections of the nucleus raphe magnus to the dorsal horn of the spinal cord, at which site opiate analgesia and pain processing are markedly influenced. The ascending serotonergic systems are involved in the regulation of emotional behavior and wide-ranging hypothalamic functions (neuroendocrine, visceral/autonomic), similar to their noradrenergic counterparts. Serotonergic neurons are involved in sleep-wakefulness cycles and, like locus coeruleus noradrenergic neurons, stop firing during rapid-eye–movement sleep. Serotonergic projections to the cerebral cortex modulate the processing of afferent inputs (e.g., from the visual cortex). The descending serotonergic neurons enhance the effects of analgesia and are essential for opiate analgesia. They also modulate preganglionic autonomic neuronal excitability and enhance the excitability of lower motor neurons. Many pharmacological agents target serotonergic neurons and their receptors, including drugs for treating depression, other cognitive and emotional behavioral states, headaches, pain, some movement disorders, and other conditions.

CLINICAL POINT

Serotonergic neurons of the raphe nuclei and adjacent reticular formation have incredibly widespread projections to virtually all subdivisions of the CNS, similar to the brain stem noradrenergic neurons. Serotonergic systems can modulate the excitability of other neural systems and are involved in the regulation of emotional behavior, neuroendocrine secretion and circadian rhythms, and widespread visceral functions (e.g., food intake, pain sensitivity, sexual behavior, and sleep-wake cycles). During rapid-eye-movement (REM) sleep, some raphe neurons cease their electrical firing. Many early physiological studies of the serotonergic and noradrenergic systems revealed that both systems help to regulate many of the same functions. Serotonin systems have been implicated in some patients with depression. Early consideration of tricyclic antidepressants focused on their ability to block reuptake of norepinephrine, but some of the most efficacious tricyclic compounds also blocked the reuptake of serotonin. The discovery of serotonin-specific reuptake inhibitors such as fluoxetine led to their use for depression; they are therapeutically successful in a subset of individuals with major (unipolar) depression. It is not surprising that some side effects of their enhancing effects on central serotonin activity include diminished libido and eating disorders involving significant weight gain.

Striatum

Nucleus accumbens

Hypothalamus

Ventral tegmental area
Entorhinal cortex
Substantia nigra pars compacta
Locus coeruleus

13.33 DOPAMINERGIC PATHWAYS

DA neurons are found in the midbrain and hypothalamus. In the midbrain, neurons in the substantia nigra pars compacta (A9) project axons (along the nigrostriatal pathway) mainly to the striatum (caudate nucleus and putamen) and to the globus pallidus and subthalamus. This nigrostriatal projection is involved in basal ganglia circuitry that aids in the planning and execution of cortical activities, the most conspicuous of which involve the motor system. Damage to the nigrostriatal system results in Parkinson's disease, a disease characterized by resting tremor, muscular rigidity, bradykinesia (difficulty initiating movements or stopping them once they are initiated), and postural deficits. The antiparkinsonian drugs such as levodopa target this system and its receptors. Dopamine neurons in the ventral tegmental area and mesencephalic RF (A10) send mesolimbic projections to the nucleus accumbens, the amygdala, and the hippocampus, and they send mesocortical projections to the frontal cortex and some cortical-association areas. The mesolimbic pathway to the nucleus accumbens is involved in motivation, reward, biological drives, and addictive behaviors, particularly substance abuse. The DA projections to limbic structures can induce stereotyped, repetitive behaviors and activities. The mesocortical projections influence cognitive functions in the planning and carrying out of frontal cortical activities, and in attention mechanisms. The mesolimbic and mesocortical DA systems and their receptors are the targets of neuroleptic and antipsychotic agents that influence behaviors in schizophrenia, obsessive-compulsive disorder, attention deficit–hyperactivity disorder, Tourette's syndrome, and

other behavioral states. Dopamine neurons in the hypothalamus form the tuberoinfundibular dopamine pathway, which projects from the arcuate nucleus to the contact zone of the median eminence, where dopamine acts as prolactin inhibitory factor. Intrahypothalamic dopamine neurons also influence other neuroendocrine and visceral/autonomic hypothalamic functions.

CLINICAL POINT

Several discrete DA systems are found in the brain. The midbrain nigrostriatal DA system projects from the substantia nigra pars compacta to the striatum; these neurons degenerate in Parkinson's disease. The tuberoinfundibular and intrahypothalamic DA systems are involved in neuroendocrine regulation. A midbrain mesolimbic and mesocortical system sends widespread projections to the forebrain. The mesolimbic pathway to the nucleus accumbens regulates motivation, reward, biological drives, and addictive behaviors, playing an important role in substance abuse. Activation of this circuit can induce stereotyped, repetitive behaviors and activities. The mesolimbic and mesocortical DA systems are involved in many psychiatric disorders, including schizophrenia, obsessive-compulsive disorders, attention deficit–hyperactivity disorder, Tourette's syndrome, and other behavioral states. The use of neuroleptic and antipsychotic medications, which are D2 receptor antagonists, to treat schizophrenia led to the hypothesis that schizophrenia is related to the regulation of dopamine. The current hypothesis is that this disease may involve excessive activity in the mesolimbic DA system and a relative decrease in activity in the mesocortical DA system in the frontal lobes. Use of neuroleptic agents must be monitored carefully because chronic D2 receptor antagonism may lead to tardive dyskinesia, permanent drug-induced movements.

Medial septal nucleus

Nucleus basalis (of Meynert)

Hippocampus

Brain stem tegmental cholinergic group

13.34 **CENTRAL CHOLINERGIC PATHWAYS**

Central cholinergic neurons are found mainly in the nucleus basalis (of Meynert) and in septal nuclei. Nucleus basalis neurons project cholinergic axons to the cerebral cortex, and the septal cholinergic neurons project to the hippocampal formation. These cholinergic projections are involved in cortical activation and memory function, particularly consolidation of short-term memory. They often appear to be damaged in patients with Alzheimer's disease (AD). Drugs that enhance cholinergic function are used for improvement of memory. Other cholinergic neurons found in the brain stem tegmentum project to structures in the thalamus, brain stem, and cerebellum. The projections to the thalamus modulate arousal and the sleep-wake cycle and appear to be important in the initiation of REM sleep. Cholinergic interneurons are present in the striatum and may participate in basal ganglia control of tone, posture, and initiation of movement or selection of wanted patterns of activity. In some cases, pharmacological agents are targeted at reducing cholinergic activity in the basal ganglia in Parkinson's disease, as a complementary approach to enhancing DA activity. Acetylcholine also is used as the principal neurotransmitter in all preganglionic autonomic neurons and lower motor neurons in the spinal cord and brain stem.

CLINICAL POINT

Central cholinergic neurons are found in the basal forebrain (nucleus basalis of Meynert and nucleus of the diagonal band) and medial septum. The nucleus basalis cholinergic neurons are found in the substantia innominata and also along the ventral extent of the forebrain. The nucleus basalis and the nucleus of the diagonal band cholinergic neurons provide the major cholinergic input to the cerebral cortex. Cholinergic neurons of the medial septum send axons through the fornix to innervate the hippocampal formation. In patients with AD, a loss of cholinergic neurons (positive for choline acetyltransferase, the rate-limiting enzyme for acetylcholine synthesis) is most closely correlated with cognitive impairment. AD patients also show a loss of muscarinic and nicotinic cholinergic receptors and high-affinity choline uptake. Pharmacological agents such as the cholinesterase inhibitor tetrahydroaminoacridine (tacrine) have targeted cholinergic neurons in AD, and some data show a slowing in short-term memory dysfunction. Because choline is recycled for resynthesis of acetylcholine, some studies have used choline or lecithin in an attempt to boost precursor availability for added synthesis of acetylcholine; this approach has not met with great success. It may reflect the fact that AD alters many other neurotransmitter systems in the CNS in addition to the cholinergics, such as substance P, CRF, somatostatin, norepinephrine, and neuropeptide Y.

A. Lateral wall

Anterior ethmoidal nerve
- Internal nasal branch (lateral ramus)
- External nasal branch

Olfactory bulb
Olfactory nerves
Cribriform plate of ethmoid bone
Olfactory tract
Lateral posterior superior nasal branches
Maxillary nerve
Pterygopalatine ganglion and branches
Nerve of pterygoid canal
Greater petrosal nerve
Deep petrosal nerve
Pharyngeal branch
Nasopalatine nerve (passing to septum)
Posterior inferior nasal branch
Lesser (minor) palatine nerves
Greater (major) palatine nerve and branches

B. Nasal septum

Cribriform plate of ethmoid bone
Internal nasal branch (medial ramus) of anterior ethmoidal nerve
Nasopalatine nerve
Incisive canal

Olfactory bulb
Olfactory nerves
Olfactory tract

13.35 THE OLFACTORY NERVE AND NERVES OF THE NOSE

The olfactory nerves and their projections into the CNS are important components of forebrain function. Bipolar cells in the olfactory epithelium are the primary sensory neurons. The peripheral axon, a chemosensory transducer, responds to the unique chemical stimuli of airborne molecules entering the nose. The central axons of the bipolar neurons aggregate into groups of approximately 20 slender olfactory nerves that traverse the cribriform plate and end in glomeruli of the ipsilateral olfactory bulb. These nerves are vulnerable to tearing, which results in anosmia. Unlike neurons in other sensory systems, these bipolar neurons can proliferate and regenerate. After processing information in the olfactory bulb, mitral neurons and tufted neurons project via the olfactory tract directly and indirectly to limbic forebrain structures, including septal nuclei and amygdaloid nuclei. These projections bypass the thalamus, have immediate access to limbic forebrain structures, and directly influence the hypothalamus and its regulation of neuroendocrine and visceral/autonomic function. The olfactory system is essential for survival in many species and is involved in territorial recognition and defense,

food and water acquisition, social behavior, reproductive behavior, and signaling of danger.

CLINICAL POINT

The olfactory nerves possess receptors that can detect a wide range of unique odorants. This information is conveyed through the olfactory bulb to central forebrain sites, particularly those in the limbic forebrain, bypassing the thalamus, usually a processing zone for sensory projections to the forebrain. Olfaction is particularly important in recognizing the taste of food. What many people interpret as taste actually has a major olfactory component. Even very strong-tasting substances cannot be readily discerned by most people when the olfactory system is blocked, perhaps explaining the reduced gustatory experience of a good meal when someone has a cold. Clearly, both taste and smell must work together for full appreciation of food. Several regions of the brain have been identified as important sites for the interpretation of smell, including the orbitofrontal cortex and its major interconnected thalamic nucleus (medial dorsal) as well as the anterior temporal lobe. Ablation of the anterior temporal lobe, particularly on the dominant side, leads to olfactory agnosias. The involvement of the temporal lobe in the interpretation and processing of olfaction is further emphasized by olfactory auras of highly aversive or foul smells during temporal lobe seizures.

Section III: **SYSTEMIC NEUROSCIENCE**

14

SENSORY SYSTEMS

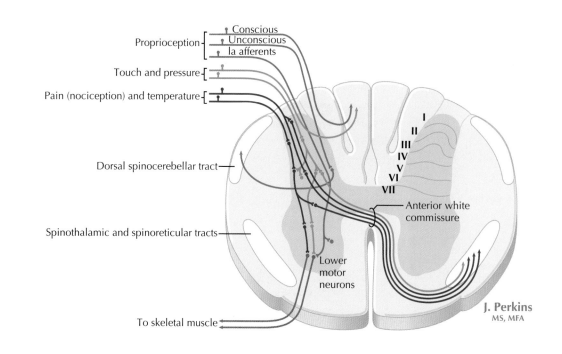

SOMATOSENSORY SYSTEMS

14.1 SOMATOSENSORY AFFERENTS TO THE SPINAL CORD

Unmyelinated (UNM) and small myelinated (M) axons that convey nociception and temperature sensation terminate in lamina I and V (origin of the spinothalamic tract). Other UNM axons terminate in the dorsal horn, from which neurons for polysynaptic reflexes and for the spinoreticular system originate. M axons for touch and pressure terminate in the dorsal horn, from which additional reflex connections, spinothalamic projections, and supplementary epicritic projections to the dorsal column (DC) nuclei originate. M axons also project directly into fasciculi gracilis and cuneatus, destined for nuclei gracilis and cuneatus; these lemniscal pathways process epicritic information for conscious interpretation. M proprioceptive axons (Ia afferents) terminate directly on lower motor neurons (LMNs) and on the Ia interneuronal pool. Additional M axons terminate in the dorsal horn on neurons of origin for the spinocerebellar tracts.

CLINICAL POINT

Primary afferents include both epicritic afferents (mainly larger diameter M axons that convey fine, discriminative touch, vibratory sensation, and joint position sense) and protopathic afferents (mainly small M or UNM axons that convey mainly nociceptive information and temperature sensation). These axons can be affected differentially in neuropathies. Some peripheral neuropathies can affect all modalities, leading to a total loss of sensation; other peripheral neuropathies affect selected populations of axons and their related modalities. Selective loss of protopathic modalities may occur in leprosy, in amyloid neuropathy, and in some cases of diabetic neuropathy, leading to insensitivity to pain and temperature. Selective loss of epicritic sensation may occur in some distal symmetrical polyneuropathies, neuropathy with

vitamin B_{12} deficiency, Guillain-Barré syndrome, and others, accompanied by paresthesias (numbness and tingling, "pins and needles," abnormal sensations), dysesthesias (disagreeable or abnormal sensations in the absence of stimulation), hyperesthesia (increased sensation with stimulation), or hypesthesia (diminished sensation with stimulation). Some neuropathic conditions also are accompanied by allodynia (pain evoked by normally nonpainful stimuli) and burning, stabbing, radiating pain. Peripheral neuropathies that affect larger diameter, M axons often can also affect the motor axons, leading to weakness and hyporeflexia or areflexia. Some small fiber neuropathies, especially diabetic neuropathies, may affect small autonomic axons to bowel, bladder, reproductive organs, and peripheral blood vessels, leading to orthostatic hypotension, bladder dysfunction, chronic gastrointestinal problems, or erectile dysfunction.

CLINICAL POINT

The monosynaptic reflex (the muscle stretch reflex) is tested in a clinical neurological examination. Specific muscle tendons are tapped, with the expected result of contraction of the homonymous muscle (e.g., tapping of the patellar tendon resulting in contraction of the ipsilateral quadriceps muscle). The muscle stretch reflexes routinely tested in a neurological examination include the biceps reflex, triceps reflex, brachioradialis reflex, patellar (knee-jerk) reflex, and the ankle-jerk reflex on both sides. The reflexes are graded on a numerical scale ranging from hyporeflexic to normoreflexic to hyperreflexic; normal physiological reflexes may vary in responsiveness, so the result of reflex testing must be considered in conjunction with other clinical signs and symptoms. For example, hyperreflexia in a pathological state such as stroke or spinal cord injury may be accompanied by hypertonia of the affected muscle, spasticity, abnormal reflexes (extensor plantar response), and repetitive hyperreflexic responses (clonus). In contrast, hyporeflexia or areflexia accompanying peripheral neuropathy may be accompanied by muscle weakness and flaccidity and diminished sensation of epicritic modalities, protopathic modalities, or both. More formal testing of reflexic responses can be done with electromyography and conduction velocity studies.

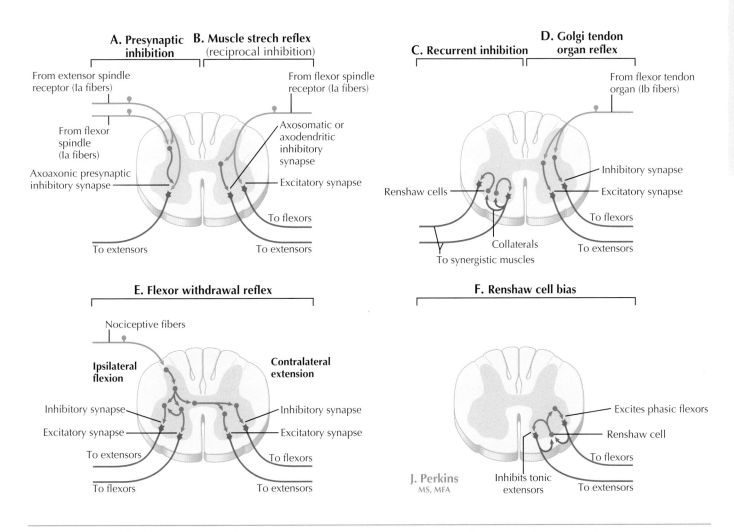

A. Presynaptic inhibition

From extensor spindle receptor (Ia fibers)

From flexor spindle (Ia fibers)

Axoaxonic presynaptic inhibitory synapse

To extensors

B. Muscle strech reflex (reciprocal inhibition)

From flexor spindle receptor (Ia fibers)

Axosomatic or axodendritic inhibitory synapse

Excitatory synapse

To flexors

To extensors

C. Recurrent inhibition

Renshaw cells

Collaterals

To synergistic muscles

D. Golgi tendon organ reflex

From flexor tendon organ (Ib fibers)

Inhibitory synapse

Excitatory synapse

To flexors

To extensors

E. Flexor withdrawal reflex

Nociceptive fibers

Ipsilateral flexion

Contralateral extension

Inhibitory synapse

Excitatory synapse

To extensors

To flexors

Inhibitory synapse

Excitatory synapse

To flexors

To extensors

F. Renshaw cell bias

Excites phasic flexors

Renshaw cell

To flexors

Inhibits tonic extensors

To extensors

J. Perkins
MS, MFA

14.2 SPINAL SOMATIC REFLEX ACTIONS AND PATHWAYS

A, Presynaptic inhibition. Some interneurons synapse on the terminal arborizations of other axons, as in the case of some afferent pools associated with muscle stretch reflexes. These axoaxonic contacts permit the modulation of neurotransmitter release from the second (target) axon terminal by depolarization of the terminal membrane, altering the influx of Ca^{++}. **B,** Muscle stretch reflex. In the muscle stretch reflex, Ia afferents excite the homonymous LMN pool directly and inhibit the antagonist LMN pool reciprocally via Ia inhibitory interneurons. **C,** Recurrent inhibition. Some interneurons receive recurrent collaterals from axons (e.g., LMN axons) and project back onto the dendrites or cell body of origin of that axon, usually inhibiting that neuron. This process can help to regulate the excitability and timing of excitation of the target neurons. Collaterals of LMN axons excite Renshaw cells (large interneurons), which inhibit the LMN of origin as well as LMNs projecting to synergistic muscles. Renshaw inhibition permits wiping the slate clean, after original excitation, of pools of LMNs, requiring additional incoming stimulation in order to excite these LMNs again. **D,** Golgi tendon organ reflex. Ib axons from Golgi tendon organs in muscle tendons terminate on pools of interneurons that inhibit LMNs to the homonymous muscle disynaptically and excite LMNs to the

antagonist muscle reciprocally. The action of this reflex as a protective mechanism to prevent damage to a muscle during generation of maximal tension on the tendon is seen in attempted passive stretch of a spastic muscle; the resultant inhibition of the homonymous LMN pool is called a clasp-knife reflex. **E,** Flexor withdrawal reflex. A flexor reflex (also called a withdrawal reflex or a nociceptive reflex) occurs when afferents derived from a noxious stimulus terminate on pools of interneurons that excite appropriate pools of LMNs (often flexor LMNs) to bring about a protective withdrawal from the source of the noxious stimulus. These interneurons also inhibit the antagonist LMNs through reciprocal inhibition. Flexor reflexes can extend throughout the spinal cord, as happens when one touches a hot stove with a finger; the result is the removal of the entire arm, or even the entire body, away from the source of heat. These flexor reflexes may involve both sides of spinal cord. **F,** Renshaw cell bias. Some reflex responses such as Renshaw reflexes (see part C) may result in the distribution of influence (bias) in a manner that favors a particular type of action. Renshaw cells receive inputs from axon collaterals of both flexor and extensor LMNs, but their projections are directed mainly toward the inhibition of extensor LMNs (and through reciprocal inhibition with the excitation of flexor LMNs). Thus, the Renshaw cell response favors flexor movements and helps to inhibit extensor movements.

Cerebellum

Superior cerebellar peduncle

Pons

Cerebellum

Medulla

Cuneocerebellar tract

Inferior cerebellar peduncle

Lateral (accessory) cuneate nucleus

Rostral spinocerebellar tract (RSCT)

Upper Body
(above T6)

Ia (to cuneocerebellar tract)
Ib (to RSCT)

Ventral spinocerebellar tract (VSCT)

Dorsal spinocerebellar tract (DSCT)

Lower Body
(below T6)

Ia (to DSCT)
Ib (to VSCT)

J. Perkins
MS, MFA

Anterior white commissure

14.3 SOMATOSENSORY SYSTEM: SPINOCEREBELLAR PATHWAYS

Proprioceptive primary somatosensory axons from joints, tendons, and ligaments (represented in this figure by Ib afferents from Golgi tendon organs) terminate on neurons of origin (border cells, dorsal horn) of the ventral spinocerebellar tract (VSCT) and the rostral spinocerebellar tract (RSCT) from the lower and upper body, respectively (level T6 is the cut-off point). Proprioceptive primary somatosensory axons from muscle spindles (represented in this figure by Ia afferents) terminate on neurons of origin (Clarke's nucleus, lateral {external} cuneate nucleus of the medulla) of the dorsal spinocerebellar tract (DSCT) and the cuneocerebellar tract from the lower and upper body, respectively (level T6 is the cut-off point). The DSCT, RSCT, and cuneocerebellar tracts remain ipsilateral. The VSCT crosses twice, once in the anterior commissure of the spinal cord and again in the cerebellum.

CLINICAL POINT

The dorsal and ventral spinocerebellar pathways travel in a conspicuous site at the lateral edge of the lateral funiculus throughout most of its length; these pathways are vulnerable to lesions that impinge on this zone of the spinal cord. They include tumors, radiculopathies with accompanying myelopathies, combined-system degeneration, demyelinating diseases, vascular infarcts in the anterior circulation of the cord, Brown-Séquard lesions, and other pathologies. Such a lesion, if superficial in the lateral funiculus, results in ipsilateral ataxia, dysmetria, clumsiness, and mild hypotonia, with impaired ability to perform heel-to-shin testing and tandem walking. However, lesions of the lateral funiculus often also involve the descending upper motor axons of the lateral corticospinal tract and the rubrospinal tract. Lesions that involve these tracts cause ipsilateral spastic hemiparesis or monoparesis, depending on the level of the lesion. The resulting spastic weakness, hyperreflexia, and hypertonus predominate in the clinical picture, thus masking the spinocerebellar symptomatology. Thus, an initial picture of spinocerebellar damage may give way to a progressive picture of spastic paresis on the same side.

Cerebrum

Cerebral cortex: postcentral gyrus

Posterior limb of internal capsule

Ventral posterolateral (VPL) nucleus of thalamus

Intralaminar nucleus

J. Perkins
MS, MFA

Midbrain

Medial lemniscus

Pons

Medial lemniscus

Gracile nucleus
Cuneate nucleus

Lower medulla

Internal arcuate fibers (decussation of the medial lemniscus)

Fasciculus gracilis
Fasciculus cuneatus

Lateral cervical nucleus (C1-C2 only)

Cervical spinal cord

Proprioception, position
Touch, pressure, vibration

Spinocervical tract

Lumbar spinal cord

Proprioception, position
Touch, pressure, vibration

14.4 SOMATOSENSORY SYSTEM: THE DORSAL COLUMN SYSTEM AND EPICRITIC MODALITIES

Primary somatosensory myelinated axons conveying fine, discriminative touch, pressure, vibratory sensation, and consciousness of joint position project directly into the DC system (fasciculus gracilis for lower body, below T6, and fasciculus cuneatus for upper body, T6 and above), where they are topographically organized. They terminate in nuclei gracilis and cuneatus, respectively, from which the medial lemniscus originates. This tract crosses (decussates) in the medulla and projects to the ventroposterolateral (VPL) nucleus of the thalamus. Axons of neurons in the VPL nucleus terminate in the primary sensory cortex topographically. The entire DC/medial lemniscal system is topographically organized; the lower body is represented medially in the primary somatosensory cortex, and the upper body (and face from trigeminal projections) is represented laterally. This representation is sometimes drawn proportionally (the resultant figure is called a homunculus); information from the fingers and hands has far greater representation in the cerebral cortex than information from the back. The spinocervical system is a small supplement to the DC system. Primary afferent projections terminate in the medial part of the dorsal horn; these neurons project to the lateral cervical nucleus (in C1 and C2 only). This nucleus contributes additional crossed axons with polysynaptic mechanoreceptive information.

Cerebrum

Cerebral cortex:
postcentral gyrus

Posterior limb of
internal capsule

Ventral posterolateral
(VPL) nucleus of
thalamus

Nonspecific
thalamic nuclei
(centromedian)

J. Perkins
MS, MFA

Midbrain

Deep layers of
superior colliculus and
periaqueductal gray

Pons

Lower medulla

Lateral reticular formation

Spinothalamic/spinoreticular
system (from all spinal levels)

Cervical spinal cord

Anterior white commissure

Pain, temperature
Pain

Lumbar spinal cord

Anterior white commissure

Pain, temperature
Pain

Somatosensory System: The Spinothalamic and Spinoreticular Systems and Protopathic Modalities

14.5 SOMATOSENSORY SYSTEM: THE SPINOTHALAMIC AND SPINORETICULAR SYSTEMS AND PROTOPATHIC MODALITIES (continued)

Primary somatosensory unmyelinated (C fibers) and small myelinated (A delta fibers) that convey nociceptive information (fast, localizing pain), temperature sensation, and light, moving touch terminate on neurons in lamina I and V. These dorsal horn neurons send crossed axons into the spinothalamic tract, projecting to neurons in the VPL nucleus of the thalamus *(red)*. This pool of neurons in the VPL nucleus is different from the pool receiving input from nuclei gracilis and cuneatus from the DC system. These thalamic neurons in the VPL nucleus project to the second somatosensory cortex (SII) as well as to the primary sensory cortex. Primary sensory C fibers also terminate in the dorsal horn and contribute to a large, cascading network for bilateral projections into the spinoreticular tract *(blue)*. This system ends mainly in the reticular formation, from which polysynaptic projections lead to nonspecific, medial dorsal, and anterior thalamic nuclei. Some spinoreticular fibers also terminate in the deeper layers of the superior colliculus (spinotectal pathway) and in the periaqueductal gray. Cortical regions such as the cingulate, insular, and prefrontal regions then process and interpret nociceptive information related to slow, agonizing, excruciating pain.

CLINICAL POINT

The spinothalamic tract conveys lemniscal information from primary afferents for nociception and temperature sensation to secondary sensory neurons in lamina I and V of the dorsal horn of the spinal cord. These dorsal horn neurons then project contralateral spinothalamic tract axons to the VPL nucleus of the thalamus, which in turn sends some information about "fast pain" (not outlasting the duration of the stimulus) to sensory cortices I and II in the parietal lobe. This is the principal protopathic system tested in the neurological examination, using light pin prick and touching the body with test tubes containing water of various temperatures. This spinothalamic tract system does not convey chronic, agonizing, deep pain that characterizes many chronic diseases; such chronic "slow" pain is conveyed through a vast polysynaptic network through the dorsal horn of the spinal cord and then the lateral reticular formation of the brain. This processed information eventually reaches the nonspecific thalamic nuclei (such as the centromedian) and is conveyed to limbic structures for more subjective, interpretative aspects of pain. This latter spinoreticular network can be influenced by a host of other inputs, including the cortex, the limbic system, the descending forebrain and diencephalic systems, and collaterals of the DC system. Collaterals of the DC system can gate nociceptive processing through the dorsal horn by activating neurons that dampen transmission of information through the cascading dorsal horn network. This process is evoked in a simple fashion by light rubbing adjacent to an injured part of the body. In a more chronic fashion, DC stimulation (by a transcutaneous electrical nerve stimulation unit) can electrically activate large-diameter axons which then gate the painful stimuli bombarding the dorsal horn nociceptive axons.

CLINICAL POINT

The DC system consists of fasciculus gracilis (lower half of the body, with T6 cutoff) and fasciculus cuneatus (upper half of the body). These pathways consist of primary sensory axons conveying fine, discriminative touch sensation, vibratory sensation, and joint-position sense (the epicritic sensations) toward the first synapse in the secondary sensory nuclei gracilis and cuneatus in the caudal medulla. These epicritic sensations are called primary DC modalities, the basic information coded mainly by large-diameter myelinated axons. Additional DC modalities are sometimes tested if the primary modalities are intact, including two-point discrimination, stereognosis (knowing what an object is just by touch), and graphesthesia (interpreting a number drawn into the palm of the hand). These are considered cortical modalities of the DC system; they require that the primary DC modalities be intact and also require the ability of the sensory cortices to interpret the information conveyed and to draw conclusions about that information. If the primary modalities are impaired, there is no reason to attempt to test the cortical modalities that depend on unimpaired primary modalities. Pure lesions of the DC system do not entirely eliminate the primary epicritic modalities, they just remove some interpretive capabilities; such a patient may realize that a vibratory stimulus is being applied to the upper extremity but may be unable to distinguish vibratory stimuli of different frequencies. The dorsal portion of the lateral funiculus carries additional epicritic information to the DC nuclei from the spinal cord dorsal horn. A lesion of both the DC and the dorsal portion of the lateral funiculus results in total loss of epicritic sensation on the affected side.

Gating Mechanism   **Spinal Mechanisms of Nociceptive Processing**

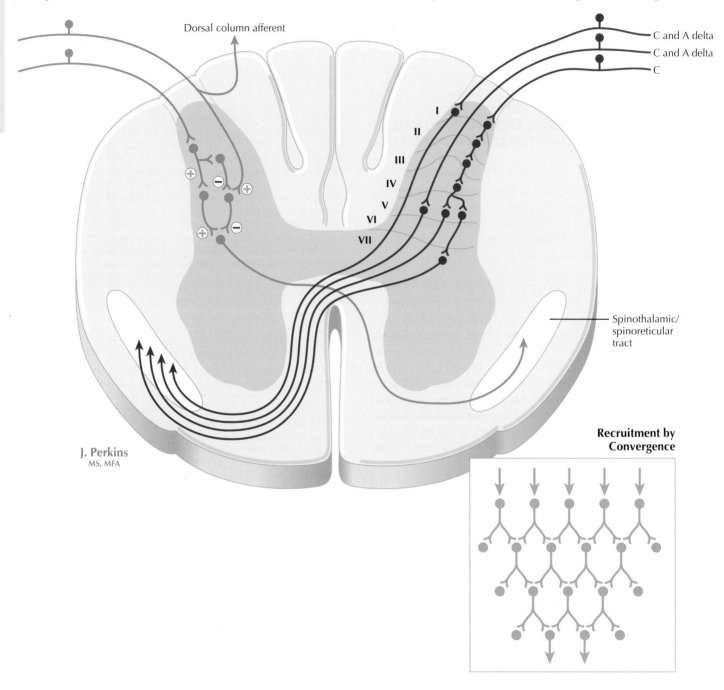

Dorsal column afferent

C and A delta
C and A delta
C

I
II
III
IV
V
VI
VII

Spinothalamic/
spinoreticular
tract

J. Perkins
MS, MFA

Recruitment by Convergence

14.6 SPINOTHALAMIC AND SPINORETICULAR NOCICEPTIVE PROCESSING IN THE SPINAL CORD

Primary afferents (C and A delta fibers) conveying fast, localized pain and temperature sensation terminate in laminae I and V of the dorsal horn of the spinal cord, from which the crossed spinothalamic axons originate. Unmyelinated primary afferents (C fibers) also terminate on neurons in the dorsal horn, from which a cascading system involving recruitment, convergence, and polysynaptic interconnections originates. This system contributes to the spinoreticular tract (mainly crossed, but some are uncrossed), which projects into the RF and continues polysynaptically to nonspecific, medial dorsal and anterior thalamic nuclei. This system contributes to perception of excruciating pain and its emotional connotation via cortical regions such as the cingulate, insular, and prefrontal cortices. The gating mechanism, shown on the left, allows primary DC axon collaterals to dampen pain processing in the dorsal horn via inhibitory interneuronal connections that inhibit the flow of information through the cascading dorsal horn system that contributes to the spinoreticular pathway.

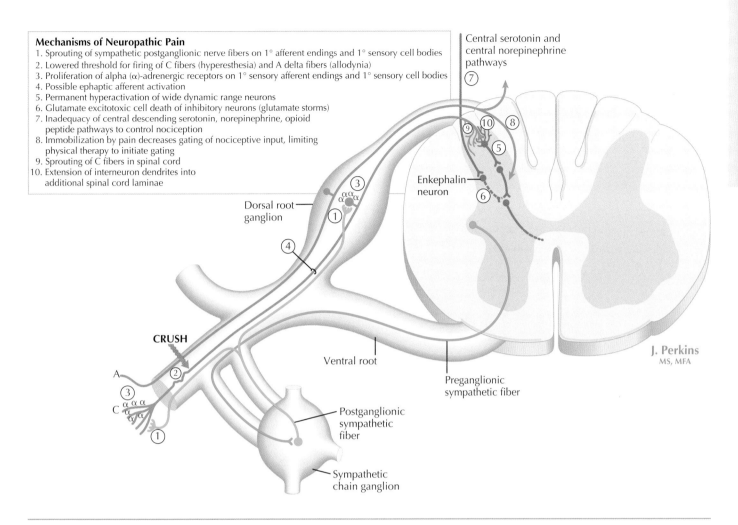

Mechanisms of Neuropathic Pain
1. Sprouting of sympathetic postganglionic nerve fibers on 1° afferent endings and 1° sensory cell bodies
2. Lowered threshold for firing of C fibers (hyperesthesia) and A delta fibers (allodynia)
3. Proliferation of alpha (α)-adrenergic receptors on 1° sensory afferent endings and 1° sensory cell bodies
4. Possible ephaptic afferent activation
5. Permanent hyperactivation of wide dynamic range neurons
6. Glutamate excitotoxic cell death of inhibitory neurons (glutamate storms)
7. Inadequacy of central descending serotonin, norepinephrine, opioid peptide pathways to control nociception
8. Immobilization by pain decreases gating of nociceptive input, limiting physical therapy to initiate gating
9. Sprouting of C fibers in spinal cord
10. Extension of interneuron dendrites into additional spinal cord laminae

Central serotonin and central norepinephrine pathways

Enkephalin neuron

Dorsal root ganglion

CRUSH

A

C

Ventral root

Postganglionic sympathetic fiber

Preganglionic sympathetic fiber

Sympathetic chain ganglion

J. Perkins
MS, MFA

14.7 MECHANISMS OF NEUROPATHIC PAIN AND SYMPATHETICALLY MAINTAINED PAIN

The cascading dorsal horn system receives primary afferent C fibers of nociceptive origin and projects into the spinoreticular system for the conscious interpretation of excruciating pain and neuropathic pain, shown in this illustration. Connections from the sympathetic nervous system can innervate terminals and cell bodies of primary nociceptive neurons directly. In neuropathic pain syndromes such as complex regional pain syndrome (CRPS), formerly called reflex sympathetic dystrophy (RSD), sympathetic postganglionic neurons may activate receptors on greatly sensitized primary afferent nerve terminals and cell bodies, either directly (on synapses) or indirectly (through secretion of norepinephrine into the blood); such activation may exacerbate the perception of the neuropathic pain. Multiple mechanisms are thought to contribute to sensitization of pain-related neurons and presence of chronic, agonizing neuropathic pain in CRPS and related syndromes. These mechanisms are noted in this illustration as numbered sites. Descending central noradrenergic and serotonergic projections are thought to play an important modulatory role in the processing of neuropathic and non-neuropathic pain.

CLINICAL POINT

In some cases of nerve damage or compression, particularly that associated with a sprain, a crush injury, a direct injection into a nerve, or even relatively minor trauma, a pathological reaction of primary afferents can result in a chronic, neuropathic pain syndrome called reflex sympathetic dystrophy, more recently renamed CRPS). It is related to the type of chronic, agonizing central pain experienced in phantom limb syndrome. CRPS affects the hand, arm, and shoulder to a greater extent than the lower extremity. Intense burning or stabbing pain is felt, with allodynia and hyperesthesia (extreme sensitivity to touch and painful stimuli, respectively). When this phenomenon affects one nerve (perhaps following a bullet wound) it is sometimes called causalgia. The primary afferents involved in CRPS appear to proliferate alpha-adrenergic receptors on their sensory receptor endings and on the dorsal root ganglion cell body and often show extraordinary sensitivity to catecholamines, which provoke a lower threshold for response to nociceptive stimuli. Permanent destruction of dorsal horn inhibitory interneurons (by glutamate excitotoxicity) and permanently altered thresholds for wide dynamic-range spinoreticular neurons also have been observed. Sympathetic-related characteristics may be noted in CRPS, such as changes in skin appearance due to vascular flow changes (vasomotor), atrophic skin and nails (trophic changes), altered sweating and skin temperature (sudomotor), and altered bone density on a tri-phasic bone scan. Treatment must occur quickly after detection and must employ simultaneous vigorous therapeutic approaches. Treatment choices normally include analgesics, tricyclic or other antidepressants to alter pain threshold in the spinal cord, membrane-stabilizing agents (e.g., Neurontin), physical therapy, and nerve stimulation.

From cerebral cortex and limbic forebrain

From hypothalamus (includes beta-endorphin axonal projections)

Stimuli from higher centers (psychological, placebo effect, etc.)

From sensory cortex

Enkephalin-containing neuron

Periaqueductal gray matter

Midbrain

Locus coeruleus

Afferent pain fibers in trigeminal nerve

Spinal trigeminal tract and nucleus

Lateral reticular formation

Medulla

Enkephalin-containing neuron

Brain stem tegmental noradrenergic cell groups

Descending norepinephrine pathway

Serotonin pathway

Corticonuclear fibers

Spinoreticular pathway

Decussation of the pyramids

Posterolateral funiculus

Anterolateral funiculus

Enkephalin-containing neuron

Afferent pain neuron of dorsal root ganglion

Spinal cord

Spinoreticular neuron

14.8 DESCENDING CONTROL OF ASCENDING SOMATOSENSORY SYSTEMS

The processing of nociceptive information in the dorsal horn of the spinal cord can be modulated by descending connections from the cerebral cortex; limbic forebrain structures; the hypothalamus (paraventricular nucleus); the periarcuate beta-endorphin neurons; the periaqueductal gray; the RF of the brain stem; the central noradrenergic neurons (of locus coeruleus and other brain stem tegmental groups); and the serotonergic (5HT) neurons (nucleus raphe magnus). The central descending noradrenergic and 5HT pathways, modulated by the periaqueductal gray, and other higher centers, are particularly important for endogenous and exogenous (i.e., opioid) modulation of pain.

CLINICAL POINT

Several regions of the central nervous system (CNS) send projections, direct and indirect, to regulate nociceptive processing through the dorsal horn of the spinal cord for the body and the descending nucleus of V for the face. These areas include regions of cerebral cortex, limbic forebrain areas, hypothalamic regions including endorphin nuclei, and sensory cortical centrifugal connections. Some of these projections use endogenous opiates. Enkephalin and dynorphin interneurons are found in pain-processing regions, particularly in the dorsal horn of the spinal cord and the descending nucleus of V, and in many hypothalamic and limbic sites that may be involved in the subjective interpretation of pain. The beta-endorphin neurons of the periarcuate region of the hypothalamus send connections to the periaqueductal gray, locus coeruleus and brain stem noradrenergic nuclei, the raphe nuclei, and many limbic regions. The periaqueductal gray is particularly important for opioid activation of the nucleus raphe magnus and other descending monoamine pathways that activate enkephalins and assist in opiate analgesia. The periaqueductal gray–raphe connection is essential for full functionality of opioid analgesia. Systemic administration of synthetic opiates activates neurons of the periarcuate region of the hypothalamus and periaqueductal gray, resulting in analgesia.

Cerebral cortex: postcentral gyrus

Centromedian nucleus (intralaminar)

Ventral posteromedial (VPM) nucleus of thalamus

Internal capsule

Midbrain

Dorsal trigeminal lemniscus (dorsal trigeminothalamic tract)

Ventral trigeminal lemniscus (ventral trigeminothalamic tract)

Pontine reticular formation

Pons

Trigeminal mesencephalic nucleus

Trigeminal motor nucleus

Principal sensory trigeminal nucleus

Touch, pressure ————

Pain, temperature ————

Proprioception - from muscle spindles ————

Trigeminal (semilunar) ganglion

Ophthalmic nerve

Maxillary nerve

Sensory root and motor root of mandibular nerve

Medullary reticular formation:
  Lateral reticular formation
  Medial reticular formation

Ventral trigeminal lemniscus

Spinal (descending) trigeminal tract

Spinal (descending) trigeminal nucleus

Dorsolateral fasciculus (of Lissauer)

Cervical spinal cord

Facial (VII) nerve

Glosso-pharyngeal (IX) nerve

Vagus (X) nerve

Substantia gelatinosa (lamina II)

J. Netter M.D.
with
J. Perkins
MS, MFA

TRIGEMINAL SENSORY SYSTEM

14.9 TRIGEMINAL SENSORY AND ASSOCIATED SENSORY SYSTEMS

Axons of primary (1°) sensory neurons enter the brain stem, travel in the descending (spinal) tract of V, and terminate in the descending (spinal) nucleus of V. Axons of the trigeminal ganglion (V) supply the face, anterior oral cavity, and teeth and gums; axons of the geniculate ganglion (VII) and jugular ganglion (X) supply a small zone of the external ear. Axons of the petrosal ganglion (IX) supply general sensation to the posterior oral cavity and pharynx. Axons (mainly crossed) of the descending nucleus of V project into the ventral trigeminal lemniscus (ventral trigeminothalamic tract) and terminate in the ventral posteromedial (VPM) nucleus of the thalamus. The VPM nucleus projects to the lateral primary sensory cortex and to intralaminar thalamic nuclei, which are associated with nociceptive processing. The caudal descending nucleus

also sends contralateral projections to the RF for processing of excruciating pain (similar to the spinoreticular system). Primary sensory axons carrying fine, discriminative modalities from V (similar to the DC system) terminate in the rostral portion of the descending nucleus of V and in the main (chief) sensory nucleus of V, which contribute to the ventral trigeminothalamic tract. A portion of the main sensory nucleus also projects ipsilaterally to the VPM nucleus via the dorsal trigeminothalamic tract. Although most of the trigeminal system is represented on the lateral portion of the contralateral primary sensory cortex (postcentral gyrus), part of the epicritic trigeminal projections as well as taste are represented in the ipsilateral sensory cortex. The mesencephalic nucleus of V is the only primary sensory nucleus found inside the CNS; these neurons supply muscle spindles for masticatory and extraocular muscles and mediate associated muscle spindle reflexes. See page 386 for a Clinical Point.

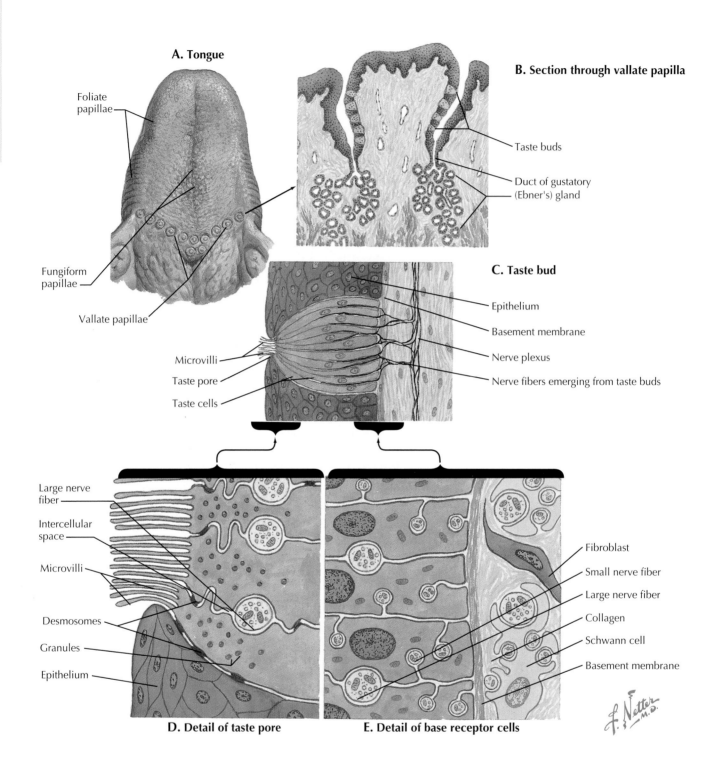

A. Tongue

Foliate papillae

Fungiform papillae

Vallate papillae

B. Section through vallate papilla

Taste buds

Duct of gustatory (Ebner's) gland

C. Taste bud

Epithelium

Basement membrane

Nerve plexus

Nerve fibers emerging from taste buds

Microvilli

Taste pore

Taste cells

Large nerve fiber

Intercellular space

Microvilli

Desmosomes

Granules

Epithelium

Fibroblast

Small nerve fiber

Large nerve fiber

Collagen

Schwann cell

Basement membrane

D. Detail of taste pore

E. Detail of base receptor cells

SENSORY SYSTEM FOR TASTE

14.10 ANATOMY OF TASTE BUDS AND THEIR RECEPTORS

Taste buds are chemosensory transducers that consist of bundles of columnar cells that lie within the epithelium. They translate individual molecular configurations or combinations of molecules for salty, sweet, sour, and bitter sensations into action potentials of both large and small primary sensory axons. The taste buds are found on the anterior and posterior regions of the tongue and, less frequently, on the palate and epiglottis, mainly in children. Nerve fibers for taste show complex responses of electrical activity across populations of many nerve fibers. The integrative interpretation of taste takes place in the CNS.

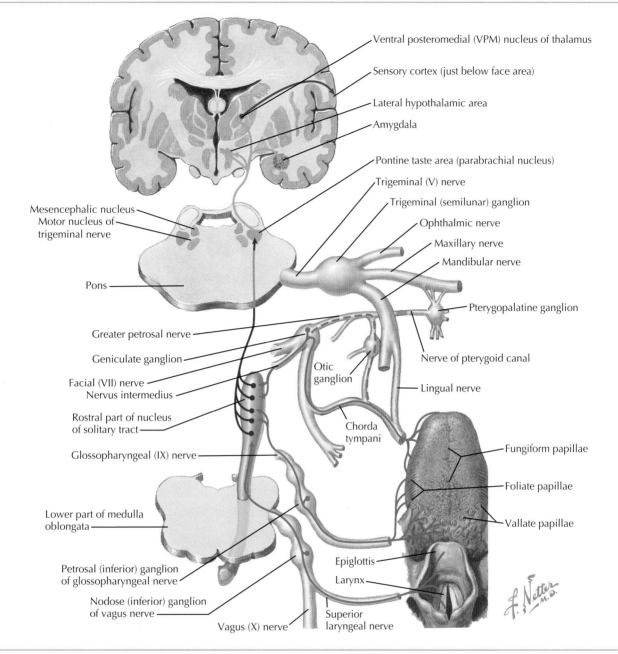

Ventral posteromedial (VPM) nucleus of thalamus

Sensory cortex (just below face area)

Lateral hypothalamic area

Amygdala

Pontine taste area (parabrachial nucleus)

Trigeminal (V) nerve

Trigeminal (semilunar) ganglion

Ophthalmic nerve

Maxillary nerve

Mandibular nerve

Pterygopalatine ganglion

Nerve of pterygoid canal

Lingual nerve

Fungiform papillae

Foliate papillae

Vallate papillae

Epiglottis

Larynx

Superior laryngeal nerve

Vagus (X) nerve

Nodose (inferior) ganglion of vagus nerve

Petrosal (inferior) ganglion of glossopharyngeal nerve

Lower part of medulla oblongata

Glossopharyngeal (IX) nerve

Rostral part of nucleus of solitary tract

Facial (VII) nerve
Nervus intermedius

Geniculate ganglion

Greater petrosal nerve

Chorda tympani

Otic ganglion

Pons

Mesencephalic nucleus
Motor nucleus of trigeminal nerve

14.11 **TASTE PATHWAYS**

Primary sensory axons of neurons of the geniculate ganglion (VII), petrosal ganglion (IX), and nodose (inferior) ganglion (X), supply taste buds on the anterior two thirds of the tongue, the posterior one third of the tongue, and the epiglottis and palate, respectively. These axons terminate in the rostral part of nucleus solitarius (nucleus of the solitary tract), which sends ipsilateral projections mainly to the parabrachial nucleus in the pons (and a few projections to nucleus VPM of the thalamus). The parabrachial nucleus projects fibers to nucleus VPM of the thalamus, to the hypothalamus (lateral hypothalamic area, paraventricular nucleus), and to amygdaloid nuclei. These nonthalamic projections are associated with the emotional, motivational, and behavioral aspects of taste and food intake.

one third), and X (epiglottis). The taste buds detect sweet, salty, bitter, and sour tastes; each taste bud appears to be associated mainly with one such modality. Combined taste receptor activation can code for a tremendous array of subtle tastes and flavors. Olfaction plays a major role in the discrimination of what an individual perceives to be taste. The primary taste afferents terminate in the rostral nucleus solitarius, which projects mainly to a pontine parabrachial nucleus and then to the parvicellular part of the VPM nucleus of the thalamus, several hypothalamic sites, and the amygdaloid complex. Some cortical areas, such as the anterior portion of the insular cortex and a lateral zone of the posterior orbitofrontal cortex, are involved in subjective aspects of taste and the gustatory experience. These pathways are mainly ipsilateral. Chemical influences can also have a profound effect on taste. Smoking may blunt taste. Many illnesses, including severe nasal congestion, liver dysfunction, autonomic problems, postradiation responses, some vitamin deficiencies, and some medications, may distort or alter the tastes of foods or may leave a lingering, unpleasant, distinctive taste. Many chemotherapeutic agents also profoundly alter taste sensation, perhaps accounting in part for loss of appetite in such individuals.

CLINICAL POINT

Taste pathways arise from primary receptors, the taste buds, which are associated with cranial nerves VII (anterior two thirds), IX (posterior

Frontal section

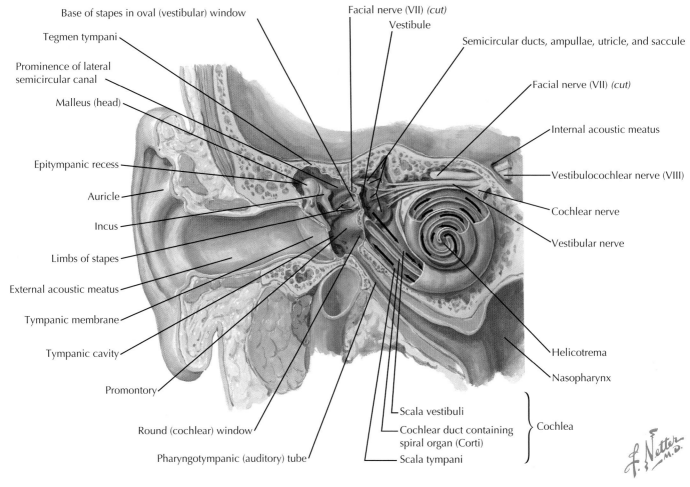

Base of stapes in oval (vestibular) window

Tegmen tympani

Prominence of lateral semicircular canal

Malleus (head)

Epitympanic recess

Auricle

Incus

Limbs of stapes

External acoustic meatus

Tympanic membrane

Tympanic cavity

Promontory

Round (cochlear) window

Pharyngotympanic (auditory) tube

Facial nerve (VII) *(cut)*

Vestibule

Semicircular ducts, ampullae, utricle, and saccule

Facial nerve (VII) *(cut)*

Internal acoustic meatus

Vestibulocochlear nerve (VIII)

Cochlear nerve

Vestibular nerve

Helicotrema

Nasopharynx

Scala vestibuli

Cochlear duct containing spiral organ (Corti)   } Cochlea

Scala tympani

AUDITORY SYSTEM

14.12 PERIPHERAL PATHWAYS FOR SOUND RECEPTION

The sound transduction process involves complex mechanical transduction of sound waves through the external ear and the external acoustic meatus and across the tympanic membrane; there it is leveraged as a mechanical force by the bones of the middle ear (ossicles) via the oval window to produce a fluid wave in the cochlear duct. This fluid wave causes differential movement of the basilar membrane, stimulating hairs on the apical portion of hair cells to release neurotransmitters that stimulate primary sensory axons of neurons of the cochlear (spiral) ganglion. The basilar membrane in the cochlea shows maximal displacement spatially according to the frequency of impinging tones, with low frequencies maximally stimulating the apex (helicotrema) and high frequencies maximally stimulating the base. The eustachian (pharyngotympanic) tube permits pressure equilibrium between the middle ear and the outside world.

CLINICAL POINT

Hearing loss may be partial or total and can involve virtually any range of detectable frequencies. The most devastating for human communication is a loss in the frequencies of speech (300 to 3000 Hz) of 40 or more decibels. In general, hearing loss can be subdivided into two categories: sensorineural and conductive. Sensorineural hearing loss involves damage to the hair cells, the auditory nerve, or central auditory pathways. Because of the neural damage, both air conduction and bone conduction are diminished. Conductive hearing loss involves damage to the outer or middle ear. Air conduction is impaired because the sound is not properly transduced into the inner ear, but bone conduction is normal. These two types of hearing loss can be tested for at the bedside by using a tuning fork of 512 Hz. The Weber test involves placing the vibrating tuning fork on the center of the forehead. Normally, the patient hears the fork equally in both ears. With sensorineural loss, the sound is heard best in the unaffected ear; with conductive loss, the sound is heard best in the affected ear. The Rinne test involves holding the vibrating tuning fork against the mastoid bone. When the fork is no longer heard, it is immediately placed just outside the external auditory meatus. Normally, air conduction is more effective than bone conduction, and the fork will again be heard when moved adjacent to the external auditory meatus (air conducting sound better than bone). If conductive hearing loss is present, once bone conduction is no longer heard, air conduction also will not be heard (bone conducting sound better than air). If sensorineural hearing loss is present, air conduction may be greater than bone conduction, although both may be diminished.

Bony and membranous labyrinths

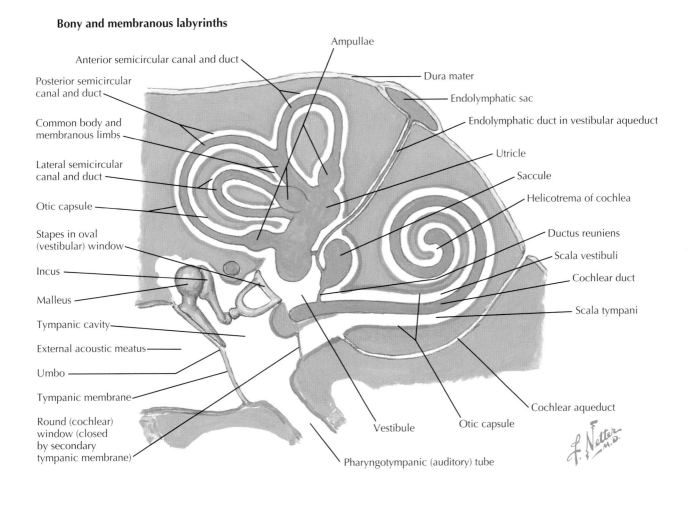

14.13 **BONY AND MEMBRANOUS LABYRINTHS**

The relationship between the cochlea and the vestibular apparatus (utricle, saccule, semicircular canals, and ducts) and the bony labyrinth that surrounds them is illustrated. The ossicles (malleus, incus, stapes) leverage the movement of the tympanic membrane to produce movement of the oval window. Movement of the oval window causes a fluid wave to move through the scala vestibuli and the scala tympani of the cochlea and ricochet onto the round window. The three semicircular canals are located at 90-degree angles to each other, representing tilted X, Y, and Z axes.

CLINICAL POINT

The semicircular canals (ducts) contain the ampullae that have hair cells that respond to angular acceleration. The utricle contains the otolith organ in the macula that responds to linear acceleration and detects gravitation. The saccule responds best to vibratory stimuli. The cochlea contains the hair cells that respond to fluid movements in the scalae vestibuli and tympani, brought about by the leveraging of the ossicles against the oval window; this movement affects hair cells in the cochlear duct.

The activity of the utricle can sometimes become distorted when debris moves away from the hairs and induces activation of the hair cells in the ampulla of the posterior semicircular canal. This produces vertigo and nystagmus that are associated with a specific position of the head (benign postural or positional vertigo). This disorder is the most common cause of vertigo seen in neurological practice. These attacks commonly occur when the patient is lying down, moving to a particular position, or tilting the head back; they may recur either briefly or for a longer period of days or weeks. Attacks can be induced by an examiner through the Hallpike maneuver (tilting the patient's head back and then 30 degrees to the side), resulting in a brief attack of vertigo and nystagmus. No pharmacological treatment is available. Attempts to reposition the debris by deliberate Hallpike-like head movements have met with some success.

Section through turn of cochlea

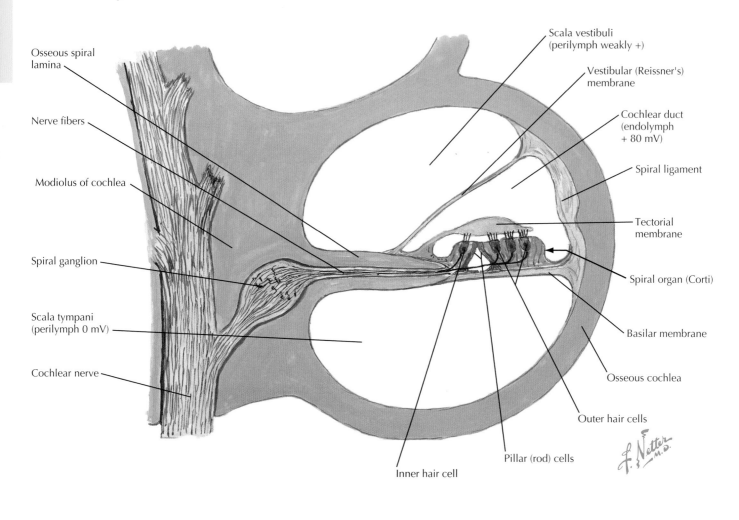

Osseous spiral lamina

Nerve fibers

Modiolus of cochlea

Spiral ganglion

Scala tympani (perilymph 0 mV)

Cochlear nerve

Inner hair cell

Pillar (rod) cells

Scala vestibuli (perilymph weakly +)

Vestibular (Reissner's) membrane

Cochlear duct (endolymph + 80 mV)

Spiral ligament

Tectorial membrane

Spiral organ (Corti)

Basilar membrane

Osseous cochlea

Outer hair cells

14.14 VIII NERVE INNERVATION OF HAIR CELLS OF THE ORGAN OF CORTI

Primary sensory axons of the spiral (cochlear) ganglion inner-vate inner and outer hair cells of the organ of Corti, located on the basilar membrane. The axons are activated by release of neurotransmitters from the hair cells, which occurs when the hairs on the apical surface are moved by shearing forces resulting from movement of the basilar membrane (fluid wave through the scalae vestibuli and tympani) in relation to the more rigidly fixed tectorial membrane. This represents the complex transduction process of the conversion of external sound waves to action potentials in spiral ganglion axons. The ionic potentials (in mV) are indicated for the scala tympani and vestibuli (perilymph) and the cochlear duct (endolymph). These potential differences contribute to the excitability of the hair cells.

CLINICAL POINT

Hair cells in the organ of Corti respond to fluid movements in the scalae vestibuli and tympani that induce shearing motion of the tecto-rial membrane relative to the basilar membrane. Each region of the spiraled cochlea contains hair cells that respond optimally to move-ment of the basilar membrane; low frequencies stimulate hair cell movement in the apex (helicotrema), and high frequencies stimulate hair cell movement in the basilar coils of the cochlea. The hair cells can be damaged by many pathological processes, such as viral infections (e.g., mumps); drugs (e.g., quinine); antibiotics; exposure to sustained loud noise; and age-related deterioration caused by free-radical dam-age. Exposure to loud noises above 85 decibels can selectively dam-age hair cells, especially those in the basilar coils of the cochlea that transduce high-frequency sounds. High-pitched machinery noise (jet engines), gunfire without ear protection, exposure to loud music at concerts or by earphones, and loud ambient noise in construction or industrial sites can induce temporary damage that can become perma-nent with repeated exposure. Environmental protection regulations now require ear protection in personnel working at such sites.

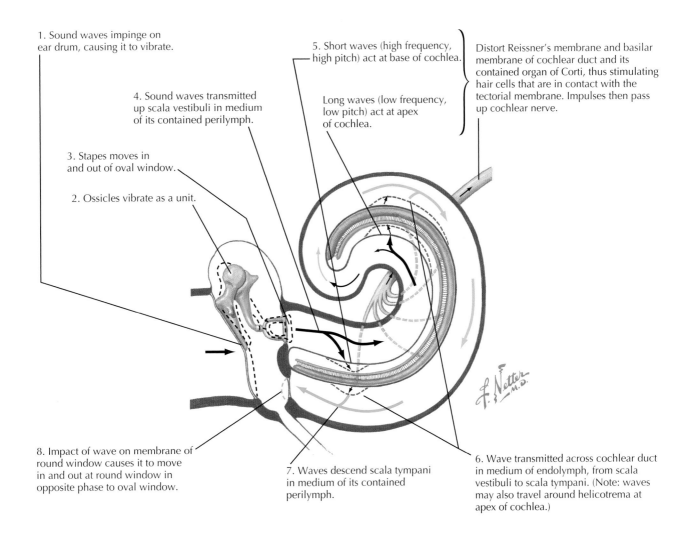

1. Sound waves impinge on ear drum, causing it to vibrate.

4. Sound waves transmitted up scala vestibuli in medium of its contained perilymph.

3. Stapes moves in and out of oval window.

2. Ossicles vibrate as a unit.

5. Short waves (high frequency, high pitch) act at base of cochlea.

Long waves (low frequency, low pitch) act at apex of cochlea.

Distort Reissner's membrane and basilar membrane of cochlear duct and its contained organ of Corti, thus stimulating hair cells that are in contact with the tectorial membrane. Impulses then pass up cochlear nerve.

8. Impact of wave on membrane of round window causes it to move in and out at round window in opposite phase to oval window.

7. Waves descend scala tympani in medium of its contained perilymph.

6. Wave transmitted across cochlear duct in medium of endolymph, from scala vestibuli to scala tympani. (Note: waves may also travel around helicotrema at apex of cochlea.)

14.15 COCHLEAR RECEPTORS

Fluid movement through scala vestibuli, around the helicotrema, and back through the scala tympani differentially moves the basilar membrane on which the organ of Corti and its hair cells reside. Movement of hairs on the apical portion of the hair cells by shearing forces of the tectorial membrane results in their depolarization and the release of neurotransmitters. This release stimulates action potentials in the primary afferent axons of spiral ganglion cells. Efferent axons from the olivocochlear bundle, controlled by descending central auditory pathways, can modulate the excitability of hair cells and the sensory transduction process.

Acoustic area of temporal lobe cortex

Medial geniculate body

Brachium of inferior colliculus

Inferior colliculus

Midbrain

Correspondence between cochlea and acoustic area of cortex:

Low tones

Middle tones

High tones

Lateral lemnisci

Nuclei of lateral lemnisci

Medulla oblongata

Superior olivary complex

Dorsal cochlear nucleus

Inferior cerebellar peduncle

Ventral cochlear nucleus

Cochlear division of vestibulocochlear nerve

Intermediate acoustic stria

Reticular formation

Dorsal acoustic stria

Trapezoid body (ventral acoustic stria)

Spiral ganglion

Inner

Outer

Hair cells

Afferent Auditory Pathways

14.16 AFFERENT AUDITORY PATHWAYS

Central axon projections of the spiral ganglion neurons terminate in dorsal and ventral cochlear nuclei in several tonotopic maps (receptor origination shown in the cochlea in colors). These cochlear nuclei project into the lateral lemniscus via acoustic striae; many of these projections remain ipsilateral. The lateral lemniscus terminates in the nucleus of the inferior colliculus, which in turn projects via the brachium of the inferior colliculus to the medial geniculate body (nucleus) of the thalamus. The thalamus sends tonotopical projections to the primary auditory cortex on the transverse gyrus of Heschl. Several accessory auditory brain stem nuclei (the superior olivary nucleus for lateral sound localization, the nuclei of the trapezoid body [not shown], and the lateral lemniscus) send both crossed and uncrossed projections through the lateral lemniscus. Sound is represented throughout the afferent auditory pathways bilaterally; thus, a unilateral lesion in the lateral lemniscus, the auditory thalamus, the auditory radiations, or the auditory cortex does not produce contralateral deafness. With such a lesion, there is a diminution in hearing and auditory neglect contralateral to the lesion with bilateral simultaneous stimulation.

CLINICAL POINT

The cochlear nerve contains axons that innervate the hair cells of the organ of Corti in the spirals of the cochlea. Primary cochlear axons enter the lateral portion of the caudal pons, terminating in the dorsal and ventral cochlear nuclei with several tonotopically representative maps of the auditory frequency world. The auditory nerve can be damaged by infections, tumors (e.g., acoustic Schwannoma), and traumas, particularly those associated with the petrous portion of the temporal bone. Irritation of auditory nerve fibers can produce tinnitus, a sense of ringing in the ears (or buzzing, humming, clicking, or other sounds). When the nerve is actually destroyed, the tinnitus stops and hearing loss ensues. Auditory nerve damage has symptoms that are present on the ipsilateral side with respect to the damage. In the brain stem, the acoustic striae project axons to a host of nuclei in bilateral fashion, including the superior olivary nuclei, the nuclei of the trapezoid body, the nuclei of the lateral lemnisci, and the inferior colliculi. The inferior colliculi, a mandatory synaptic processing site for central auditory processing, receive information from both ears. These projections proceed to the medial geniculate nucleus and then via the auditory radiations to the auditory cortex (transverse gyrus of Heschl). Damage in the interior of the brain stem or, more likely, in the temporal lobe, generally caused by a vascular infarct, tumor or abscess, or trauma, may result in diminished hearing but not unilateral deafness.

Excitatory endings → → →
Inhibitory endings → → →
Intermediate endings ⇢ ⇢

14.17 CENTRIFUGAL (EFFERENT) AUDITORY PATHWAYS

Descending pathways travel from the auditory cortex, the medial geniculate body of the thalamus, the inferior colliculus, and accessory auditory nuclei of the brain stem to terminate in caudal structures in the pathway, such as the cochlear nuclei and the superior olivary nucleus. These centrifugal connections permit descending control of incoming auditory information. The olivocochlear bundle, from the superior olivary nuclei, projects back to the hair cells in the organ of Corti and modulates the transduction process between the hair cells and the primary afferent axons. The motor nuclei of V and VII send LMN axonal projections to the tensor tympani and stapedius muscles, respectively, for reflex dampening of the ossicles in the presence of sustained loud noise.

A. Membranous labyrinth

Vestibular and cochlear divisions of vestibulocochlear nerve

Vestibular ganglion

Saccule

Utricle

Superior semicircular canal

Horizontal semicircular canal

Cochlear duct (scala media)

Macula

Cristae within ampullae

Posterior semicircular canal

B. Position within base of skull

Canals: Superior

Posterior

Plane of horizontal canal and utricle

30°

60°

Plane of saccule

Plane of superior canal

Superior

Horizontal

90°

Posterior

Plane of posterior canal

C. Section of crista

Opposite wall of ampulla

Gelatinous cupula

Hair tufts

Hair cells

Nerve fibers

Basement membrane

E. Structure and innervation of hair cells

Excitation

Inhibition

Kinocilium

Stereocilia

Cuticle

Basal body

Kinocilium

Stereocilia

Cuticle

Basal body

Hair cell (type I)

Supporting cells

Afferent nerve calyx

Efferent nerve ending

Basement membrane

Myelin sheath

Hair cell (type II)

Supporting cells

Efferent nerve ending

Afferent nerve calyx

Myelin sheath

D. Section of macula

Otoconia

Gelatinous otolithic membrane

Hair tuft

Hair cell

Supporting cells

Basement membrane

Nerve fibers

VESTIBULAR SYSTEM

14.18 VESTIBULAR RECEPTORS

The vestibular receptors include hair cells in the cristae ampullaris of the utricle (linear acceleration or gravity) and saccule (low frequency vibration) and in the maculae of the orthogonally oriented semicircular canals (angular acceleration or movement of the head). Hair tufts from the cristae ampullaris and the maculae are embedded in a gelatinous substance, which is moved when gravity (utricle) exerts force on the calcium carbonate crystals (otoliths) resting on top of the hairs or when fluid movement occurs in a semicircular canal (head movement). Bending of the kinocilium in the hair tufts depolarizes the hair cell, causing the release of neurotransmitters that stimulate action potentials in primary sensory axons of the vestibular (Scarpa's) ganglion. Additional efferent projections from the CNS modulate this transduction process, similar to centrifugal regulation of auditory transduction.

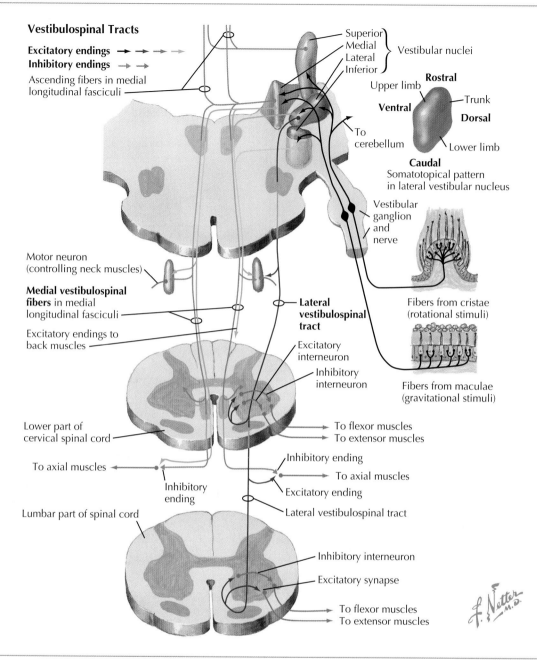

Vestibulospinal Tracts

Excitatory endings →→ →→ →→ →→

Inhibitory endings →→ →→

Ascending fibers in medial longitudinal fasciculi

Superior
Medial
Lateral
Inferior
} Vestibular nuclei

Upper limb   **Rostral**

Ventral   Trunk

Dorsal

To cerebellum   Lower limb

Caudal
Somatotopical pattern in lateral vestibular nucleus

Vestibular ganglion and nerve

Motor neuron (controlling neck muscles)

Medial vestibulospinal fibers in medial longitudinal fasciculi

Excitatory endings to back muscles

Lateral vestibulospinal tract

Excitatory interneuron

Inhibitory interneuron

Fibers from cristae (rotational stimuli)

Fibers from maculae (gravitational stimuli)

Lower part of cervical spinal cord

To flexor muscles
To extensor muscles

To axial muscles

Inhibitory ending

Inhibitory ending
To axial muscles
Excitatory ending

Lumbar part of spinal cord

Lateral vestibulospinal tract

Inhibitory interneuron

Excitatory synapse

To flexor muscles
To extensor muscles

14.19 VESTIBULAR PATHWAYS

Primary afferent vestibular axons from the vestibular ganglion terminate in the four vestibular nuclei (superior, inferior, medial, and lateral) and directly in the cerebellum (deep nuclei and cortex). Descending axons are sent from the medial vestibulospinal tract (medial nucleus) to spinal cord LMNs that regulate head and neck movements. Descending axons are sent from the lateral vestibulospinal tract (lateral nucleus) to all levels of spinal cord LMNs to activate extensor movements. Multiple vestibular nuclei project to the cerebellum to modulate and coordinate muscle activity for basic tone and posture and to extraocular LMNs via the medial longitudinal fasciculus to coordinate eye movements with head and neck movements. Some ascending axons from the vestibular nuclei may reach the thalamus (near the VPM and posterior nuclei), with thalamic projections to the lateral postcentral gyrus (area 2, motion perception and spatial orientation) and to the insular cortex and temporoparietal cortex.

CLINICAL POINT

The vestibular nerve consists of axons that supply the hair cells of the cristae in the ampullae of the semicircular canals, as well as the maculae of the utricle and saccule. These primary vestibular axons terminate in the four vestibular nuclei and directly in the vestibular-cerebellum (part of the vermis and flocculonodular lobe). The vestibular nuclei send axonal projections to the LMNs of the spinal cord (vestibulospinal tracts), the cerebellum, the extraocular nuclei (medial longitudinal fasciculus), and the RF. The peripheral vestibular and auditory apparatus can be damaged by increased endolymphatic pressure that gradually destroys hair cells in both the vestibular and auditory peripheral systems. This condition, called Meniere's disease, is characterized by abrupt attacks of severe vertigo that can last for as long as several hours. The attacks are incapacitating and immobilizing and produce nausea and vomiting. The vestibular symptoms are accompanied by auditory symptoms, including tinnitus and progressive sensorineural deafness. Most cases are unilateral, but bilateral disease does occur. After many episodes, some remission is occasionally seen, but the disease can progress to the point where the hearing loss and vestibular damage are almost total.

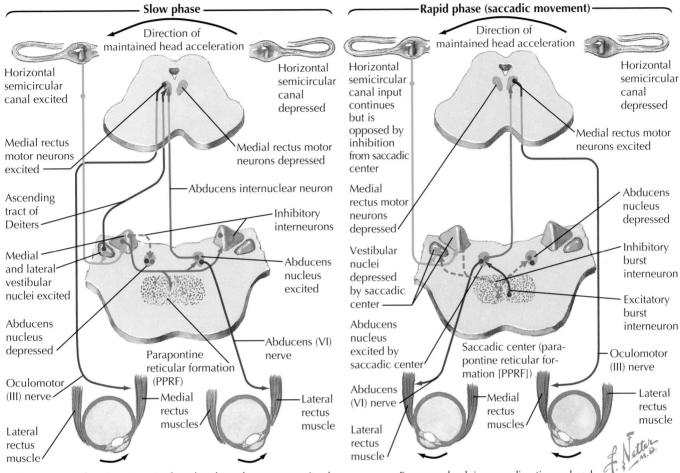

Slow phase

Direction of maintained head acceleration

Horizontal semicircular canal excited

Horizontal semicircular canal depressed

Medial rectus motor neurons excited

Medial rectus motor neurons depressed

Ascending tract of Deiters

Abducens internuclear neuron

Inhibitory interneurons

Medial and lateral vestibular nuclei excited

Abducens nucleus excited

Abducens nucleus depressed

Parapontine reticular formation (PPRF)

Abducens (VI) nerve

Oculomotor (III) nerve

Medial rectus muscles

Lateral rectus muscle

Lateral rectus muscle

Eyes move in direction opposite from head; tend to preserve visual fixation; rate determined by degree of horizontal canal excitation.

Rapid phase (saccadic movement)

Direction of maintained head acceleration

Horizontal semicircular canal input continues but is opposed by inhibition from saccadic center

Horizontal semicircular canal depressed

Medial rectus motor neurons excited

Medial rectus motor neurons depressed

Abducens nucleus depressed

Vestibular nuclei depressed by saccadic center

Inhibitory burst interneuron

Excitatory burst interneuron

Abducens nucleus excited by saccadic center

Saccadic center (parapontine reticular formation [PPRF])

Oculomotor (III) nerve

Abducens (VI) nerve

Medial rectus muscles

Lateral rectus muscle

Lateral rectus muscle

Eyes snap back in same direction as head.

14.20 NYSTAGMUS

Nystagmus is repetitive, alternating back-and-forth movements of the eye, requiring central coordination of extraocular LMNs and eye movements. Optokinetic nystagmus is a normal process of visually activated movement of the eyes via tracking mechanisms, with the eyes returning to a forward position by means of visual association cortex projections through the superior colliculus to extraocular LMNs. Vestibular nystagmus results from asymmetrical input from receptors in the semicircular canals or from damage to vestibular nuclei or the vestibular cerebellum and is mediated by vestibular projections via the medial longitudinal fasciculus to extraocular nuclei (LMNs); the asymmetrical input provokes the slow phase (or drift) of vestibular nystagmus, eliciting eye movements as if the head were turning. The fast phase (saccadic movement) is the return of the eyes to a forward position, which is provoked when the slow phase moves the eyes to a maximal position.

Horizontal section

Scleral venous sinus (Schlemm's canal)
Scleral spur
Zonular fibers (suspensory ligament of lens)
Ciliary body and ciliary muscle
Ciliary part of retina
Tendon of lateral rectus muscle
Optic (visual) part of retina
Choroid
Perichoroidal space
Sclera
Fascial sheath of eyeball (Tenon's capsule)
Episcleral space
Fovea centralis in macula
Outer sheath of optic nerve
Subarachnoid space

Iris
Lens
Capsule of lens
Cornea
Anterior chamber
Posterior chamber
Iridocorneal angle
Ciliary processes
Bulbar conjunctiva
Ora serrata
Tendon of medial rectus muscle
Vitreous body
Hyaloid canal
Lamina cribrosa of sclera
Optic nerve (II)
Central retinal artery and vein

VISUAL SYSTEM

14.21 ANATOMY OF THE EYE

The eye consists of three major layers, or tunics. The outer fibrous layer, the fibrous tunic, consists of the protective cornea (transparent) and the sclera (opaque). The middle layer, the vascular tunic (uveal tract), consists of the choroid, the ciliary body, and the iris. The transparent biconvex lens, with its surrounding capsule of zonular fibers, is suspended from the ciliary process of the ciliary body. The inner layer, or tunic, consists of the neuroretina, the non-pigment epithelium of the ciliary body, and the pigment epithelium of the posterior iris. The retina contains the photoreceptors for transduction of photon energy from light into neuronal activity. Aqueous humor is secreted from blood vessels of the iris into the posterior chamber and flows through the aperture of the pupil into the anterior chamber, where it is absorbed into the trabecular meshwork into Schlemm's canal at the iridocorneal angle. Blockage of this absorption of aqueous humor results in glaucoma. The vitreous humor fills the interior of the eyeball.

CLINICAL POINT

When light impinges on the eye, it is refracted to focus on the photoreceptors of the retina to permit interpretation of the outside visual world. A vast proportion (close to 90%) of the refraction of light is accomplished by the cornea. A smaller percentage (approximately 10%) of the refraction is accomplished by the lens; however, this smaller percentage can be regulated neurologically, via CN III and its influence on accommodation to near vision. If the cornea is opacified (e.g., following abrasion that results in vascularization) it may impede the light pathway and cause a distortion of vision. Accommodation to near vision occurs when one tries to look at an object that is close rather than distant and usually involves simultaneous convergence, constriction (pupil), and accommodation. Accommodation involves a portion of the nucleus of Edinger-Westphal, which acts through CN III axonal projections to the ciliary ganglion. This portion provides postganglionic parasympathetic cholinergic innervation to the ciliary muscle. When this parasympathetic system is activated, the ciliary muscle lifts up and in, releasing tension on the zonular fibers that suspend the lens, permitting the lens to bunch up (fatten) and refract light. Accommodation commonly diminishes with age (presbyopia). A CN III palsy damages both pupillary constriction (resulting in a fixed, dilated pupil) and accommodation to near vision. Accommodation also can be damaged by trauma, diabetes, viral infections, and other pathology. If accommodation is impaired, corrective lenses are needed to allow proper focusing of light on the retina.

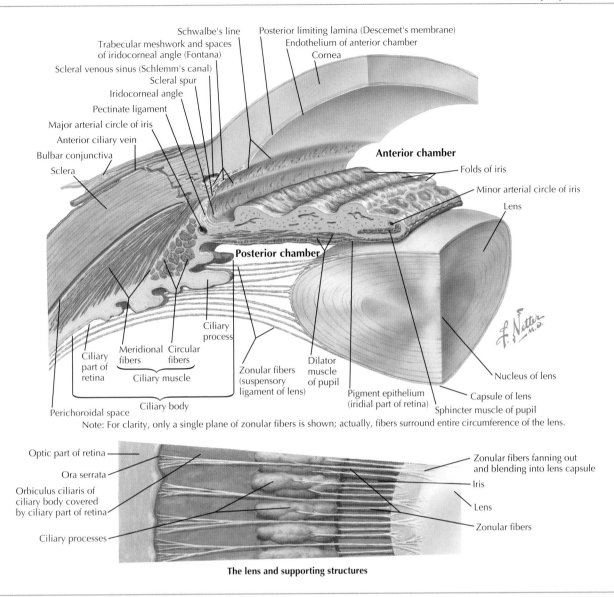

Schwalbe's line
Trabecular meshwork and spaces
of iridocorneal angle (Fontana)
Scleral venous sinus (Schlemm's canal)
Scleral spur
Iridocorneal angle
Pectinate ligament
Major arterial circle of iris
Anterior ciliary vein
Bulbar conjunctiva
Sclera

Posterior limiting lamina (Descemet's membrane)
Endothelium of anterior chamber
Cornea

Anterior chamber

Folds of iris
Minor arterial circle of iris
Lens

Posterior chamber

Ciliary
process

Ciliary
part of
retina

Meridional   Circular
fibers   fibers

Ciliary muscle

Zonular fibers
(suspensory
ligament of lens)

Dilator
muscle
of pupil

Pigment epithelium
(iridial part of retina)

Nucleus of lens
Capsule of lens
Sphincter muscle of pupil

Perichoroidal space   Ciliary body

Note: For clarity, only a single plane of zonular fibers is shown; actually, fibers surround entire circumference of the lens.

Optic part of retina
Ora serrata
Orbiculus ciliaris of
ciliary body covered
by ciliary part of retina
Ciliary processes

Zonular fibers fanning out
and blending into lens capsule
Iris
Lens
Zonular fibers

The lens and supporting structures

14.22 ANTERIOR AND POSTERIOR CHAMBERS OF THE EYE

The ciliary muscle and the pupillary constrictor muscle are supplied by parasympathetic postganglionic myelinated nerve fibers from the ciliary ganglion (innervated by preganglionics in the nucleus of Edinger-Westphal in CN III). Contraction of the ciliary muscle reduces the tension on zonular fibers and causes the lens to curve or bunch, which induces accommodation for near vision. The pupillary constrictor muscle also is supplied by parasympathetic postganglionic fibers from the ciliary ganglion. In the pupillary light reflex, light shone into one eye stimulates photoreceptors and related neurons in the retina; retinal ganglion cells send neural projections via the optic (II) nerve (afferent limb), which terminate in the pretectum. Neurons of the pretectum project bilaterally (crossed axons through the posterior commissure) to the Edinger-Westphal nucleus. This nucleus projects to the ciliary ganglion via CN III (efferent limb), which causes both direct (ipsilateral) and consensual (contralateral) pupillary constriction. The pupillary dilator muscle is supplied by sympathetic postganglionic unmyelinated nerve fibers from the superior cervical ganglion (innervated by preganglionics in T1 and T2). Schlemm's canals are conspicuous at the iridocorneal angle.

The lens is surrounded by a capsule anchored and suspended by an array of zonular fibers fanning out in circular fashion to attach to the ciliary processes of the ciliary body. Some interior zonular fibers extend along the ciliary body to the junction at the ora serrata.

CLINICAL POINT

Aqueous humor is secreted from the vasculature of the ciliary apparatus into the posterior chamber. It circulates through the pupillary aperture into the anterior chamber. From the anterior chamber, the aqueous humor is resorbed into the scleral venous sinuses, called the canals of Schlemm. If the canals of Schlemm are blocked, preventing absorption of aqueous humor, increased ocular pressure occurs; this results in pressure on the optic nerve head, cupped discs, atrophy, and defective vision of increasing severity, including total blindness. Glaucoma, the most common cause of optic nerve damage, occurs in more than 1% of the population over 40 years of age. This condition can be detected through ophthalmoscopy and tonometry. The principal type of glaucoma is called wide-angle glaucoma, which involves gradual sclerosis of the canals of Schlemm. A far less common type of glaucoma is narrow-angle (acute or closed-angle) glaucoma, a medical emergency in which bunching of the dilator muscle or narrowing of the iridocorneal angle blocks resorption of aqueous humor. The eye is red, swollen, and painful, sometimes causing a headache. It can be precipitated by pupillary dilation during an ophthalmological examination and must be reversed by means of pharmacological pupillary constriction.

Section through retina

Retinal Layers

- Nerve fiber layer
- Ganglion cell layer
- Inner plexiform layer
- Inner nuclear layer
- Outer plexiform layer
- Outer nuclear layer
- Photoreceptor layer
- Pigment epithelium

Cells

- Inner limiting membrane
- Axons at surface of retina passing via optic nerve, chiasm, and tract to lateral geniculate body
- Ganglion cell
- Müller cell (supporting glial cell)
- Bipolar cell
- Amarcine cell
- Horizontal cell
- Rod
- Cone
- Pigment cells of choroid

14.23 THE RETINA: RETINAL LAYERS

The retina is a tissue-paper-thin piece of CNS tissue that contains the photoreceptors; it is attached to the vascular tunic at the ora serrata. The layers of the retina in the interior of the eyeball are oriented from outer to inner. The pigment epithelium is at the outer margin, followed by the outer nuclear layer (photoreceptors), the inner nuclear layer (bipolar neurons, amacrine and horizontal cells), and the ganglion cell layer. The outer and inner plexiform layers are the zones of synaptic connectivity. The ganglion cell axons form an inner nerve fiber layer projecting centrally toward the optic nerve head, into which they collect as the optic nerve, CN II. The outer segments of the photoreceptors, the rods and cones, are embedded in a pigment epithelium in the outer part of the interior eyeball to prevent backscatter of light. The rods and cones connect synaptically with bipolar cells in the outer plexiform layer; these bipolar neurons connect with the ganglion cells of the retina in the inner plexiform layer. The retinal ganglion cells are the equivalent of secondary sensory nuclei for other sensory modalities. Horizontal and amacrine cells provide horizontal interconnections in the retina, mainly at the outer plexiform layer and the inner plexiform layer, respectively. These cells modulate the central flow of information from the photoreceptors to the bipolar neurons to the retinal ganglion cells. The central point for visual focusing is the fovea centralis (0.4 mm in diameter) in the macula (3 mm in diameter), which is found temporally and slightly below the geometric midpoint. The fovea consists purely of cones for color vision (photopic); these cone projections to ganglion cells involve very little convergence. In the fovea, there is close to a one-to-one-to-one relationship among the cones, bipolar neurons, and ganglion cells. The peripheral retinal photoreceptors are mainly rods, for night vision (scotopic); there is huge convergence of rods onto bipolar neurons, which in turn converge onto single ganglion cells. Thus, acuity is best achieved in the fovea, the region for color vision.

CLINICAL POINT

Cones permit color vision and are concentrated in the macula of the retina, the point of focus for high-acuity vision. The center of the macula, the fovea centralis, consists entirely of cones. These cones are connected with bipolar retinal cells, which in turn contact retinal ganglion cells, resulting in conveyance of visual information via the optic nerve into other CNS structures (superior colliculus, pretectum, hypothalamus, lateral geniculate nucleus). The macular pathway is essential for photopic (color, high-acuity) vision. The peripheral retina contains rods as the main photoreceptors; rods massively converge onto bipolar neurons. This peripheral retinal pathway is active in scotopic (night) vision. The macula can undergo a gradual process of depigmentation and degeneration in elderly individuals, leading to the loss of central vision and reading capability. Although there is no immediate cure for macular degeneration, carotenoid supplements of lutein and zeaxanthin appear to replenish the macula with these important depleted carotenoids, slowing the degenerative process. Although macular degeneration is mainly a disease of the elderly, some young individuals with inherited storage diseases (Tay-Sachs) or infectious processes may experience macular degeneration.

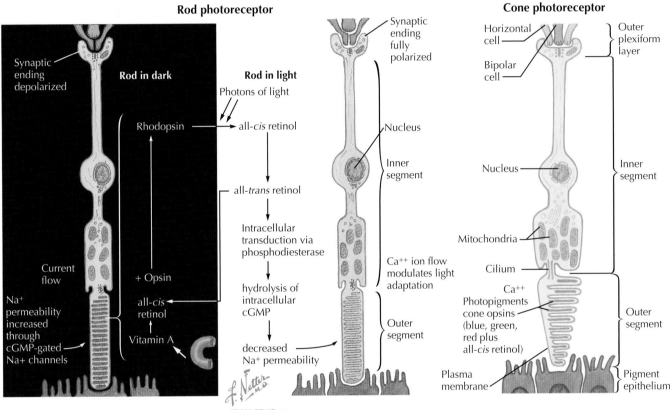

Rod photoreceptor

Synaptic ending depolarized

Rod in dark

Rod in light

Photons of light

Rhodopsin → all-*cis* retinol

all-*trans* retinol

Intracellular transduction via phosphodiesterase

hydrolysis of intracellular cGMP

decreased Na⁺ permeability

+ Opsin

all-*cis* retinol

Vitamin A

Current flow

Na⁺ permeability increased through cGMP-gated Na+ channels

Synaptic ending fully polarized

Nucleus

Inner segment

Ca⁺⁺ ion flow modulates light adaptation

Outer segment

Cone photoreceptor

Horizontal cell

Bipolar cell

Outer plexiform layer

Nucleus

Inner segment

Mitochondria

Cilium

Ca⁺⁺ Photopigments cone opsins (blue, green, red plus all-*cis* retinol)

Plasma membrane

Outer segment

Pigment epithelium

14.24 THE RETINA: PHOTORECEPTORS

Rods use the photopigment rhodopsin to achieve transduction of photons of energy from light into neurotransmitter release that can activate electrical activity in bipolar neurons. Rod light transduction involves conversion of all-*cis*-retinol (from rhodopsin) to an all-*trans* form, provoking calcium influx and a decrease in sodium conductance with hyperpolarization. This process is outlined in detail in the first two parts of the figure, a rod in the dark and a rod in light. When a rod is activated by light, it hyperpolarizes rather than depolarizes. A cone uses opsin photopigments for blue, green, and red, as well as all-*cis* retinal; these cone pigments permit color vision.

A. Topography of retinal nerve fibers

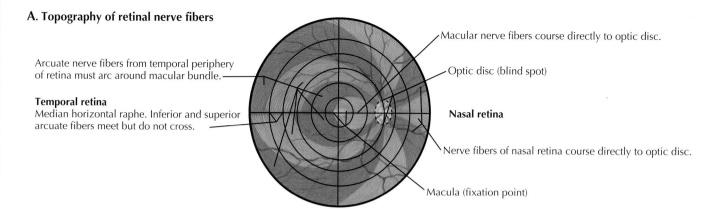

Arcuate nerve fibers from temporal periphery of retina must arc around macular bundle.

Temporal retina
Median horizontal raphe. Inferior and superior arcuate fibers meet but do not cross.

Macular nerve fibers course directly to optic disc.

Optic disc (blind spot)

Nasal retina

Nerve fibers of nasal retina course directly to optic disc.

Macula (fixation point)

B. Anatomy of optic nerve

Retinal nerve fibers
Retina
Choroid
Sclera
Central retinal vessels
Vascular circle of Zinn-Haller
Short posterior ciliary artery
Lamina cribrosa
Nerve fiber bundles
Pial layer
Arachnoid layer
Dura mater

Optic nerve layers

Nerve fiber layer

Prelaminar layer

Laminar layer

Retrolaminar layer

14.25 THE RETINA: OPTIC NERVE

A, The retina is topographically organized; a representation of the visual world (referred to as a visual field) is mapped onto the retina of each eye. Because the eye acts like a camera, the visual world is inverted as it projects onto the retina. The temporal (lateral) visual field falls on the nasal hemiretina, and the nasal (medial) visual field falls on the temporal hemiretina. The upper visual field falls on the lower hemiretina, and the lower visual field falls on the upper hemiretina. When viewing the retina directly using ophthalmoscopy, the macula is located nasally and slightly inferiorly to the geometric midpoint of the retina. The optic disc (zone of optic nerve fibers, sometimes called the blind spot) is located temporally and slightly below (inferior to) the geometric midpoint. The precise retinotopic organization is maintained throughout the projections of the main visual pathway (the retino-geniculo-calcarine pathway).

B, The optic nerve (CN II) is a CNS tract that consists of myelinated axons of the ganglion cells of the retina. These axons collect across the innermost layer of the neuroretina and form the optic nerve, which exits from the eyeball nasally, slightly above the horizontal midline. These optic nerve fibers are myelinated by oligodendroglia. The optic nerve is surrounded by meninges, as part of the CNS. A subarachnoid space containing cerebrospinal fluid is present between the arachnoid and pial layers of the meninges. Elevated intracranial pressure can exert pressure on the optic nerve head (where the ganglion cell axons first form the optic nerve), forcing it inward; this phenomenon is called papilledema and is evidence of increased intracranial pressure; approximately 24 hours are required for increased intracranial pressure to cause papilledema. Major retinal vessels from the central retinal artery and vein travel in the optic nerve.

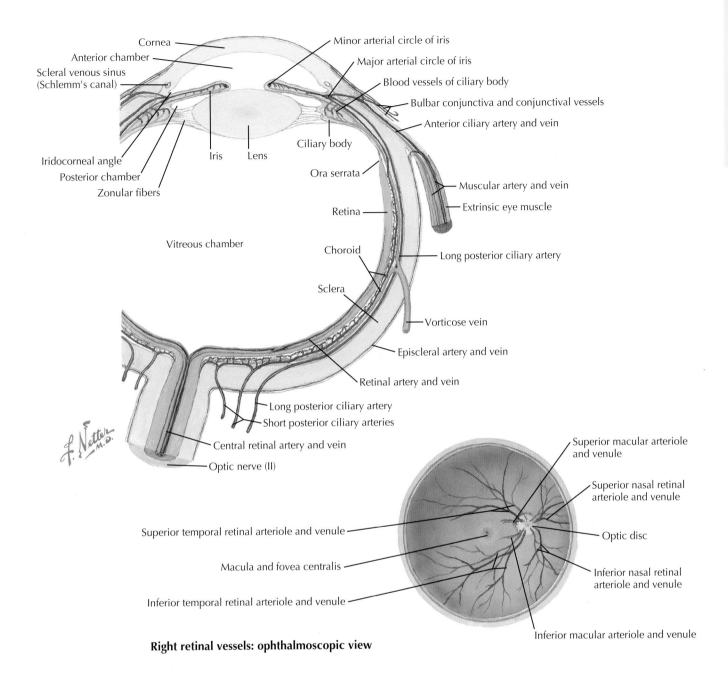

Right retinal vessels: ophthalmoscopic view

14.26 ARTERIES AND VEINS OF THE EYE

The central retinal artery and its branches supply blood to the retina. This arterial system, derived from the ophthalmic artery (the first branch off the internal carotid artery), is commonly the first site where ischemic or embolic events (transient ischemic attacks) herald the presence of serious vascular disease and high risk for a future stroke. Ciliary arteries supply the middle vascular tunic, which also contributes partial blood supply to the retina; this component of blood supply can be disrupted by a detached retina. Blood vessels enter and exit the retina at the optic disc (nerve head), located nasally and slightly inferiorly from the geometric midpoint of the eyeball. The macula is located temporally and slightly inferiorly from this midpoint.

CLINICAL POINT

The central retinal artery is a common site of emboli in impending cerebrovascular disease; such emboli are forerunners of stroke and indications of carotid atherosclerosis or occlusion. An embolus in the central retinal artery may produce temporary (fleeting) blindness in the affected eye, called amaurosis fugax, which lasts for several minutes but less than an hour; such an episode is called a transient ischemic attack. An infarct in the central retinal artery produces characteristic ophthalmologic findings, such as loss of opalescence in the fovea (a so-called cherry-red spot). If the central retinal vein is occluded, a hemorrhage is seen, and the resultant visual loss may be significant. In addition to hemorrhages, edema and exudates may be present, indicative of hypertension or diabetic problems. If the retina becomes detached, it may be separated from part of its blood supply from the ciliary arteries in the middle vascular tunic, which also results in loss of vision.

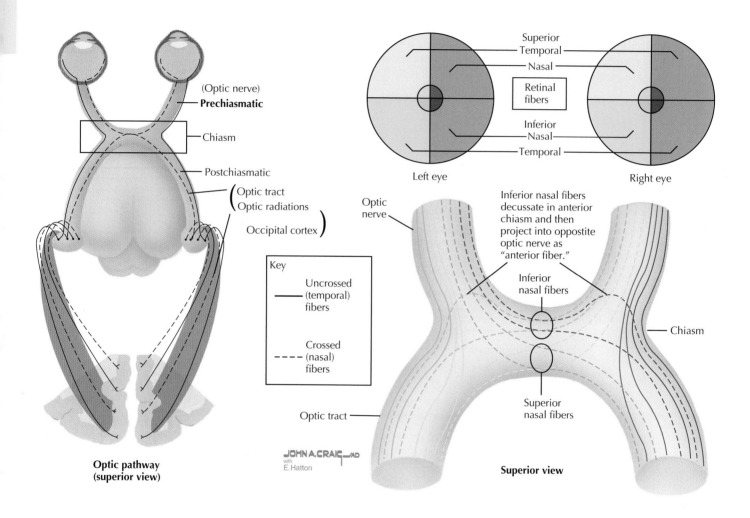

(Optic nerve)
Prechiasmatic

Chiasm

Postchiasmatic

(Optic tract
Optic radiations

Occipital cortex)

Key

Uncrossed
(temporal)
fibers

Crossed
(nasal)
fibers

**Optic pathway
(superior view)**

Superior
Temporal
Nasal

Retinal
fibers

Inferior
Nasal
Temporal

Left eye

Right eye

Optic
nerve

Inferior nasal fibers
decussate in anterior
chiasm and then
project into opposite
optic nerve as
"anterior fiber."

Inferior
nasal fibers

Chiasm

Superior
nasal fibers

Optic tract

JOHN A. CRAIG
with
E. Hatton

Superior view

14.27 ANATOMY AND RELATIONSHIPS OF THE OPTIC CHIASM

Axons from ganglion cells in the temporal hemiretinas (carrying information from the nasal visual fields) travel into the optic nerve and remain ipsilateral in the optic chiasm; they synapse in the ipsilateral lateral geniculate body or nucleus. Axons from ganglion cells in the nasal hemiretinas (carrying information from the temporal visual fields) travel into the optic nerve and cross the midline in the optic chiasm; they synapse in the contralateral lateral geniculate body. Therefore, crossing axons in the optic chiasm carry information from the temporal visual fields, which are derived from retinal ganglion cells in the nasal hemiretinas. These crossing axons are susceptible to disruption by a pituitary adenoma; such a lesion can produce a bitemporal hemianopia, starting first as an upper visual quadrant defect and progressing to full hemianopia. The optic tract contains axons from the ipsilateral temporal hemiretina and the contralateral nasal hemiretina, representing the contralateral visual field; disruption of the optic tract results in contralateral hemianopia.

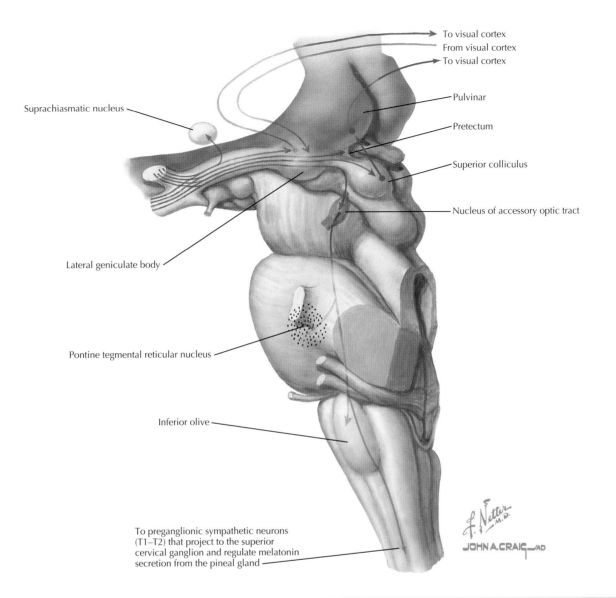

Suprachiasmatic nucleus

To visual cortex
From visual cortex
To visual cortex

Pulvinar

Pretectum

Superior colliculus

Nucleus of accessory optic tract

Lateral geniculate body

Pontine tegmental reticular nucleus

Inferior olive

To preganglionic sympathetic neurons (T1–T2) that project to the superior cervical ganglion and regulate melatonin secretion from the pineal gland

14.28 VISUAL PATHWAYS: RETINAL PROJECTIONS TO THE THALAMUS, HYPOTHALAMUS, AND BRAIN STEM

Retinal projections travel through the optic nerve, chiasm, and tract and terminate in several regions, including the lateral geniculate body or nucleus, the upper layers of the superior colliculus, the pretectum, the hypothalamus (suprachiasmatic nucleus), and the nucleus of the accessory optic tract. The lateral geniculate body mediates conscious visual interpretation of visual input via the retino-geniculo-calcarine (area 17) pathway. The superior colliculus provides a second visual pathway through the pulvinar to the associative visual cortex (areas 18 and 19), providing localizing information for visual stimuli. It also provides descending contralateral connections (tectospinal tract) to cervical LMNs to mediate reflex visual effects on head and neck movements. The pretectum mediates the pupillary light reflex. The suprachiasmatic nucleus of the hypothalamus integrates light flux and regulates circadian rhythms and diurnal cycles. The nucleus of the inferior accessory optic tract may help to mediate brain stem responses

for visual tracking and may interconnect with sympathetic preganglionic neurons in T1 and T2 (regulating the superior cervical ganglion).

CLINICAL POINT

Ganglion cells of the retina (the neural equivalents of the secondary sensory nuclei in other sensory systems, such as the nuclei gracilis and cuneatus) send projections through the optic nerve, chiasm, and tract to terminate in the superior colliculus, the lateral geniculate nucleus of the thalamus, the pretectum, the suprachiasmatic nucleus of the hypothalamus, and some brain stem sites. However, they all require the projection of axons through the optic nerve, chiasm, and tract. If the optic nerve is damaged (by multiple sclerosis, glaucoma, inflammatory disorder, trauma, vascular pathology), there is visual loss in a selected area (scotoma) or in the entire ipsilateral eye (monocular blindness). If the optic chiasm is damaged, usually by a pituitary tumor, the growth of the tumor impinges on the crossing fibers in a manner that disrupts the outer visual fields (bitemporal hemianopia), usually from the upper to the lower fields (much like pulling down the shades.). If the optic tract is damaged, axons from the ipsilateral temporal hemiretina and the contralateral nasal hemiretina are disrupted, producing a contralateral visual field deficit (homonymous contralateral hemianopia).

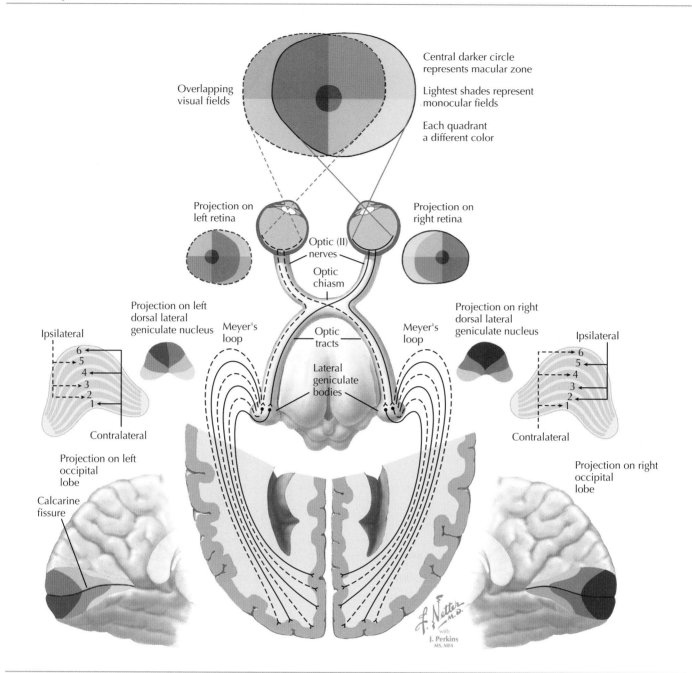

Overlapping visual fields

Central darker circle represents macular zone

Lightest shades represent monocular fields

Each quadrant a different color

Projection on left retina

Projection on right retina

Optic (II) nerves

Optic chiasm

Projection on left dorsal lateral geniculate nucleus

Meyer's loop

Optic tracts

Meyer's loop

Projection on right dorsal lateral geniculate nucleus

Ipsilateral

Lateral geniculate bodies

Ipsilateral

Contralateral

Contralateral

Projection on left occipital lobe

Calcarine fissure

Projection on right occipital lobe

14.29 VISUAL PATHWAY: THE RETINO-GENICULO-CALCARINE PATHWAY

The retino-geniculo-calcarine pathway conveys information about fine-grained conscious visual analysis of the outside world. It is organized topographically (retinotopic) throughout its course to the calcarine cortex in the occipital lobe. The nasal hemiretinal ganglion cell axons cross the midline in the optic chiasm, whereas the temporal hemiretinal ganglion cell axons remain ipsilateral. Thus, each optic tract conveys information from the contralateral visual world (or visual field); damage to the optic tract produces contralateral hemianopia. The optic tract terminates in the lateral geniculate body or nucleus and is organized in 6 layers, as shown. However, binocular convergence does not take place here; ganglion cell axons from the ipsilateral temporal hemiretina terminate in layers 2, 3, and 5, and ganglion cell axons from the contralateral nasal hemiretina terminate in layers 1, 4, and 6. The optic radiations project to the calcarine (striate) cortex (area 17). A portion of the optic radiations loops through the temporal lobe (Meyer's loop) and can be damaged by a tumor or mass, resulting in contralateral upper quandrantanopia. Bilateral convergence from right and left retinas first takes place in the primary visual cortex, area 17.

CLINICAL POINT

Meyer's loop consists of axons of the lateral geniculate nucleus that loop downward through the temporal lobe before extending posteriorly to synapse on cortical neurons in layer 4 of the lower bank of the ipsilateral calcarine fissure (area 17, primary visual cortex). The temporal lobe is a site at which tumor or abscess formation is far more likely than it is in the parietal or occipital lobes. If such a mass lesion damages fibers of Meyer's loop, the individual loses vision in the upper quadrant of the contralateral visual field (upper contralateral quadrantanopia), reflecting the persistent "retinotopic" organization of the entire retino-geniculo-calcarine pathway that is depicted in this illustration.

Frontal lobe

Parietal lobe

Spatial visual pathway: positional relationships among objects in visual scene, analysis of motion

Middle temporal area: direction selective and motion responsive

Occipital lobe

MT

V3
V2

V4

V3
V2

V1

JOHN A.CRAIG—AD

V4: shape and color perception

Temporal lobe

Object recognition pathway: high resolution and form

14.30 VISUAL PATHWAYS IN THE PARIETAL AND TEMPORAL LOBES

Neurons in the primary visual cortex (V1, area 17) send axons to association visual cortices (V2 and V3, areas 18 and 19). V2 and V3 also receive input from the superior colliculus via the pulvinar. V1, V2, and V3 project to the middle temporal area and V4. Middle temporal neurons are direction selective and motion responsive, and further project into the parietal lobe for spatial visual processing. The parietal neurons provide analysis of motion and positional relationships among objects in the visual field. V4 neurons are involved in shape and color perception. Neurons in V4 project into the temporal lobe, in which further neuronal processing provides high-resolution object recognition, including faces, animate objects, and the classification and orientation of objects. Small infarcts in the temporal lobe may produce specific agnosias, inability to recognize specific types of objects, such as faces or animate objects.

CLINICAL POINT

The retino-geniculo-calcarine pathway projects to area 17, the primary visual cortex; subsequent axonal projections are sent to areas 18 and 19. In these visual-association cortices, feature extraction from simple to complex to hypercomplex cells occurs, giving form to new visual information. A parietal cortical pathway further processes information related to the direction and motion of objects—a spatial visual pathway. A temporal cortical pathway conveys further information about the shape, color, and form of objects. Some discrete lesions in these parietal and temporal cortical pathways can produce distinctive visual deficits. Visual agnosias occur when an individual cannot recognize objects that are viewed but has full visual acuity. This can happen with lesions in the occipito-temporal visual pathway. Visual agnosias are particularly common with lesions in the dominant mesial portion of the occipital cortex; they accompany a right homonymous hemianopia. Cortical color agnosias (cortical color blindness) also can occur with lesions in the occipito-temporal visual pathway, through V4. Some specific lesions of the occipito-temporal pathway, especially when bilateral, can result in prosopagnosia, the inability to recognize faces. Some lacunar infarcts in this pathway also may result in the inability to distinguish between animate and inanimate objects. Lesions in the occipito-parietal visual pathway, particularly in the nondominant hemisphere, can cause visual-spatial disorientation, appearing clinically as impaired ability to see.

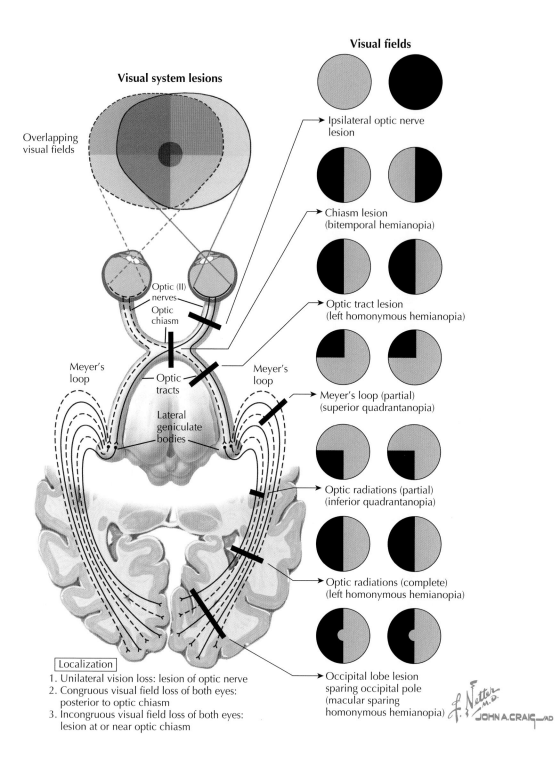

Visual system lesions

Overlapping visual fields

Optic (II) nerves

Optic chiasm

Meyer's loop

Optic tracts

Lateral geniculate bodies

Meyer's loop

Visual fields

Ipsilateral optic nerve lesion

Chiasm lesion (bitemporal hemianopia)

Optic tract lesion (left homonymous hemianopia)

Meyer's loop (partial) (superior quadrantanopia)

Optic radiations (partial) (inferior quadrantanopia)

Optic radiations (complete) (left homonymous hemianopia)

Occipital lobe lesion sparing occipital pole (macular sparing homonymous hemianopia)

Localization
1. Unilateral vision loss: lesion of optic nerve
2. Congruous visual field loss of both eyes: posterior to optic chiasm
3. Incongruous visual field loss of both eyes: lesion at or near optic chiasm

14.31 VISUAL SYSTEM LESIONS
Lesions of the optic nerve, optic chiasm, optic tract, Meyer's loop in the temporal lobe, optic radiations, and visual cortex produce specific visual-field deficits, as shown in this figure.

15

MOTOR SYSTEMS

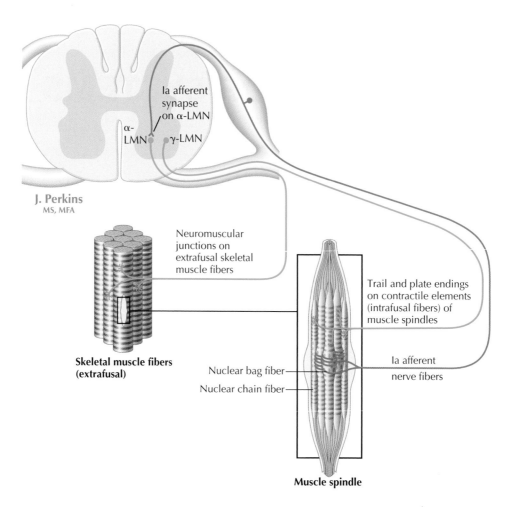

J. Perkins
MS, MFA

Ia afferent
synapse
on α-LMN

α-
LMN   γ-LMN

Neuromuscular
junctions on
extrafusal skeletal
muscle fibers

Trail and plate endings
on contractile elements
(intrafusal fibers) of
muscle spindles

**Skeletal muscle fibers
(extrafusal)**

Nuclear bag fiber

Nuclear chain fiber

Ia afferent
nerve fibers

Muscle spindle

LOWER MOTOR NEURONS

15.1 ALPHA AND GAMMA LOWER MOTOR NEURONS

All lower motor neuron (LMN) groups except the facial nerve nucleus that supplies the muscles of facial expression consist of both alpha LMNs that supply the skeletal muscle fibers (extrafusal fibers) and gamma LMNs that supply the small contractile elements in the muscle spindles (intrafusal fibers). The muscles of facial expression do not have muscle spindles and are not supplied by gamma LMNs. The alpha LMNs regulate contraction of the skeletal muscles to produce movement. The gamma LMNs regulate the sensitivity of the muscle spindles for group Ia and group II afferent modulation of alpha LMN excitability.

CLINICAL POINT

An alpha LMN supplies motor axons to a variable number of skeletal muscle fibers (extrafusal fibers), ranging from just a few (e.g., extraocular muscles) to several thousand (large muscles such as the quadriceps). The LMN and its innervated skeletal muscle fibers are called a motor unit. Supporting cells (such as Schwann cells) and myocytes produce trophic factors to maintain the nerve-muscle association; when nerve injury occurs, growth factors help to attract motor axonal regrowth to reestablish the prior nerve-muscle association. When motor axons degenerate, the neuromuscular junctions (NMJs) disappear, and the nicotinic cholinergic receptors spread across the

membrane of the denervated skeletal muscle fibers. This results in denervation hypersensitivity to nicotinic cholinergic stimulation, noted as random individual muscle fiber twitches (fibrillation), best observed by electromyography. If motor nerves are attracted back to the muscle fibers and NMJs are restored, the nicotinic cholinergic receptors are again restricted to the secondary folds of the NMJ. If the motor axon that was lost cannot regrow, neighboring motor axons of other motor units that supply adjacent skeletal muscle fibers may send sprouts to the denervated muscle fibers and incorporate them into the motor unit; the consequence is a larger motor unit and a greater demand on the LMN cell body that now supplies a greater than normal number of skeletal muscle fibers. This mechanism may account for recovery of physiological function in some LMN diseases such as polio. If the alpha-LMN cell body itself is damaged or is in the process of dying (e.g., in amyotrophic lateral sclerosis), the axon may produce aberrant action potentials (agonal bursts of electrical activity) that result in muscle fiber contraction throughout the motor unit, called a fasciculation, which is visually observable. A denervated muscle fiber must be reinnervated within 1 year or so if it is to restore relatively normal function; a longer period leads to permanent changes that preclude proper reinnervation. Many experimental approaches are seeking to restore innervation or attract a more robust nerve supply to denervated muscle fibers by applying or inducing gene expression of growth factors and trophic factors. Denervated skeletal muscle fibers are flaccidly paralyzed, lack muscle tone, cannot be induced to contract with muscle stretch reflexes, and undergo atrophy; these are classic characteristics of LMN syndrome.

A. Cytoarchitecture of the spinal cord gray matter

Nuclear cell columns   **Laminae of Rexed**

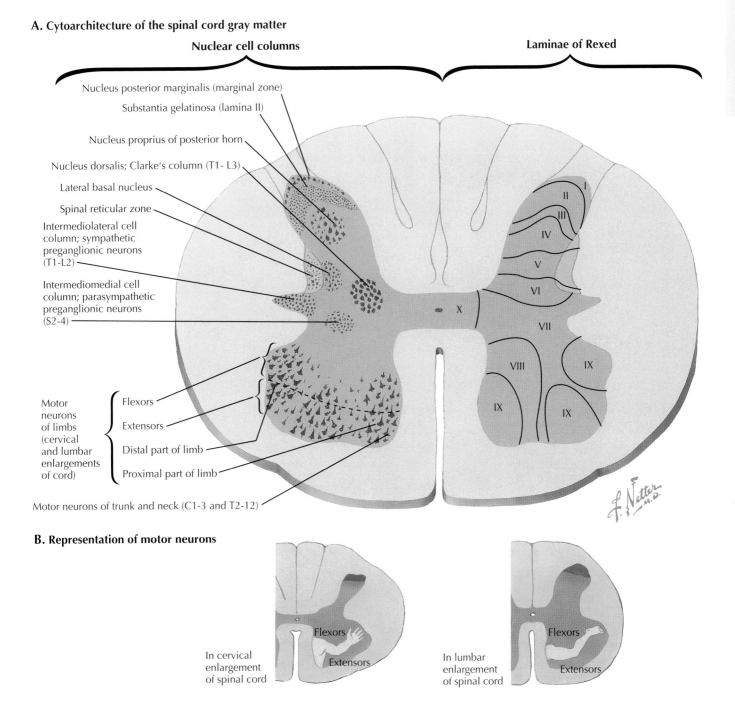

Nucleus posterior marginalis (marginal zone)

Substantia gelatinosa (lamina II)

Nucleus proprius of posterior horn

Nucleus dorsalis; Clarke's column (T1- L3)

Lateral basal nucleus

Spinal reticular zone

Intermediolateral cell column; sympathetic preganglionic neurons (T1-L2)

Intermediomedial cell column; parasympathetic preganglionic neurons (S2-4)

Motor neurons of limbs (cervical and lumbar enlargements of cord)

Flexors

Extensors

Distal part of limb

Proximal part of limb

Motor neurons of trunk and neck (C1-3 and T2-12)

I
II
III
IV
V
VI
VII
VIII
IX
IX
IX
X

B. Representation of motor neurons

In cervical enlargement of spinal cord

Flexors

Extensors

In lumbar enlargement of spinal cord

Flexors

Extensors

15.2 DISTRIBUTION OF LOWER MOTOR NEURONS IN THE SPINAL CORD

LMNs are found as clusters of neurons in the anterior (ventral) horn of the spinal cord, represented as lamina IX of Rexed. Distinct clusters of LMNs supply distinct skeletal muscles with motor innervation. These LMN groups are organized topographically; LMNs distributing to trunk and neck muscles are found medially, and LMNs distributing to muscles of distal extremities are found laterally. Within spinal cord segments, LMNs distributing to flexor muscle groups are found dorsally, and LMNs distributing to extensor muscle groups are found ventrally.

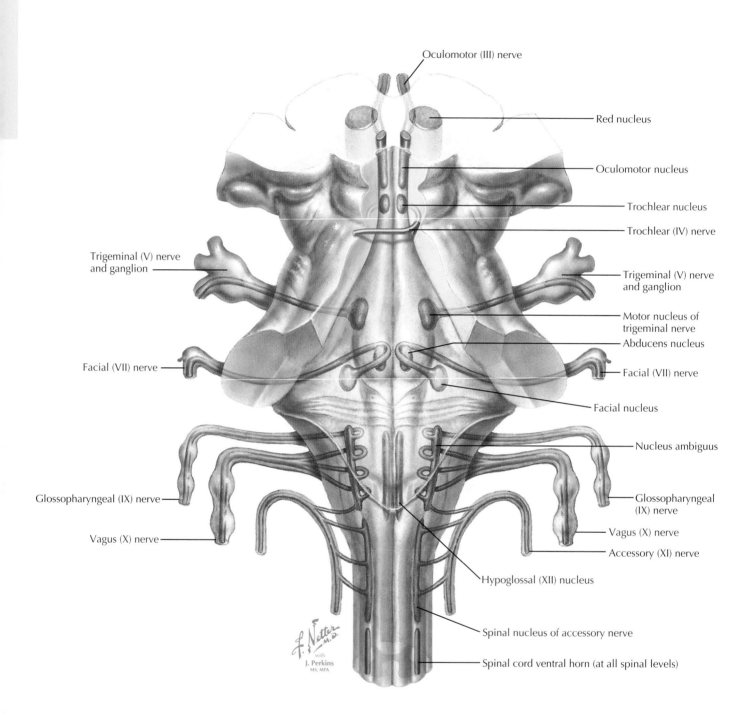

Oculomotor (III) nerve

Red nucleus

Oculomotor nucleus

Trochlear nucleus

Trochlear (IV) nerve

Trigeminal (V) nerve and ganglion

Trigeminal (V) nerve and ganglion

Motor nucleus of trigeminal nerve

Abducens nucleus

Facial (VII) nerve

Facial (VII) nerve

Facial nucleus

Nucleus ambiguus

Glossopharyngeal (IX) nerve

Glossopharyngeal (IX) nerve

Vagus (X) nerve

Vagus (X) nerve

Accessory (XI) nerve

Hypoglossal (XII) nucleus

Spinal nucleus of accessory nerve

Spinal cord ventral horn (at all spinal levels)

15.3 DISTRIBUTION OF LOWER MOTOR NEURONS IN THE BRAIN STEM

LMNs are found in medial and lateral columns in a longitudinal view of the brain stem. The medial column (LMNs of the oculomotor nucleus, trochlear nucleus, abducens nucleus, and hypoglossal nucleus) derives from the general somatic efferent system, and the lateral column (LMNs of motor nucleus V, facial nucleus, nucleus ambiguus, and spinal accessory nucleus) derives from the special visceral efferent system. LMNs in the spinal cord are found in a longitudinal column coursing through the anterior horn at all levels.

Cerebral Cortex: Efferent Pathways

From frontal cortex to thalamus, basal ganglia, pontine nuclei, and reticular formation

Corticobulbar, corticorubral, corticonuclear, and corticospinal pathways

Caudate nucleus

Anterior limb of internal capsule

Lentiform nucleus { Globus pallidus / Putamen

From frontal eye fields to interstitial nucleus of Cajal

Cerebral peduncle

Red nucleus

Corticospinal axons

Corticonuclear axons

Pons

For pontocerebellar connections

Facial nerve nucleus of opposite side for lower face

Upper part of medulla oblongata

Pyramids

Lower part of medulla oblongata

Decussation of pyramids

Anterior (direct) corticospinal tract

Spinal cord

Anterior (ventral) horns

From parietal cortex to thalamus, pontine nuclei and reticular formation

Thalamus

Posterior limb of internal capsule

From occipital eye fields to superior colliculus

From auditory cortex to inferior colliculus

Superior colliculi

Interstitial nucleus of Cajal

Inferior colliculus

Trigeminal sensory nucleus

Trigeminal motor nucleus

Reticular formation

Solitary tract nucleus

Nucleus ambiguus

Dorsal motor nucleus of vagus and glossopharyngeal nerves

Hypoglossal nucleus

Reticular formation

Cuneate nucleus

Gracile nucleus

Reticular formation

Lateral (crossed) corticospinal tract

Posterior (dorsal) horn

AWC

UPPER MOTOR NEURONS

15.4 CORTICAL EFFERENT PATHWAYS

Cortical neurons in the motor cortex (area 4) and the supplemental and premotor cortices (area 6) send axons to the basal ganglia (caudate nucleus and putamen), the thalamus (ventral anterior [VA], and ventral lateral [VL] nuclei), the red nucleus, the pontine nuclei, the cranial nerve (CN) motor nuclei on both sides, and the spinal cord ventral horn, mainly on the contralateral side. These axons form the corticospinal tract, corticobulbar tract, corticostriatal projections, corticopontine projections, corticothalamic projections, and cortical connections to the upper motor neurons (UMNs) of the brain stem (reticular formation [RF] motor areas, red

nucleus, superior colliculus). Neurons of the sensory cortex (areas 3, 1, 2) send axons mainly to secondary sensory nuclei (corticonuclear fibers) to regulate incoming lemniscal sensory projections destined for conscious interpretation. Neurons in the frontal eye fields (area 8) project to the superior colliculus, the horizontal and vertical gaze centers of the brain stem, and the interstitial nucleus of Cajal to coordinate voluntary eye movements and associated head movements. Other regions of sensory cortex project axons to thalamic and brain stem structures that regulate incoming lemniscal sensory information. Some cortical efferent fibers project to limbic forebrain regions, such as the amygdaloid nuclei, hippocampal formation, and septal nuclei.

Lateral/oblique view

Cortical efferent fibers

Cortical efferent fibers

Midline fibers, corpus callosum

Superior cerebellar peduncle

Pyramids

15.5 **COLOR IMAGING OF CORTICAL EFFERENT PATHWAYS**

This diffusion tensor image shows the cortical efferent pathways in a lateral oblique section. These pathways, shown in blue, channel from widespread areas of the cerebral cortex to structures in the forebrain, the thalamus, the brain stem, the cerebellum, and the spinal cord. Additional cortical association pathways are depicted in green (running in anterior-posterior direction) and commissural pathways are shown in red (running in left-right direction).

Primary motor cortex (Area 4)

Neck
Brow
Eyelid
Nares
Lips
Tongue
Larynx

Posterior limb

Internal capsule

Anterior limb

Midbrain

III
IV

Pons

VI
V
VII upper
VII lower

Medulla

XII

Nucleus ambiguus (IX, X, XI)

Area 6   Area 4
Hip
Trunk
Arm
Hand
Face

Lateral aspect of cerebral cortex to show topographic projection of motor centers on precentral gyrus and premotor and supplemental motor cortex

III   III (ipsilateral and contralateral)
IV   IV (ipsilateral and contralateral)

VI   VI   VI (ipsilateral and contralateral)
V   V   V (ipsilateral and contralateral)
Upper   VII to upper face (ipsilateral and contralateral)
Lower   VII to lower face (contralateral only)
VII   VII

XII   XII   XII (ipsilateral and contralateral)

IX, X, and XI (ipsilateral and contralateral)
IX, X, XI   IX, X, XI

15.6 CORTICOBULBAR TRACT

The corticobulbar tract (CBT) arises mainly from the lateral portion of the primary motor cortex (area 4). CBT axons project through the genu of the internal capsule into the cerebral peduncle, the basis pontis, and the medullary pyramids on the ipsilateral side. The axons distribute to CN motor nuclei on the ipsilateral and contralateral sides except for the portion of the facial nerve nucleus (CN VII) that supplies the muscles of facial expression for the lower face, which receives exclusively contralateral projections. The CBT projections to the hypoglossal nucleus are mainly contralateral; CBT projections to the spinal accessory nucleus are mainly ipsilateral. CBT lesions result mainly in contralateral drooping lower face that is paretic to attempted movements from voluntary commands (central facial palsy), in contrast to Bell's palsy (CN VII palsy), in which the entire ipsilateral face is paralyzed.

Primary motor cortex (Area 4)

Hip
Knee
Trunk
Shoulder
Elbow
Wrist
Fingers
Thumb
Ankle
Toes

Posterior limb

Internal capsule

Anterior limb

Midbrain

Pons

Medulla

Decussation of pyramids (approximately 80% of CST fibers)

Spinal cord

Lateral (crossed) corticospinal tract

Anterior (direct) corticospinal tract

Area 6   Area 4
Hip
Trunk
Arm
Hand
Face

Lateral aspect of cerebral cortex showing topographic localization of motor centers on precentral gyrus and premotor and supplemental motor cortex

Posterior

Visual and auditory
Temporopontine
Sensory
Corticospinal
Corticobulbar
Frontopontine
Frontothalamic

Horizontal section through internal capsule showing location of principal pathways

Anterior

Ventral aspect of brain stem showing decussation of pyramids

Decussation

Corticospinal Tract

15.7 CORTICOSPINAL TRACT

The motor portion of the corticospinal tract (CST) originates from neurons of many sizes, mainly from the primary motor cortex (area 4) and the supplemental and premotor cortices (area 6). The primary sensory cortex (areas 3, 1, 2) contributes axons into the CST, but these axons terminate mainly in secondary sensory nuclei to regulate the processing of incoming lemniscal sensory information. The CST travels through the posterior limb of the internal capsule, the middle region of the cerebral peduncle, numerous fascicles of axons in the basis pontis, and the medullary pyramid on the ipsilateral side. Most of the CST axons (approximately 80%, but variable from individual to individual) cross the midline in the decussation of the pyramids at the medullary-spinal cord junction. These crossed fibers descend in the lateral CST in the lateral funiculus of the spinal cord and synapse on alpha and gamma LMNs, both directly and indirectly through interneurons. CST axons that do not decussate continue as the anterior CST in the anterior funiculus of the spinal cord and then decussate at the appropriate level through the anterior white commissure to terminate directly and indirectly on alpha and gamma LMNs contralateral to the cortical cells of origin. Only a very small portion of the motor connections of the corticospinal tract terminate on LMNs on the ipsilateral side of the spinal cord.

CLINICAL POINT

The motor portion of the CST arises mainly from neurons in the primary motor cortex (area 4) and the supplemental and premotor cortices (area 6). The primary sensory cortex and superior parietal lobule contribute corticospinal axons (corticonuclear fibers) to secondary sensory nuclei in the lower brain stem and spinal cord. Approximately 80% of the CST axons cross in the decussation of the pyramids and terminate directly and indirectly with alpha and gamma LMNs that control movements of the distal extremities, especially the hands and fingers. At least 10% of the CST terminates monosynaptically on alpha LMNs, especially those associated with hand and finger musculature. A lesion in the internal capsule damages the CST, corticorubral fibers, and corticoreticular fibers, resulting in contralateral hemiplegia. Initially, the hemiplegia is flaccid, with loss of tone and reflexes. Within days to a week or so, the hemiplegia becomes spastic, with hyperreflexia and hypertonus. The affected musculature shows initial resistance to attempted passive movement, followed by a dissipation or "melting" of tone (the clasp-knife reflex), perhaps because of high threshold Ib Golgi tendon organ inhibitory influences on the homonymous LMNs. The initial suspected mechanism of classical UMN syndrome was disinhibition of dynamic gamma LMNs, which drives initial resistance to passive stretch, mediated via subsequent Ia afferent influences over alpha LMNs; this mechanism was reinforced by observations that dorsal root sectioning diminished spasticity in UMN syndromes. Further studies have revealed additional potential mechanisms, including diminished reciprocal inhibition, recurrent Renshaw inhibition, and presynaptic inhibition on Ia afferents, all suggestive of major changes in interneurons of the spinal cord following a classic UMN lesion. In UMN syndrome, the plantar reflexes are extensor (reverting to a developmentally early stage in the absence of the CST), and abdominal reflexes are absent on the affected side. Clonus (repetitive alternating flexor and extensor muscle stretch reflexes) also may occur and is possibly attributable to interneuronal changes such as diminished Renshaw inhibition.

CLINICAL POINT

The CBT arises mainly from the lateral portion of the primary motor cortex; it descends through the genu of the internal capsule and the cerebral peduncle (medial to the corticospinal tract fibers) ipsilaterally, and it distributes both bilaterally to the motor CN nuclei (CNN) of the brain stem, except to the facial nucleus for the lower face, which receives almost exclusively contralateral projections. The corticobulbar axons terminate mainly on interneurons that regulate LMN output. Originally, *corticobulbar* was a term reserved for cortical projections to LMNs of the medulla (bulb), but it now has been expanded to include CNN for V, VII, nucleus ambiguus, XII, and the spinal accessory (XI) nucleus. A lesion in the genu of the internal capsule (embolic or thrombotic stroke, or hemorrhage of the middle cerebral artery or its branches) or the cerebral peduncle (Weber's syndrome, compression of the peduncle against the free edge of the tentorium cerebelli with transtentorial herniation) results mainly in a drooping face (central facial palsy) on the contralateral side. The intact hemisphere can control voluntary movement of the LMNs in the CNN for all other brain stem motor nuclei. In some individuals, a predominance of contralateral fibers to LMNs for the soft palate or the tongue is noted, resulting in a temporary contralateral palsy; or a predominance of ipsilateral fibers to LMNs of XI may be noted, resulting in an ipsilateral palsy of the sternocleidomastoid and upper trapezius muscles. This central paresis occurs without atrophy. Bilateral corticobulbar lesions result in profound paralysis of voluntary movement in all muscles supplied by CNN, with preservation of muscle bulk, reflex responses, and some emotional responses using those LMNs. The LMNs in CNN III, IV, and VI receive cortical input from the frontal eye fields (area 8) and parietal eye fields of both sides.

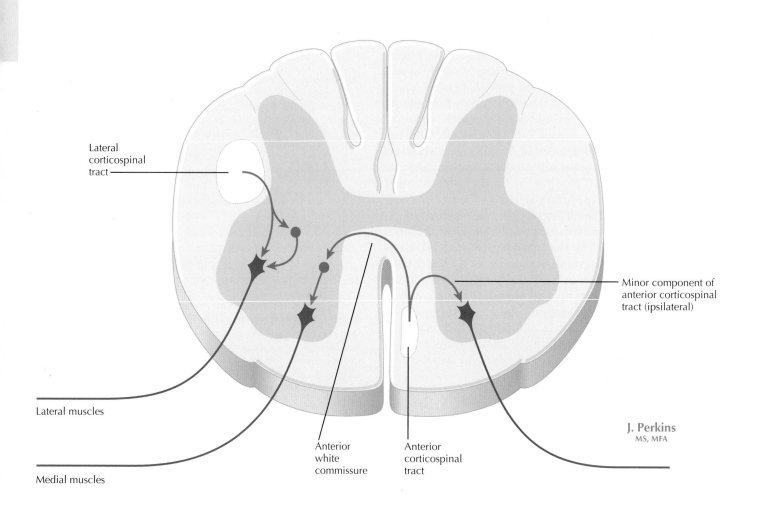

Lateral corticospinal tract

Lateral muscles

Medial muscles

Anterior white commissure

Anterior corticospinal tract

Minor component of anterior corticospinal tract (ipsilateral)

J. Perkins
MS, MFA

15.8 CORTICOSPINAL TRACT TERMINATIONS IN THE SPINAL CORD

Crossed axons in the lateral CST, intermixed with axons of the rubrospinal tract, travel in the lateral funiculus. These CST axons terminate directly and indirectly mainly on LMNs associated with distal musculature, especially for skilled hand and finger movements. The uncrossed anterior CST axons decussate predominantly in the anterior white commissure and terminate directly and indirectly mainly on LMNs that supply medial musculature. A small number of anterior CST axons terminate ipsilateral to the cortical cells of origin. An isolated lesion in the CST in the medullary pyramids results in weakness of contralateral fine, dexterous hand and finger movements. All other lesions involving the CST, intermixed with other descending motor systems (internal capsule, cerebral peduncle, pons), produce contralateral spastic hemiplegia with hypertonus, hyperreflexia, and plantar extensor responses as long-term consequences. Lesions in the lateral CST produce similar symptoms ipsilateral to the damaged lateral funiculus below the level of the lesion.

Rubrospinal Tract

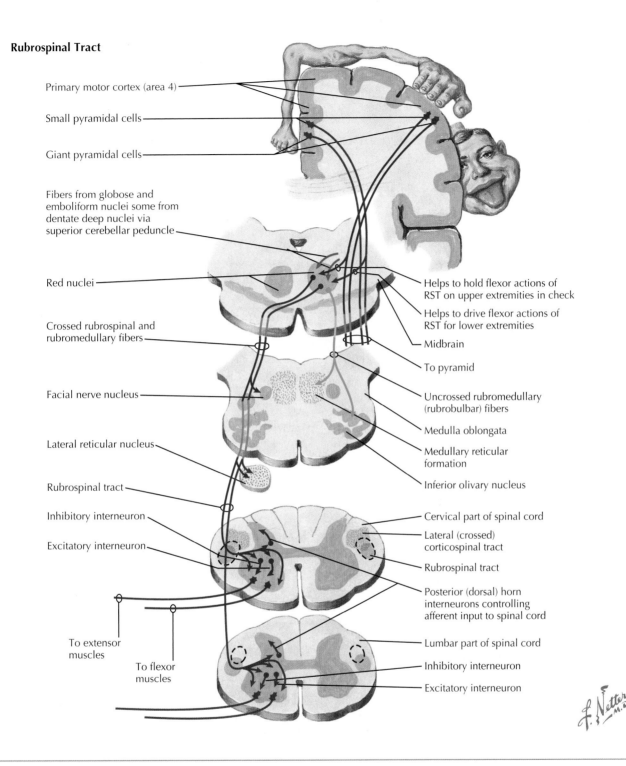

Primary motor cortex (area 4)

Small pyramidal cells

Giant pyramidal cells

Fibers from globose and emboliform nuclei some from dentate deep nuclei via superior cerebellar peduncle

Red nuclei

Crossed rubrospinal and rubromedullary fibers

Facial nerve nucleus

Lateral reticular nucleus

Rubrospinal tract

Inhibitory interneuron

Excitatory interneuron

To extensor muscles

To flexor muscles

Helps to hold flexor actions of RST on upper extremities in check

Helps to drive flexor actions of RST for lower extremities

Midbrain

To pyramid

Uncrossed rubromedullary (rubrobulbar) fibers

Medulla oblongata

Medullary reticular formation

Inferior olivary nucleus

Cervical part of spinal cord

Lateral (crossed) corticospinal tract

Rubrospinal tract

Posterior (dorsal) horn interneurons controlling afferent input to spinal cord

Lumbar part of spinal cord

Inhibitory interneuron

Excitatory interneuron

15.9 RUBROSPINAL TRACT

The cortico-rubro-spinal system is an indirect corticospinal system that regulates spinal cord LMNs. The red nucleus in the midbrain receives topographically organized ipsilateral connections from the primary motor cortex (area 4). Axons of the rubrospinal tract (RST) decussate in the ventral tegmental decussation and descend in the lateral brain stem and the lateral funiculus of the spinal cord, where they are intermixed extensively with axons of the lateral CST. The RST terminates directly and indirectly on alpha and gamma LMNs in the spinal cord, particularly those associated with flexor movements of the extremities. The RST helps to drive flexor movements of the upper extremity and helps to hold in check flexor movements of the lower extremity. RST lesions usually occur in conjunction with the CST in the spinal cord; corticorubral lesions also occur in conjunction with the CST in the internal capsule and cerebral peduncle. These lesions result in contralateral spastic hemiplegia as long-term consequences. Brain stem lesions caudal to the red nucleus result in decerebration (extensor spasticity), reflecting the removal of the flexor drive of the rubrospinal tract to LMNs supplying the upper limbs. See page 386 for a Clinical Point.

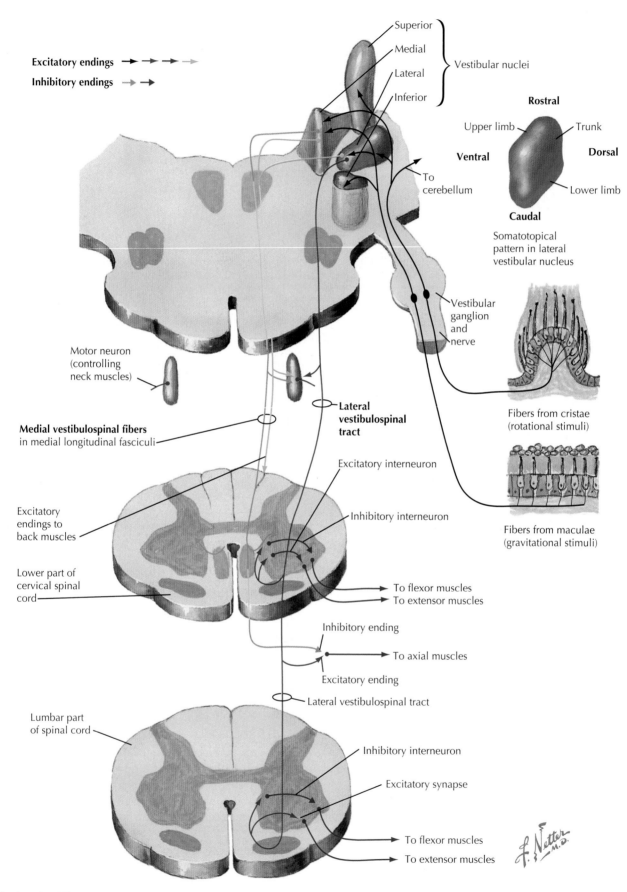

Excitatory endings →→→→

Inhibitory endings →→

Superior

Medial

Lateral

Inferior

Vestibular nuclei

Rostral

Upper limb — Trunk

Ventral **Dorsal**

Lower limb

Caudal

Somatotopical pattern in lateral vestibular nucleus

To cerebellum

Vestibular ganglion and nerve

Fibers from cristae (rotational stimuli)

Fibers from maculae (gravitational stimuli)

Motor neuron (controlling neck muscles)

Lateral vestibulospinal tract

Medial vestibulospinal fibers in medial longitudinal fasciculi

Excitatory interneuron

Inhibitory interneuron

Excitatory endings to back muscles

To flexor muscles
To extensor muscles

Lower part of cervical spinal cord

Inhibitory ending

To axial muscles

Excitatory ending

Lateral vestibulospinal tract

Lumbar part of spinal cord

Inhibitory interneuron

Excitatory synapse

To flexor muscles
To extensor muscles

Vestibulospinal Tracts

15.10 **VESTIBULOSPINAL TRACTS**

The lateral vestibulospinal tract arises from the lateral vestibular nucleus and terminates directly and indirectly on ipsilateral alpha- and gamma-LMNs associated with extensor musculature, especially proximal musculature. If this powerful antigravity extensor system were not kept in check by descending connections from the red nucleus and by connections from the cerebellum, it would produce a constant state of extensor hypertonus. Removal of these influences can occur with lesions caudal to the red nucleus, producing decerebration with powerful extensor posturing. The medial vestibulospinal tract arises from the medial vestibular nucleus and provides inhibition of alpha- and gamma-LMNs controlling neck and axial musculature. The medial vestibulospinal tract terminates mainly on interneurons in the cervical spinal cord ventral horn. These two vestibulospinal tracts stabilize and coordinate the position of the head, neck, and body and provide important reflex and brain stem control over tone and posture. The vestibulospinal tracts work with the reticulospinal tracts to control tone and posture.

CLINICAL POINT

Primary vestibular input from both the maculae of the utricle and the cristae of the ampullae of the semicircular canals terminates in the vestibular nuclei of the medulla and pons, including the cells of origin of the vestibular UMN tracts, the lateral and medial vestibular nuclei. This allows influences from the direction of the gravitational field (linear acceleration) and head movement (angular acceleration) to affect the firing of neurons in the vestibular nuclei. The lateral vestibular nuclei give rise to a powerful vestibulospinal antigravity system that terminates mainly indirectly on alpha- and gamma-LMNs in the medial part of the ventral horn, which is associated with proximal extensor musculature. This system, if left unchecked and uninhibited, would drive the neck and body into marked extensor posturing, called decerebration (or decerebrate rigidity). The lateral vestibulospinal system is inhibited mainly by the red nucleus and the anterior cerebellum. In decerebrate posturing, sectioning of the dorsal roots (dorsal rhizotomy) abolishes the extraordinary "rigidity" (it is actually spasticity, not true rigidity), suggesting the decerebration results from the unregulated activity of the reticulospinal and lateral vestibulospinal tract driving the gamma-LMNs. This is consistent with the earlier hypothesis of the mechanism of spasticity, although additional spinal interneuronal inhibition is also most likely involved in decerebrate posturing. The medial vestibulospinal tract exerts inhibitory influences on LMNs that innervate neck muscles, permitting unconscious adjustments to move the head in response to vestibular stimuli. Thus, the vestibulospinal tracts help to promote body and head movements to maintain appropriate posture with vestibular activation, particularly during movement; these systems also coordinate with projections via the medial longitudinal fasciculus that synchronize eye movements.

Reticulospinal and Corticoreticular Pathways

Excitatory endings ⟶ ⟶ ⟶

Inhibitory endings ⟶ ⟶

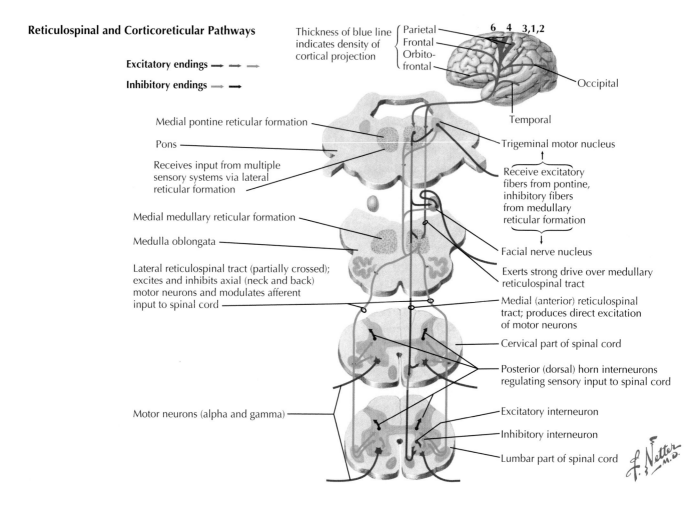

Thickness of blue line indicates density of cortical projection

Parietal
Frontal
Orbito-frontal

6   4   3,1,2

Occipital

Temporal

Medial pontine reticular formation

Pons

Receives input from multiple sensory systems via lateral reticular formation

Medial medullary reticular formation

Medulla oblongata

Lateral reticulospinal tract (partially crossed); excites and inhibits axial (neck and back) motor neurons and modulates afferent input to spinal cord

Motor neurons (alpha and gamma)

Trigeminal motor nucleus

Receive excitatory fibers from pontine, inhibitory fibers from medullary reticular formation

Facial nerve nucleus

Exerts strong drive over medullary reticulospinal tract

Medial (anterior) reticulospinal tract; produces direct excitation of motor neurons

Cervical part of spinal cord

Posterior (dorsal) horn interneurons regulating sensory input to spinal cord

Excitatory interneuron

Inhibitory interneuron

Lumbar part of spinal cord

15.11 RETICULOSPINAL AND CORTICORETICULAR PATHWAYS

The pontine reticulospinal tract (RetST) arises from neurons of the medial pontine RF (nuclei pontis caudalis and oralis). Axons descend as the pontine (medial) RetST, mainly ipsilaterally, and terminate directly and indirectly on alpha- and gamma-LMNs at all levels. This tract has a distinct extensor bias for axial musculature and reinforces the action of the lateral vestibulospinal tract. Although some cortical axons terminate in the nuclei of origin of the pontine RetST, the cortex provides minimal influence on the activity of this tract; the pontine RetST is driven primarily by polysensory input from trigeminal and somatosensory sources. The medullary RetST originates from the medial RF (nucleus gigantocellularis) and is heavily driven by cortical input, especially from the motor cortex and supplemental and premotor cortices. Axons of the medullary (lateral) RetST terminate bilaterally, directly and indirectly, on alpha- and gamma-LMNs at all levels. The medullary RetST exerts a flexor bias, reinforcing the CST and RST. The reticulospinal tracts are important regulators of basic tone and posture. They are not organized somatotopically. See page 386 for a Clinical Point.

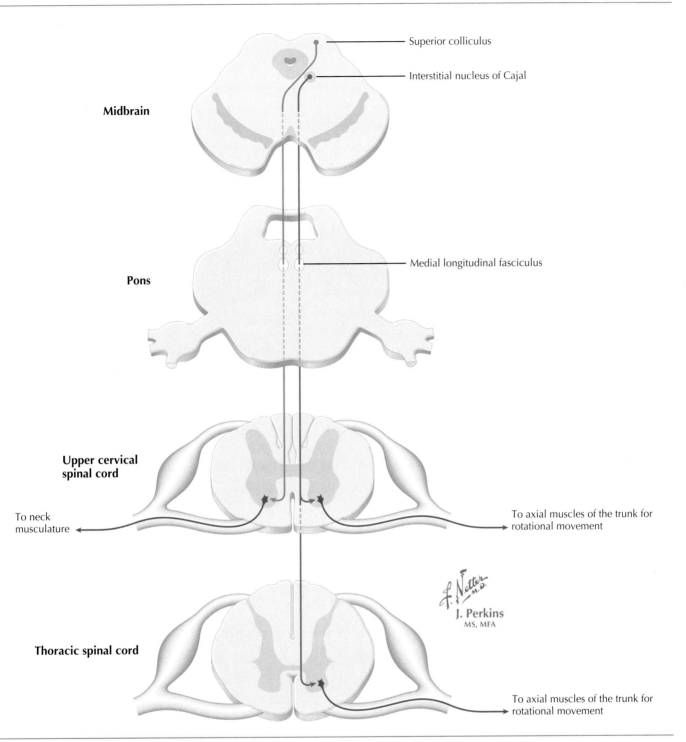

Superior colliculus

Interstitial nucleus of Cajal

Midbrain

Pons

Medial longitudinal fasciculus

**Upper cervical
spinal cord**

To neck
musculature

To axial muscles of the trunk for
rotational movement

J. Perkins
MS, MFA

Thoracic spinal cord

To axial muscles of the trunk for
rotational movement

15.12 TECTOSPINAL TRACT AND INTERSTITIOSPINAL TRACT

The tectospinal tract arises from neurons in deep layers of the superior colliculus, decussates in the dorsal tegmental decussation, descends contralaterally near the midline, and terminates directly and indirectly on alpha- and gamma-LMNs in the cervical spinal cord associated with head and neck movements. This pathway mediates reflex and visual tracking influences for positioning the head with regard to visual input. The interstitiospinal tract arises from the interstitial nucleus of Cajal, a region of the midbrain that helps to coordinate eye movements and gaze centers. The interstitiospinal tract descends ipsilaterally in the medial longitudinal fasciculus

and terminates directly and indirectly on alpha- and gamma-LMNs associated with the axial musculature of the trunk that is involved in rotational movement of the body around its central axis.

CLINICAL POINT

The superior colliculus, neurons of origin of the tectospinal tract, is responsive to input from the retina, the visual cortex, and the frontal eye fields. Of particular note is the role of tectospinal and tectobulbar projections (especially to the reticular formation) that help to coordinate movements of both the head and the eyes. Part of the tectospinal pathway may receive indirect input from the inferior colliculus and help to mediate head movements in response to loud or conspicuous sounds.

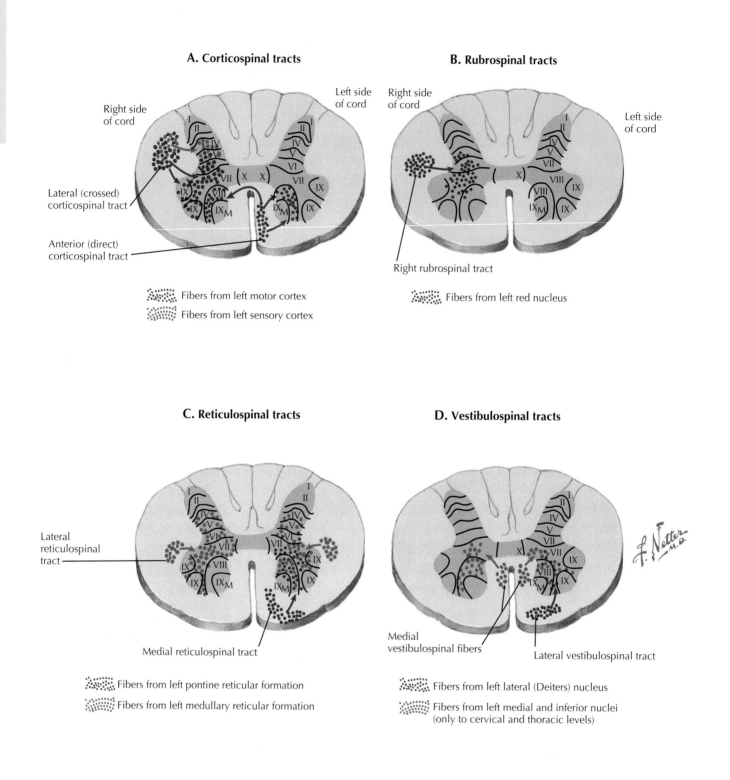

A. Corticospinal tracts

Left side of cord

Right side of cord

Lateral (crossed) corticospinal tract

Anterior (direct) corticospinal tract

Fibers from left motor cortex
Fibers from left sensory cortex

B. Rubrospinal tracts

Right side of cord

Left side of cord

Right rubrospinal tract

Fibers from left red nucleus

C. Reticulospinal tracts

Lateral reticulospinal tract

Medial reticulospinal tract

Fibers from left pontine reticular formation
Fibers from left medullary reticular formation

D. Vestibulospinal tracts

Medial vestibulospinal fibers

Lateral vestibulospinal tract

Fibers from left lateral (Deiters) nucleus
Fibers from left medial and inferior nuclei (only to cervical and thoracic levels)

15.13 SPINAL CORD TERMINATIONS OF MAJOR DESCENDING UPPER MOTOR NEURON TRACTS

The lateral corticospinal tract and the RST terminations are directed mainly toward LMNs associated with distal limb musculature. The anterior CST, the RSTs, and the vestibulospinal tracts are directed mainly toward LMNs associated with more proximal and axial musculature.

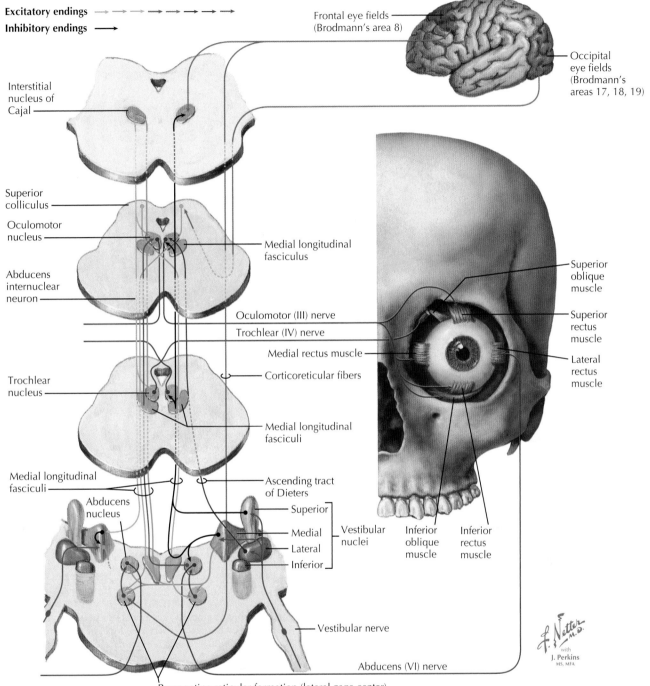

Excitatory endings →→ →→ →→ →→ →→
Inhibitory endings →

Frontal eye fields
(Brodmann's area 8)

Occipital
eye fields
(Brodmann's
areas 17, 18, 19)

Interstitial
nucleus of
Cajal

Superior
colliculus

Oculomotor
nucleus

Medial longitudinal
fasciculus

Superior
oblique
muscle

Abducens
internuclear
neuron

Oculomotor (III) nerve

Trochlear (IV) nerve

Superior
rectus
muscle

Medial rectus muscle

Lateral
rectus
muscle

Trochlear
nucleus

Corticoreticular fibers

Medial longitudinal
fasciculi

Medial longitudinal
fasciculi

Ascending tract
of Dieters

Abducens
nucleus

Superior

Medial

Vestibular
nuclei

Inferior
oblique
muscle

Inferior
rectus
muscle

Lateral

Inferior

Vestibular nerve

Abducens (VI) nerve

Parapontine reticular formation (lateral gaze center)

15.14 **CENTRAL CONTROL OF EYE MOVEMENTS**

Central control of eye movements is achieved through the coordination of extraocular motor nuclei for CNs III (oculomotor), IV (trochlear), and VI (abducens). This is achieved by the parapontine reticular formation (horizontal gaze center); it receives input from the vestibular nuclei; the deep layers of the superior colliculus (input from V1, V2, and V3); the cerebral cortex (frontal eye fields); and the interstitial nucleus of Cajal (which receives input from the vestibular nuclei and the frontal eye fields). The parapontine reticular formation supplies the ipsilateral VI nucleus for movement of the lateral rectus muscle and the contralateral III nucleus (via interneurons in VI nucleus) for movement of the medial rectus muscle, thus coordinating horizontal eye movements. The interstitial nucleus of Cajal helps to coordinate vertical and oblique eye movements. Secondary sensory vestibular projections also terminate in the extraocular motor CNN. Axons interconnecting the extraocular motor CNN travel through the medial longitudinal fasciculus. See page 386 for a Clinical Point.

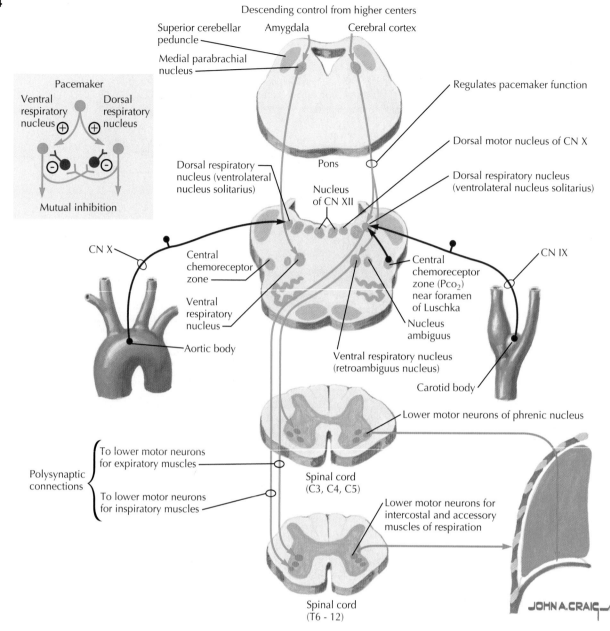

Descending control from higher centers

Superior cerebellar peduncle

Medial parabrachial nucleus

Amygdala

Cerebral cortex

Pacemaker

Ventral respiratory nucleus $\oplus$

Dorsal respiratory nucleus $\oplus$

Mutual inhibition

Regulates pacemaker function

Dorsal motor nucleus of CN X

Pons

Nucleus of CN XII

Dorsal respiratory nucleus (ventrolateral nucleus solitarius)

Dorsal respiratory nucleus (ventrolateral nucleus solitarius)

CN X

Central chemoreceptor zone

Ventral respiratory nucleus

Aortic body

Central chemoreceptor zone (Pco_2) near foramen of Luschka

Nucleus ambiguus

CN IX

Ventral respiratory nucleus (retroambiguus nucleus)

Carotid body

Lower motor neurons of phrenic nucleus

To lower motor neurons for expiratory muscles

Polysynaptic connections

To lower motor neurons for inspiratory muscles

Spinal cord (C3, C4, C5)

Lower motor neurons for intercostal and accessory muscles of respiration

Spinal cord (T6 - 12)

JOHN A. CRAIG—AD

15.15 CENTRAL CONTROL OF RESPIRATION

Inspiration and expiration are regulated by nuclei of the RF. The dorsal respiratory nucleus (lateral nucleus solitarius) sends crossed axons to terminate on cervical spinal cord LMNs of the phrenic nucleus and on thoracic spinal cord LMNs that supply intercostal muscles and accessory musculature associated with inspiration. The ventral respiratory nucleus (nucleus retroambiguus) sends crossed axons to terminate on thoracic spinal cord LMNs that supply accessory musculature associated with expiration. The dorsal respiratory nucleus receives input from the carotid body V (via CN IX); from the aortic body chemosensors (via CN X); and from central chemoreceptive zones of the lateral medulla. The dorsal respiratory nucleus and ventral respiratory nucleus mutually inhibit each other. The medial parabrachial nucleus acts as a respiratory pacemaker to regulate the dorsal respiratory nucleus and the ventral respiratory nucleus. The medial parabrachial nucleus receives input from higher centers, such as the amygdala and the cerebral cortex.

CLINICAL POINT

The dorsal respiratory nucleus (lateral nucleus solitarius) sends axonal projections to the contralateral cervical LMNs of the phrenic nucleus and thoracic LMNs of accessory respiratory muscles, regulating inspiration. The ventral respiratory nucleus (nucleus retroambiguus) sends axonal projections to contralateral thoracic LMNs that supply accessory musculature associated with expiration. The medial parabrachial nucleus functions as a pacemaker and receives input from higher levels of the central nervous system. Progressive damage to the forebrain and brain stem elicits relatively predictable changes in respiration. Progressive damage through the telencephalon and diencephalons elicits Cheyne-Stokes respiration (crescendo-decrescendo breathing; periods of hyperpnea alternating with brief periods of apnea). The hyperpnea phase is provoked by Pco_2 from the apneic phase and results in the lowering of Pco_2, again provoking apnea. If damage extends through the mesencephalon and upper pons, respiration becomes shallow, with hyperventilation, but the patient still is relatively hypoxic. If damage extends through the lower pons, respiration involves long inspiratory pauses prior to expiration, called apneustic breathing. Damage extending further into the medulla produces ataxic breathing with irregular patterns, including inspiratory gasps and periods of apnea. This pattern of breathing foreshadows total respiratory failure and death as the basic brain stem centers fail.

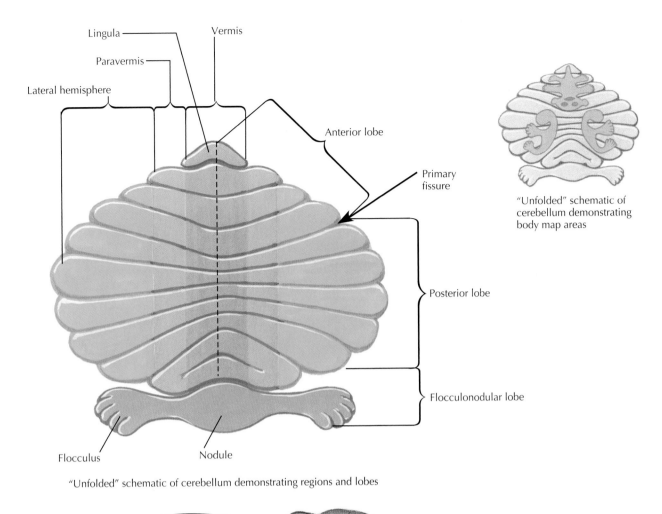

Lingula

Vermis

Paravermis

Lateral hemisphere

Anterior lobe

Primary fissure

Posterior lobe

Flocculonodular lobe

Flocculus

Nodule

"Unfolded" schematic of cerebellum demonstrating regions and lobes

"Unfolded" schematic of cerebellum demonstrating body map areas

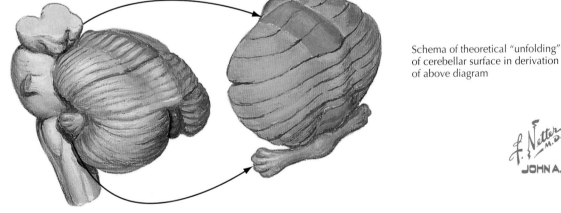

Schema of theoretical "unfolding" of cerebellar surface in derivation of above diagram

CEREBELLUM

15.16 FUNCTIONAL SUBDIVISIONS OF THE CEREBELLUM

The cerebellum is classically subdivided into anterior, middle (posterior), and flocculonodular (FN) lobes, each associated with ipsilateral syndromes, such as stiff-legged gait (anterior lobe); loss of coordination, with dysmetria, action tremor, hypotonus, ataxia, and decomposition of movement (middle lobe); and truncal ataxia (FN lobe). The cerebellum also is classified according to a longitudinal scheme that is based on cerebellar cortical regions that project to deep cerebellar nuclei, which in turn project to and coordinate the activity of specific UMN cell groups. This scheme includes the vermis and FN lobe (projecting to the fastigial nucleus and the lateral vestibular nucleus); the paravermis (projecting to the globose and emboliform nuclei); and the lateral hemispheres (projecting to the dentate nucleus). Each cerebellar subdivision is interlinked with circuitry related to specific UMN systems.

Cerebellar Cortex

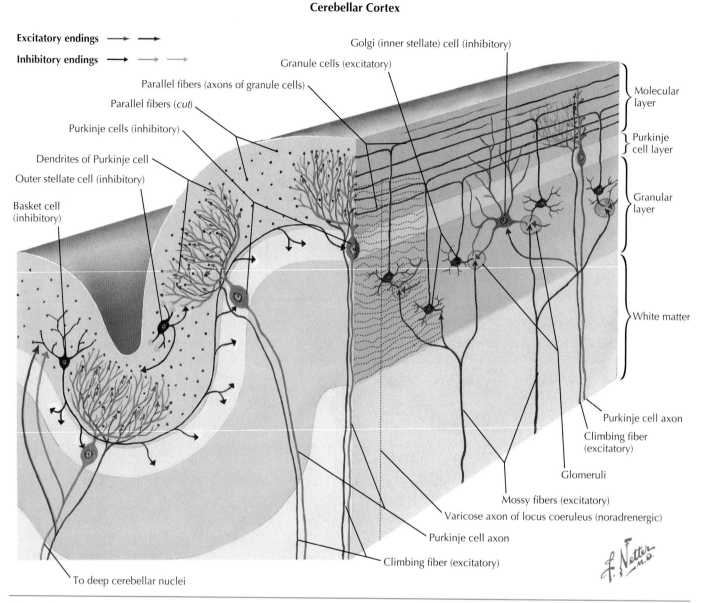

Excitatory endings →→

Inhibitory endings →→→→

Golgi (inner stellate) cell (inhibitory)

Granule cells (excitatory)

Parallel fibers (axons of granule cells)

Parallel fibers (*cut*)

Purkinje cells (inhibitory)

Dendrites of Purkinje cell

Outer stellate cell (inhibitory)

Basket cell (inhibitory)

Molecular layer

Purkinje cell layer

Granular layer

White matter

Purkinje cell axon

Climbing fiber (excitatory)

Glomeruli

Mossy fibers (excitatory)

Varicose axon of locus coeruleus (noradrenergic)

Purkinje cell axon

Climbing fiber (excitatory)

To deep cerebellar nuclei

15.17 CEREBELLAR NEURONAL CIRCUITRY

The cerebellum is organized into four parts: an outer three-layered cortex, white matter, deep cerebellar nuclei, and cerebellar peduncles that connect with the spinal cord, brain stem, and thalamus. In the cortex, the Purkinje cells (the major output neurons) have their dendritic trees in the molecular layer (arranged in parallel "plates" adjacent to each other), their cell bodies in the Purkinje cell layer, and their axons in the granular layer and deeper white matter. Inputs into the cerebellar cortex arrive as climbing fibers (from inferior olivary nuclei); mossy fibers (all other inputs except monoaminergic); or fine, highly branched, varicose arborizations (noradrenergic and other monoaminergic inputs). The mossy fibers synapse on granule cells, whose axons form an array of parallel fibers that extend through the dendritic trees of several hundred Purkinje cells. Additional interneurons modulate interconnections in the molecular layer (outer stellate cells); at the Purkinje cell body (basket cells); and at granule cell–molecular layer associations (Golgi cells). Noradrenergic axons of locus coeruleus neurons terminate in all three layers and modulate the excitability of other cerebellar connectivities.

CLINICAL POINT

The cerebellum is a target for significant adverse effects of several types of drugs, sometimes in therapeutic dose ranges and sometimes in toxic dose ranges. Many pharmaceutical agents can exert both direct effects on the cerebellum and more global neurological effects, including ischemia or hypoxia. Cerebellar damage is usually manifested first as impairment of gait, followed later by limb ataxia. These cerebellar side effects often resolve after discontinuation of the medication, but some deficits may remain. Some antiseizure agents, including phenytoin, carbamazepine, and barbiturates, can lead to cerebellar symptoms; after prolonged treatment, particularly with phenytoin, some permanent deficits such as degeneration of Purkinje cells may occur. Valproate may provoke an intention tremor. Some cancer chemotherapeutic agents also can cause adverse cerebellar effects, occasionally permanently. Treatment of psychiatric disorders by multiple pharmaceutical agents, particularly neuroleptics, also can produce adverse cerebellar effects. Toxic damage resulting from exposure to dangerous environmental agents also may damage the cerebellum. Exposure to organophosphate agents and organic solvents may induce cerebellar symptomatology. Exposure to heavy metals, including methylmercury, lead, and thallium, can induce gait disturbance and ataxia.

A. General Scheme

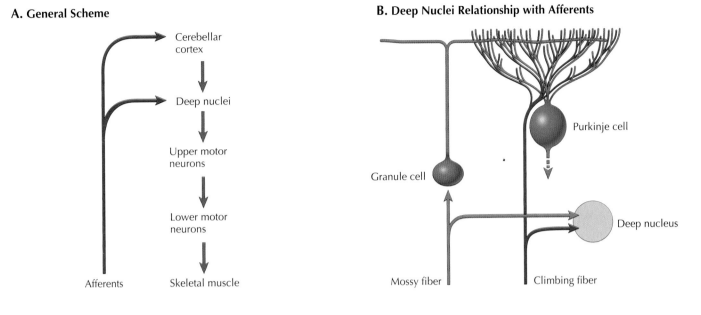

B. Deep Nuclei Relationship with Afferents

C. Circuitry of Cerebellar Neurons - Mossy Fibers

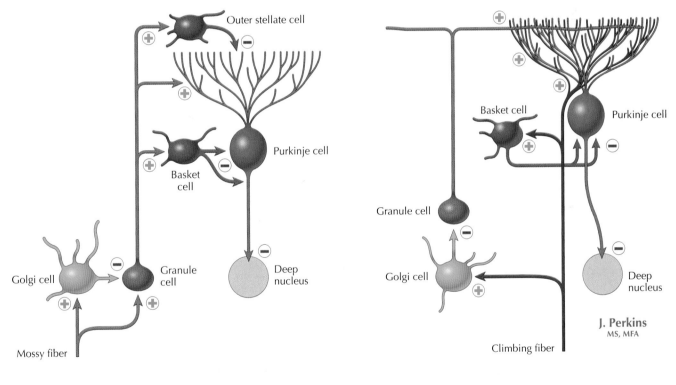

D. Circuitry of Cerebellar Neurons - Climbing Fibers

J. Perkins
MS, MFA

15.18 CIRCUIT DIAGRAMS OF AFFERENT CONNECTIONS IN THE CEREBELLUM

Afferents to the cerebellum include mossy fibers, climbing fibers, and locus coeruleus noradrenergic fibers. The mossy fibers synapse in deep nuclei and on granule cells. The climbing fibers intertwine around a Purkinje cell dendritic tree. The noradrenergic locus coeruleus axons terminate on all cell types in the cerebellar cortex. The loops and circuits in parts C and D of the figure show interneuronal modulation of afferent connections and Purkinje cell outflow. The entire circuitry of the cerebellar cortex provides fine-tuning of the original processing in the deep cerebellar nuclei. The entire Purkinje cell output to the deep nuclei is mediated by inhibition, using gamma-aminobutyric acid (GABA) as the neurotransmitter.

Cortical input

Nucleus reticularis tegmenti pontis

Pontine nuclei (contralateral)

Spinal input

Inferior olive

Upper part of medulla oblongata

Spinal input

Vestibular nerve and ganglion

Lower part of medulla oblongata

Cortical input

Lateral reticular nucleus

Spinal input

Cervical part of spinal cord

Motor interneuron

Rostral spinocerebellar tract

Spinal border cells

Motor interneuron

Lumbar part of spinal cord

Clarke's column

Ventral spinocerebellar tract

Red NUC

Trig NUC

Superior cerebellar peduncle

Middle cerebellar peduncle

To contralateral cerebellar cortex

Leg   Arm Face

Primary fissure

To nodule and flocculus

Inferior cerebellar peduncle

Vestibular nuclei

Reticulocerebellar tract

Cuneocerebellar tract

Gracile nucleus

Main cuneate nucleus (relay for cutaneous information)

External cuneate nucleus (relay for proprioceptive information)

From skin (touch and pressure)

From muscle (spindles and Golgi tendon organs)

From skin and deep tissues (pain and Golgi tendon organs)

From skin (touch and pressure) and from muscle (spindles and Golgi tendon organs)

Dorsal spinocerebellar tract

15.19 AFFERENT PATHWAYS TO THE CEREBELLUM

Afferents to the cerebellum terminate in both the deep nuclei and the cerebellar cortex in topographically organized zones. The body is represented in the cerebellar cortex in at least three separate regions. Afferents traveling through the inferior cerebellar peduncle include spinocerebellar pathways (dorsal and rostral spinocerebellar tracts, cuneocerebellar tract); the inferior olivary input; RF input from the lateral reticular nucleus and other regions; vestibular input from the vestibular ganglion and vestibular nuclei; and some trigeminal input. The middle cerebellar peduncle conveys mainly pontocerebellar axons carrying crossed corticopontocerebellar inputs. Afferents traveling through the superior cerebellar peduncle include the ventral spinocerebellar tract, visual and auditory tectocerebellar input, some trigeminal input, and noradrenergic locus coeruleus input. The dorsal spinocerebellar tract and cuneocerebellar tract derive mainly from muscle spindle afferent information, whereas the ventral and rostral spinocerebellar tracts derive mainly from Golgi tendon organ afferent information.

CLINICAL POINT

Several forms of progressive neuronal degeneration involve cerebellar neurons and connections, including Friedreich's ataxia and olivopontocerebellar atrophy. Friedreich's ataxia is an autosomal recessive disorder that begins in late childhood and progresses over several decades. The disorder commonly starts with ataxia and gait dysfunction, dysmetria and decomposition of movement, and dysarthria. Spastic motor involvement and sensory losses also may occur. Neuropathological examination reveals degeneration of primary afferents and of axons in the spinal cord white matter, especially the dorsal and lateral funiculi, including the spinocerebellar tracts. Some axonal damage also may occur in both the peripheral nervous system and the central nervous system, but the cerebellum itself is usually not a focus of direct neuronal degeneration.

Olivopontocerebellar atrophy is a progressive, mainly autosomal dominant, neurodegenerative disorder that affects adults in midlife. This disorder commonly begins with gait abnormalities and progresses to full-blown cerebellar dysfunction with limb ataxia and dysarthria. Additional symptoms, such as chorea, dystonia, and rigidity, suggest some degenerative involvement of the basal ganglia as well. Neuropathological examination usually reveals neurodegeneration of the cerebellar cortex, the inferior olivary nuclei, and the pontine nuclei. As a consequence, the inferior and middle cerebellar peduncles are diminished. Additional degenerative changes in the cerebral cortex and descending UMN pathways and in the basal ganglia also are commonly present.

Excitatory endings ⟶ ⟶

Inhibitory endings
of Purkinje cells ⟶

Motor and premotor cerebral cortex

Internal capsule

Ventral anterior and ventral lateral nuclei of thalamus

Cerebral peduncle

Mesencephalic reticular formation

Decussation of superior cerebellar peduncles

Red nucleus

Descending fibers from superior cerebellar peduncles

Fastigial nucleus

Globose nuclei

Hook bundle of Russell

Emboliform nucleus

Dentate nucleus

Cerebellar cortex

Section A–B viewed from below

Section B–C viewed from above

Vestibular nuclei

Inferior cerebellar peduncle

Inferior olive

Lateral reticular nucleus

Medulla oblongata

Pontomedullary reticular formation

Planes of
section:
red arrows
indicate
direction
of view

15.20 CEREBELLAR EFFERENT PATHWAYS

Efferents from the cerebellum derive from the deep nuclei. Projections from the fastigial nucleus exit mainly through the inferior cerebellar peduncle and terminate mainly ipsilaterally in the lateral vestibular nucleus and in other vestibular nuclei as well as in pontine and medullary reticular nuclei that give rise to the reticulospinal tracts; there, they primarily modulate the activity of the vestibulospinal and reticulospinal UMN pathways. Axons from neurons of the globose and emboliform nuclei project mainly contralaterally through the decussation of the superior cerebellar peduncle to the red nucleus, with a smaller contribution to the VL nucleus of the thalamus; primarily, they modulate activity of the RST. Axons from neurons in the dentate nucleus project mainly contralaterally through the decussation of the superior cerebellar peduncle to the VL and to a lesser extent to the VA nuclei of the thalamus; mainly, they modulate the activity of the corticospinal tract. A small projection from the dentate nucleus also distributes to the contralateral red nucleus and to brain stem reticular motor nuclei.

Cerebellovestibular pathways

Vestibulocerebellar pathways

Excitatory endings ⟶ ⟶ ⟶ ⟶
Inhibitory endings ⟶ ⟶

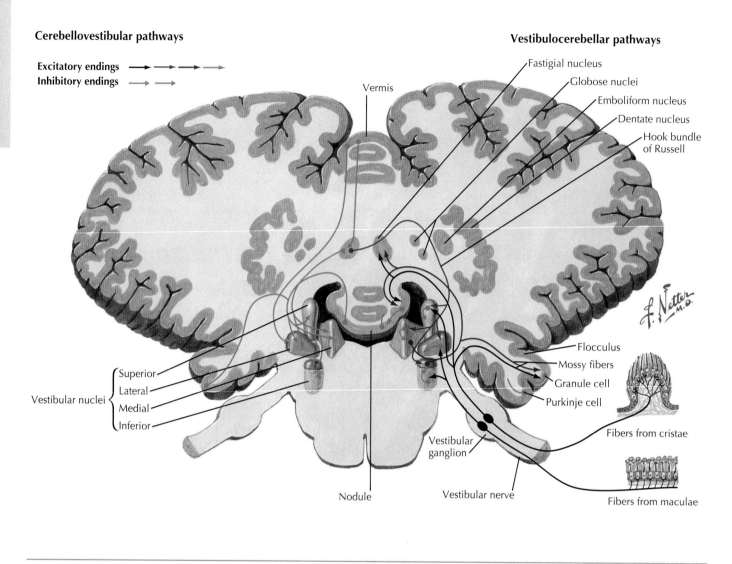

Vermis

Fastigial nucleus
Globose nuclei
Emboliform nucleus
Dentate nucleus
Hook bundle of Russell

Vestibular nuclei {
Superior
Lateral
Medial
Inferior

Flocculus
Mossy fibers
Granule cell
Purkinje cell

Fibers from cristae

Vestibular ganglion

Nodule

Vestibular nerve

Fibers from maculae

15.21 CEREBELLOVESTIBULAR AND VESTIBULOCEREBELLAR PATHWAYS

Primary sensory vestibular inputs terminate in the four vestibular nuclei and in the fastigial nucleus and the cerebellar cortex of the vermis and FN lobe. The vestibular nuclei also project to the cerebellar cortex of the vermis and FN lobe. Purkinje cells in the vermis and FN lobe, in turn, project back to the vestibular nuclei and the fastigial nucleus. The fastigial nucleus projects to the vestibular nuclei and to the pontine and medullary medial reticular formation. Thus, primary and secondary vestibular neurons project to the fastigial nucleus and cerebellar cortex, and both the cerebellar cortex and deep nuclei project back to the vestibular nuclei. This extensive reciprocal vestibulocerebellar circuitry regulates basic spatial position and body tone and posture.

CLINICAL POINT

Alcohol consumption may result in acute or chronic dysfunction of the cerebellum and its pathways. Acutely, alcohol intoxication can cause global cerebellar dysfunction, including staggering gait, limb ataxia, dysmetria, dysdiadochokinesia, dysarthria, and oculomotor dysfunction. Cerebellar testing for alcohol intoxication in the field involves tandem walking, finger-to-nose testing, speech patterns and coordination, and gait testing. These more global effects of alcohol on the cerebellum generally subside with catabolism of the alcohol. Chronic alcoholism results in more permanent damage to the cerebellum, with a particular initial predilection for the anterior lobe of the cerebellum and the vermis (paleocerebellum). The patient may show a staggering, broad-based gait with a stiff-legged movement. The mechanism of this unusual appearance of cerebellar damage (in contrast to the hypotonic, ataxic gait that occurs with global cerebellar damage, particularly in the lateral hemispheres) appears to be removal of the anterior cerebellar influence, via cerebellovestibular connections, on the lateral vestibular nucleus, disinhibiting this extensor-dominant system. This anterior cerebellar syndrome may diminish if the patient stops drinking. With further alcohol exposure, the entire cerebellum may become damaged, leading to the classic appearance of global cerebellar dysfunction, including gait disturbance, limb ataxia, dysarthria, and uncoordinated extraocular involvement. In addition to direct toxicity from alcohol, neural damage may also occur because of vitamin deficiencies, liver dysfunction, and other metabolic aspects of alcoholism. Other parts of the brain, including the cerebral cortex, also can be significantly damaged in chronic alcoholism.

15.22 SCHEMATIC DIAGRAMS OF EFFERENT PATHWAYS FROM THE CEREBELLUM TO UPPER MOTOR NEURON SYSTEMS

The lateral cerebellar hemisphere connects through the dentate nucleus with nuclei VA and VL of the thalamus; the major thalamic inputs to the cells of origin of the CST in the motor cortex, and with the supplemental and premotor cortices. The paravermal cerebellar cortex connects through the globose and emboliform nuclei with the red nucleus, cells of origin for the RST. The cerebellar connections to the cells of origin for the CST and RST are mainly crossed, and these UMN systems cross again before terminating on LMNs. Thus, the cerebellum is associated with the ipsilateral LMNs through two crossings. The vermis and FN lobe connect with the fastigial nucleus and lateral vestibular nuclei. The fastigial nucleus projects mainly ipsilaterally to cells of origin of the vestibulospinal and reticulospinal tracts, exerting mainly an ipsilateral influence on spinal cord LMNs through these UMN systems. The lateral vestibular nucleus is the source of the lateral vestibular tract, which exerts a marked extensor influence on ipsilateral LMNs of the spinal cord.

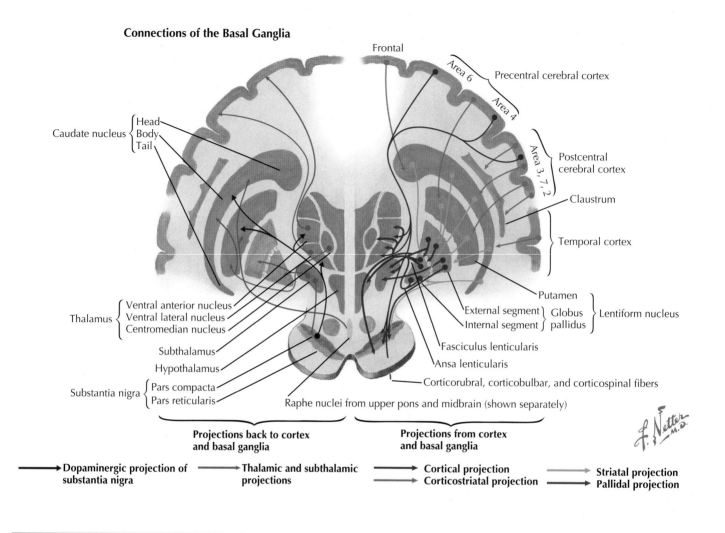

Connections of the Basal Ganglia

BASAL GANGLIA

15.23 CONNECTIONS OF THE BASAL GANGLIA

The basal ganglia consist of the striatum (caudate nucleus and putamen) and the globus pallidus. The substantia nigra (SN) and the subthalamic nucleus (STN), which are reciprocally connected with the basal ganglia, are often included as part of the basal ganglia. Inputs into the basal ganglia from the cerebral cortex, the thalamus (intralaminar nuclei), the SN pars compacta (dopaminergic input), the subthalamic nucleus, and rostral raphe nuclei (serotonergic input), are directed mainly toward the striatum. Inputs from the STN are directed mainly toward the globus pallidus. The striatum projects to the globus pallidus. The internal segment of the globus pallidus projects to the thalamus (VA, VL, and centromedian nuclei), and the external segment projects to the STN. The VA and VL thalamic nuclei provide input into the cells of origin of the corticospinal tract. Damage to basal ganglia components often results in movement disorders. Damage to the dopamine neurons in SN pars compacta results in Parkinson's disease (characterized by resting tremor, muscular rigidity, bradykinesia, and postural instability).

CLINICAL POINT

Disorders of the basal ganglia are frequently referred to as movement disorders and were previously called involuntary movement disorders. Despite the conspicuous presence of motor-related symptoms, the basal ganglia also are involved in cognitive and affective processing, particularly in assisting the cerebral cortex to select wanted subroutines of activity and to suppress unwanted patterns. The basal ganglia assist in providing a connection between motivation and emotional context on one hand and movement on the other. Observations of discrete infarcts of parts of the basal ganglia have revealed such abnormalities as abnormal positioning of parts of the body with the presence of increased tone (dystonia) and other movements such as athetosis (slow, writhing movements) or chorea (brisk, dancelike movements). With caudate nucleus damage, more cognitive and affective symptoms may occur, such as apathy and loss of initiative, slowed thinking, and blunted emotional reactivity (abulia), possibly related to the interconnections between the caudate nucleus and the prefrontal cortex. In the classic movement disorders, as in the progressive neurodegenerative diseases, there is a mixture of symptoms showing loss of action, such as bradykinesia (difficulty in initiating movements or diminished movements such as blinking), and symptoms showing an excess of action, such as rigidity, athetosis, chorea, or dystonia. As an example of excess movement, Tourette's syndrome involves tics and involuntary vocalizations, sometimes accompanied by echolalia, grunts and vocal spasms, explosive cursing, and hyperactive behavior, often starting in childhood. Treatment strategies have included use of D2 dopamine antagonists such as haloperidol.

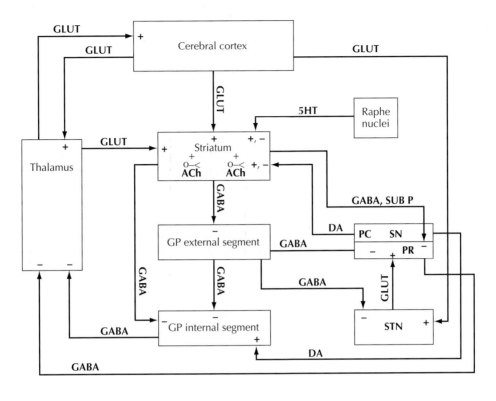

SN = Substantia nigra
STN = Subthalamic nucleus
GLUT = Glutamate
GABA = Gamma aminobutyric acid
DA = Dopamine

5HT = 5-Hydroxytryptamine (serotonin)
PC = Pars compacta
PR = Pars reticulata
ACh = Acetylcholine
GP = Globus pallidus
SUB P = Substance P

15.24 BASIC BASAL GANGLIA CIRCUITRY AND NEUROTRANSMITTERS

Inputs from the cerebral cortex and thalamus to the striatum are excitatory (glutamate). The striatopallidal connection is inhibitory (GABA), and the pallidothalamic connection is inhibitory (GABA) too, resulting in a net drive over the thalamocortical (and resultant corticospinal) output. However, extensive inhibitory and excitatory circuitry also exists through the internal segment of the globus pallidus, the substantia nigra, and the subthalamic nucleus, producing complex modulation of basal ganglia output. The dopaminergic nigrostriatal connections can exert both inhibitory and excitatory effects on the striatum. Thus, with loss of nigrostriatal dopamine axons in Parkinson's disease, both negative symptoms (bradykinesia) and positive symptoms (resting tremor, muscular rigidity, postural instability) exist side by side. Additional interneurons are found in some basal ganglia structures such as the excitatory cholinergic interneurons in the striatum.

CLINICAL POINT

In Parkinson's disease, the pars compacta of the substantia nigra shows loss of pigmented (melanin-containing) neurons that use dopamine as their major neurotransmitter. Both the substantia nigra and the target of the axonal projections, the caudate nucleus and putamen, are severely depleted of their dopamine content. By the time symptoms of Parkinson's disease are clinically evident, at least 50% (and sometimes as much as 80%) of the dopamine neurons in the pars compacta of the substantia nigra have degenerated. Neurons in the substantia nigra sometimes demonstrate Lewy inclusion bodies or neurofibrillary tangles, further evidence of the degenerative process in Parkinson's disease. The neuropathology of Parkinson's disease sometimes also includes the degeneration of dopamine neurons in the ventral tegmental area of the midbrain, of serotonergic neurons in the raphe nuclei, of cholinergic neurons in nucleus basalis, and of other pigmented neurons in regions such as the dorsal (motor) nucleus of CN X. Although the dopamine deficit in the substantia nigra is the most conspicuous pathological hallmark of Parkinson's disease, these other degenerative processes may contribute to some of the symptoms.

A. Motor loop

Cortex

Primary motor cortex
Premotor/supplemental cortex
Primary sensory cortex

STN

Thalamus

VL
VA
CM

Striatum

Putamen

GP
External segment

SN
PC

GPl, Midbrain
Internal segment
SN - PR

B. Limbic loop

Cortex

Anterior cingulate cortex
Temporal cortex
Entorhinal cortex and hippocampus
Inferior prefrontal cortex

STN

Thalamus

MD (parvo)

Striatum

Ventral striatum
Nucleus accumbens

GP
External segment

SN
PC

GPl, Midbrain
Ventral pallidum
Ventral tegmental area

C. Cognitive loop

Cortex

Dorsolateral prefrontal cortex
Lateral orbitofrontal cortex

STN

Thalamus

VA - parvo, magno
MD - parvo, magno

Striatum

Caudate nucleus – head
Dorsolateral
Ventromedial

GP
External segment

SN
PC

GPl, Midbrain
Internal segment
(lateral and medial)
SN - PR

D. Oculomotor loop

Cortex

Frontal eye fields
Posterior parietal cortex
Dorsolateral prefrontal cortex

STN

Thalamus

VA - magno
MD - paralamellar

Striatum

Caudate nucleus – body

GP
External segment

SN
PC

GPl, Midbrain
Internal segment
(central zone)
SN - PR (ventrolateral)

Midbrain

Horizontal and vertical gaze centers

Superior colliculus

CM = Centromedian nucleus
GPl = Globus pallidus internal segment
magno = Magnocellular
MD = Medial dorsal nucleus

parvo = Parvocellular
PC = Pars compacta
PR = Pars reticulata
SN = Substantia nigra

STN = Subthalamic nucleus
VA = Ventral anterior nucleus
VL = Ventrolateral nucleus

15.25 PARALLEL LOOPS OF CIRCUITRY THROUGH THE BASAL GANGLIA

The corticostriatal, striatopallidal, and pallidothalamic connections form parallel loops for motor, limbic, cognitive, and oculomotor circuitry. The motor circuitry is processed through the putamen; the limbic circuitry through the ventral pallidum and nucleus accumbens; the cognitive circuitry through the head of the caudate nucleus; and the oculomotor circuitry through the body of the caudate nucleus. Connections through the globus pallidus and the pars reticulata of the substantia nigra or ventral tegmental area then project to appropriate regions of the thalamus to link back to the cortical neurons of origin for the initial corticostriatal projections. These parallel loops through the basal ganglia and the cortex serve to modulate specific subroutines of cortical activity distinct to the appropriate function. The pars compacta of the substantia nigra may act as the principal interconnections among these parallel loops.

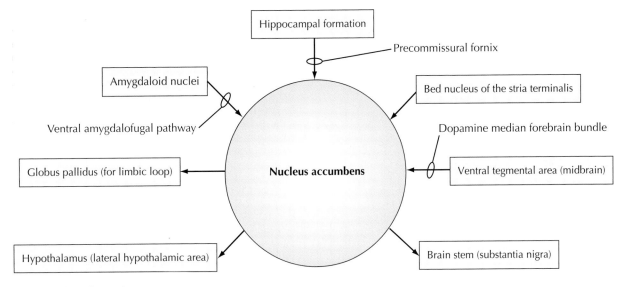

Connections of Nucleus Accumbens

15.26 CONNECTIONS OF NUCLEUS ACCUMBENS

Nucleus accumbens is located at the anterior end of the striatum in the interior of the ventral and rostral forebrain (see Figure 13.12). Inputs are derived from limbic structures (amygdala, hippocampal formation, bed nucleus of the stria terminalis) and from the ventral tegmental area of the midbrain via a rich dopaminergic projection. Nucleus accumbens is central to motivational states and addictive behaviors. It also appears to be a principal region in brain reward circuits associated with joy, pleasure, and gratification. The involvement of nucleus accumbens with a specific limbic basal ganglia loop helps to provide motor expression of emotional responses and accompanying gestures and behaviors.

CLINICAL POINT

See Fig. 14.9. The varicella-zoster virus of childhood chickenpox can reside as a latent virus in dorsal root ganglia, the trigeminal ganglia, and other ganglia. During immunosuppression (medication, cancers, chronic stressors), the reactivation of this virus can cause painful eruptions in the distribution of a sensory nerve root or a division of the trigeminal nerve; this condition is commonly known as shingles or herpes zoster (postherpetic) neuralgia. The most common sites are the thoracic nerve roots or the ophthalmic division (V_1) of the trigeminal nerve. The skin erupts with vesicles and a sharp, radiating or burning pain is felt in the region of the eruptions. Sometimes the painful sensations (dysesthesias) occur several days before the eruptions appear. A particular risk related to the ophthalmic division of CN V is corneal ulcerations and subsequent opacities. The nerve, the ganglion, and sometimes the surrounding tissues show inflammatory reactivity. Usually, with combined antiviral therapy and analgesics, the eruptions can subside within a week or so. However, the postherpetic neuralgia, with burning pain, can last for weeks to months and may require the same type of treatment that other neuropathic pain syndromes (reflex sympathetic dystrophy or complex regional pain syndrome) require, including analgesics, tricyclic antidepressants to alter the pain threshold, membrane-stabilizing agents, anti-inflammatory medication, and other approaches.

CLINICAL POINT

See Fig. 15.9. The rubrospinal tract, arising from magnocellular neurons of the red nucleus, is part of a cortico-rubro-spinal system that may represent an indirect corticospinal pathway. Rubrospinal tract connections are contralateral and have mainly indirect effects (through interneurons) on both alpha and gamma LMNs. Some authors believe that the rubrospinal tract has a minor role in humans, although observations of decorticate and decerebrate posturing suggest otherwise. In conditions of UMN pathology, the cortico-rubro-spinal system is usually damaged in conjunction with the corticospinal tract (posterior limb of the internal capsule, lateral funiculus of the spinal cord), resulting in a clinical picture of UMN syndrome. Bilateral damage to the forebrain and diencephalon, leaving only the rubrospinal tract, reticulospinal tracts, and vestibulospinal tracts intact, results in a classic UMN appearance bilaterally, with upper limbs in a flexed position and lower limbs in an extended posture (called decorticate posturing). If the lesion extends just below the red nucleus, further removing rubrospinal tract influences, the lateral vestibulospinal tracts are markedly disinhibited, resulting in decerebrate posturing with all four limbs extended. These observations suggest that the rubrospinal system particularly drives flexor activity in the upper extremities and has a lesser role in the lower extremities.

CLINICAL POINT

See Fig. 15.11. The reticulospinal tracts originate from isodendritic neurons in the medial portion of the pontine and medullary RF. The pontine RF gives rise to the pontine (medial) reticulospinal tract, which influences mainly proximal musculature. The medullary RF gives rise to the medullary (lateral) reticulospinal tract, which lies more laterally in the spinal cord and influences muscles of the extremities. The reticulospinal tracts help to regulate basic tone and postural responses, sometimes coordinating musculature supplied by LMNs at multiple spinal cord levels. These tracts also may help to direct stereotyped movements such as those involved in extending a limb toward an object. The reticulospinal tracts can selectively influence both alpha- and gamma-LMNs, thus providing a mechanism for activation of static or dynamic gamma-LMNs in conditions of damage to other descending systems, such as the corticospinal and cortico-rubro-spinal systems.

CLINICAL POINT

See Fig 15.14. Vestibular nuclei receive input from the hair cells in the ampullae of the semicircular canals and are connected with extraocular CN motor nuclei, thereby permitting vestibular reflex control of eye movements. This circuitry establishes the connections of the vestibulo-ocular reflex. When the head is rotated in one direction, the lateral semicircular canal initiates a vestibulo-ocular reflex that moves the eyes in the opposite direction, thereby maintaining the position of the eyes. Stimulation of the hair cells on one side of the vestibular apparatus with cold water in the external auditory meatus (the caloric response) provides the brain stem on that side with the neural signaling of apparent movement, and elicits eye movements that would be appropriate to an actual movement, were one occurring. This elicited movement is called caloric nystagmus; it evokes a sense of apparent movement, a tendency to fall to one side, and past-pointing. A lesion or irritative stimulation of the vestibular nerve on one side also gives the neural perception of movement, eliciting pathological nystagmus. If a person rotates in one direction to a greater extent than a simple vestibulo-ocular reflex can easily correct through compensatory eye movements, the eyes will be directed sufficiently far to one side that a quick movement (saccade) will be necessary to refocus them straight ahead. This is called rotational nystagmus, with the slow phase opposite from the direction of movement and the saccade (fast phase) in the direction of the movement; the saccade is neurally directed from the occipital lobe visual cortices. After the rotation stops, the individual will feel as if she or he is still rotating, but in the opposite direction (post-rotational nystagmus), with the saccade in the direction opposite from the original movement, and past-pointing in the direction of apparent movement. If an individual is stationary and stimuli move past the visual field (telephone poles and a person in a moving car), tracking reflexes move the eyes, and a cortically-evoked saccade corrects the eye position with a quick movement of the eyes. This normal physiologic process is called optokinetic nystagmus.

16

AUTONOMIC-HYPOTHALAMIC-LIMBIC SYSTEMS

Inputs to autonomic preganglionic neurons

Preganglionic sympathetic

Postganglionic sympathetic

Preganglionic parasympathetic

Postganglionic parasympathetic

Inputs to autonomic preganglionic neurons of sympathetic and parasympathetic nervous systems:
Limbic forebrain structures
Some cortical regions
Hypothalamic regions
Brain stem centers and nuclei
Sensory inputs

Pupillary constrictor muscle
Ciliary muscle

Ciliary ganglion

Nucleus of Edinger-Westphal

Lacrimal glands
Glands of nasal mucosa

Pterygopalatine ganglion

Oculomotor (III) nerve

Superior salivatory nucleus

Submandibular gland
Sublingual gland

Submandibular ganglion

Facial (VII) nerve

Salivary glands

Otic ganglion

Glossopharyngeal (IX) nerve

Inferior salivatory nucleus

Parotid gland

Vagus (X) nerve

Dorsal motor (autonomic) nucleus of X

Smooth muscle, cardiac muscle, secretory glands in heart, lung viscera, GI tract to descending colon

Intramural ganglia

Lateral horn (intermediolateral cell column)

To vascular smooth muscle in skin and muscles, arrector pili muscles, sweat glands in limbs

Spinal nerve

White ramus communicans

Gray ramus communicans

Ventral root

Thoracic spinal cord (T1-L2)

Secretion of epinephrine and norepinephrine into blood

Adrenal medulla

Splanchnic nerve

Sympathetic chain ganglia

To cardiac muscle, smooth muscle, secretory glands, metabolic cells (liver, fat), cells of immune system

Collateral ganglia

Intermediate gray

Ventral root

Smooth muscle, secretory glands in lower GI tract, pelvic viscera

Intramural ganglia

Pelvic nerves

Sacral spinal cord (S2-S4)

J. Netter M.D.
with J. Perkins MS, MFA

General Organization of the Autonomic Nervous System

AUTONOMIC NERVOUS SYSTEM

16.1 GENERAL ORGANIZATION OF THE AUTONOMIC NERVOUS SYSTEM

The autonomic nervous system is a two-neuron chain connecting preganglionic neurons through ganglia to visceral target tissues (cardiac muscle, smooth muscle, secretory glands, metabolic cells, cells of the immune system). The sympathetic division (sympathetic nervous system; SNS) is a thoracolumbar (T1–L2) system arising from the intermediolateral cell column of the lateral horn of the spinal cord, acting through chain ganglia and collateral ganglia; it is a system designed for fight-or-flight reactions in an emergency. The parasympathetic division (parasympathetic nervous system) is a craniosacral system arising from brain stem nuclei associated with cranial nerves (CNs) III, VII, IX, and X and from the intermediate gray in the S2–S4 spinal cord. Connections from CNs III, VII, and IX act through cranial nerve ganglia; connections from the vagal system and sacral system act through intramural ganglia in or near the target tissue. The parasympathetic nervous system is a homeostatic reparative system. Central connections from the limbic forebrain, hypothalamus, and brain stem regulating the sympathetic and parasympathetic nervous systems' outflow to the body act mainly through connections to vagal and sympathetic preganglionic neurons.

CLINICAL POINT

Preganglionic parasympathetic neurons in the brain stem and sacral spinal cord, as well as preganglionic sympathetic neurons in the thoracolumbar spinal cord, send projections to ganglion cells and use acetylcholine as the principal neurotransmitter. The ganglion cells possess mainly nicotinic cholinergic receptors for transducing fast neurotransmission responses. Postganglionic sympathetic neurons use mainly norepinephrine as their neurotransmitter, whereas postganglionic parasympathetic neurons use acetylcholine. Target tissue possesses alpha and beta adrenoceptor subclasses and cholinergic muscarinic receptor subclasses (M1–M3). In the heart, beta1 receptors increase the force and rate of contraction, increase cardiac output, and dilate coronary arteries, whereas M2 receptors decrease the force and rate of contraction and cardiac output. In vascular smooth muscle and smooth muscles of the pupil, ureters, and bladder, alpha1 receptors cause contraction. In blood vessels, alpha2 receptors also cause constriction. In smooth muscle of the tracheobronchial system, uterus, and gastrointestinal tract vasculature, beta2 receptors cause relaxation. Alpha1 receptors cause relaxation of gastrointestinal smooth muscles, and M1 receptors cause slow contraction. M3 receptors cause contraction of most parasympathetic smooth muscle target structures. In salivary glands, alpha1 receptors cause secretion and beta2 receptors cause mucus secretion. In adipose tissue, alpha1 receptors cause glycogenolysis, beta1 receptors cause lipolysis, and alpha2 receptors inhibit lipolysis. In sweat glands, alpha1 receptors cause secretion. In the kidney, alpha1 receptors enhance reabsorption of Na^+, and beta1 receptors provoke renin release. In liver and skeletal muscles, beta2 receptors cause glycogenolysis. In the pancreas, beta2 receptors stimulate insulin release, and alpha2 receptors inhibit insulin release. The balance of adrenergic and cholinergic neurotransmission determines the relative degree of activation of target tissues, and differential affinity of ligands for the various receptor subclasses helps to determine the final integrative physiological response.

1 Preoptic nuclei
2 Paraventricular nucleus
3 Anterior hypothalamic area
4 Supraoptic nucleus
5 Lateral hypothalamic area
6 Dorsal hypothalamic area
7 Dorsomedial nucleus
8 Ventromedial nucleus
9 Posterior hypothalamic area
10 Mammillary body
11 Optic chiasm
12 Lamina terminalis
13 Anterior commissure
14 Hypothalamic sulcus
15 Interthalamic adhesion
16 Fornix
17 Septum pellucidum
18 Interpeduncular fossa and region
19 Thalamus
20 Tuber cinereum
21 Optic nerve
22 Infundibulum
23 Anterior lobe of pituitary
24 Posterior lobe of pituitary

Planes of frontal sections

HYPOTHALAMUS AND PITUITARY

16.2 GENERAL ANATOMY OF THE HYPOTHALAMUS

The hypothalamus is a collection of nuclei and fiber tracts in the ventral diencephalon that regulates visceral autonomic functions and neuroendocrine functions, particularly from the anterior and posterior pituitary. Many nuclei are found between the posterior boundary (mammillary bodies) and the anterior boundary (lamina terminalis, anterior commissure) of the hypothalamus; these nuclei are subdivided into four general hypothalamic zones: (1) preoptic; (2) anterior or supraoptic; (3) tuberal; and (4) mammillary or posterior. From the medial boundary at the III ventricle to the lateral boundary, the nuclei are subdivided into three general zones or areas: (1) periventricular; (2) medial; and (3) lateral. The pituitary gland is attached at the base of the hypothalamus by the infundibulum (pituitary stalk), which possesses an important zone of neuroendocrine transduction, the median eminence.

Sections through Hypothalamus I

Plane 1

Plane 1 labels:
- Corpus callosum
- Septum pellucidum
- Anterior horn of lateral ventricle
- Head of caudate nucleus
- Septal area
- Column of fornix
- Anterior limb of internal capsule
- 3rd ventricle
- Putamen
- Globus pallidus
- Anterior commissure
- Lateral preoptic area
- Medial preoptic area
- Hippocampal formation
- Substantia innominata
- Optic chiasm

Plane 2

Plane 2 labels:
- Interventricular foramen (of Monro)
- 3rd ventricle
- Column of fornix
- Periventricular nucleus
- Ansa lenticularis
- Paraventricular nucleus
- Inferior thalamic peduncle
- Lateral hypothalamic area
- Anterior hypothalamic area
- Supraoptic nucleus
- Optic tract
- Optic chiasm

16.3 SECTIONS THROUGH THE HYPOTHALAMUS: PREOPTIC AND SUPRAOPTIC ZONES

The major nuclei in the preoptic zone include the medial and lateral preoptic areas. The organum vasculosum of the lamina terminalis (OVLT), a circumventricular organ (with no blood-brain barrier) is present in this hypothalamic area. The major nuclei in the supraoptic (anterior) zone include the supraoptic (SON) and paraventricular (PVN) nuclei, the suprachiasmatic nucleus, the anterior hypothalamic area, and the lateral hypothalamic area (LHA). Some nuclei such as the PVN have many subregions (such as the magnocellular and parvocellular regions) that contain many collections of chemically specific neurons (20 or more) that have discrete projections and functions. These groups are sometimes intermingled within one subregion of the nucleus.

CLINICAL POINT

The hypothalamus and brain stem structures are involved in regulating the sleep-wake cycle. Ablative lesions of the preoptic area result in insomnia. Some preoptic neurons appear to be maximally activated during sleep and may inhibit neurons in the posterior hypothalamus (such as tuberomammillary neurons) that contribute to wakefulness. The LHA also contains neurons involved in wakefulness through the secretion of an activating neuropeptide, hypocretin. Neurons of the LHA activate the tuberomammillary neurons as well as the locus coeruleus in the pons, a noradrenergic cell group with widespread projections to all regions of the central nervous system (CNS) and a major role in arousal and wakefulness. Early epidemics of encephalitis lethargica (sleeping sickness) demonstrated damage to the midbrain and posterior regions of the hypothalamus. This scheme is consistent with a role for the posterior hypothalamus in sympathetic activation and arousal and with a role for the anterior and preoptic hypothalamus in parasympathetic activation and quiet, reparative, homeostatic functions.

Narcolepsy is a condition of episodic periods of overwhelming daytime drowsiness and then an abrupt episode of sleep, even in the middle of an activity. The person then awakens and feels alert. Night-time sleep may be disturbed, but this is not the cause of daytime sleep episodes; patients with narcolepsy go into rapid eye movement sleep in a matter of minutes rather than hours. Many stimuli (e.g., intense emotion, excitation, laughter) may precipitate an episode of cataplexy in which the knees give out, the person falls, and an abrupt sleep episode follows. Sleep apnea is a major sleep disorder, often associated with obesity, in which patients have prolonged periods of apnea, followed by gasping and including disturbed sleep and loud snoring. It is a major risk factor for heart disease.

The suprachiasmatic nucleus (SCN) sits just above the optic chiasm and contains the major neurons of the CNS that act as a "pacemaker" system for the control of diurnal, or circadian, rhythms. The intrinsic pacemaker has a cycle that is a bit longer than 24 hours (studied in humans who lived in caves with no external light cues); however, input from the retina to the suprachiasmatic nucleus entrains the diurnal rhythms to a 24-hour period. These diurnal rhythms drive many hormone and metabolic levels (e.g., cortisol is low in the late evening, high in the morning before rising; melatonin is highest in late evening) and physiological functions (blood pressure and core body temperature are lowest in early morning, highest in late afternoon). Superimposed on these diurnal rhythms are broader factors, such as effects of the sleep-wake cycle, life stress, levels of activity, and other environmental factors. Sleep has a particularly important influence on cortisol rhythms. Disrupted or poor sleep habits can ablate the diurnal cortisol rhythm, leading to a propensity for fat to be deposited in a central abdominal location because of the effects of high cortisol levels. This can contribute to the likelihood of metabolic syndrome, with its elevated inflammatory mediators (C-reactive protein and interleukin [IL]-6) and increased risk for cardiovascular disease, stroke, type II diabetes, and many cancers. The SCN is influenced by a host of limbic and other forebrain influences superimposed on diurnal rhythms. The SCN, in turn, has axonal projections to other regions of the hypothalamus, the locus coeruleus, and limbic sites through which the diurnal regulatory control of these hormones and physiological functions is achieved.

Sections through Hypothalamus II

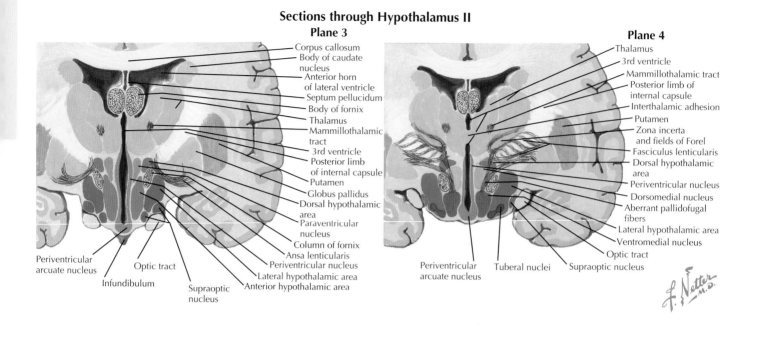

Plane 3

Corpus callosum
Body of caudate nucleus
Anterior horn of lateral ventricle
Septum pellucidum
Body of fornix
Thalamus
Mammillothalamic tract
3rd ventricle
Posterior limb of internal capsule
Putamen
Globus pallidus
Dorsal hypothalamic area
Paraventricular nucleus
Column of fornix
Ansa lenticularis
Periventricular nucleus
Lateral hypothalamic area
Anterior hypothalamic area

Periventricular arcuate nucleus
Optic tract
Infundibulum
Supraoptic nucleus

Plane 4

Thalamus
3rd ventricle
Mammillothalamic tract
Posterior limb of internal capsule
Interthalamic adhesion
Putamen
Zona incerta and fields of Forel
Fasciculus lenticularis
Dorsal hypothalamic area
Periventricular nucleus
Dorsomedial nucleus
Aberrant pallidofugal fibers
Lateral hypothalamic area
Ventromedial nucleus
Optic tract

Periventricular arcuate nucleus
Tuberal nuclei
Supraoptic nucleus

16.4 SECTIONS THROUGH THE HYPOTHALAMUS: TUBERAL ZONE

The major nuclei in the tuberal zone include the dorsomedial nucleus, the ventromedial nucleus, the periventricular area or nucleus, the arcuate nucleus, the periarcuate area (beta-endorphin cells), the tuberal nuclei, the dorsal hypothalamic area, and the LHA. Some nuclei from the supraoptic zone (PVN, SON, LHA) extend caudally into this zone. The median eminence extends from this region, and axons from releasing-factor and inhibitory-factor neurons that control the release of anterior pituitary hormone funnel down to the contact zone, where they release these factors (hormones) into the hypophyseal portal system, which bathes the cells of the anterior pituitary.

CLINICAL POINT

The secretion of hormones by the anterior pituitary gland is regulated by releasing factors (hormones) and inhibitory factors (hormones) that are produced by neurons of the hypothalamus and adjacent sites and are secreted by their axons into the hypophyseal portal vasculature for delivery in extraordinarily high concentrations to cells of the anterior pituitary. The best known of these factors is corticotropin-releasing hormone, produced by parvocellular neurons of the paraventricular nucleus, which regulates subsequent secretion of adrenocorticotropic hormone (ACTH) and cortisol. Another important releasing hormone, growth hormone–releasing hormone, is produced by neurons in the arcuate nucleus and delivered by their axons to the hypophyseal portal system. Somatostatin is a growth hormone–inhibitory hormone and is produced by other neurons in the arcuate nucleus as well as elsewhere. These hormones are regulated by neural connections, hormonal influences, and metabolic factors.

Growth hormone (GH) is released in pulsatile bursts during stage 3 and stage 4 sleep, accounting for 70% of GH release. GH release also is stimulated by exercise, acute stressors, hypoglycemia, and intake of protein, and is suppressed by intake of glucose and many fatty acids. Children who experience emotional deprivation secrete low levels of GH and may fail to grow. Recent studies have shown that mirthful laughter associated with viewing humorous videos markedly stimulates GH secretion and diminishes cortisol and epinephrine secretion. Even more remarkable, when subjects anticipate viewing something humorous, the anticipation itself provokes GH secretion that is as great as or greater than the GH secretion seen in stage 3 and stage 4 sleep.

Sex steroid hormones influence brain development. In a male fetus, the developing testes provide androgens (converted in the brain to estradiol) that influence CNS development in a male pattern during critical developmental periods. All developing fetuses are exposed to maternal estrogen as well as some placental hormones, but the estrogen is bound by alpha-fetoprotein, which protects the female fetus from masculinization by the CNS. One important consequence of fetal exposure to sex steroids is the subsequent hypothalamic control of follicle-stimulating hormone (FSH) and leuteinizing hormone (LH) from the anterior pituitary gland. In females, these hormones are released in a cyclic fashion. In males, FSH and LH are released in steady amounts, a phenomenon dependent upon CNS exposure to estradiol via androgens during fetal development. In the CNS, FSH and LH secretion is controlled by gonadotropin-releasing hormone (GnRH), formerly called leuteinizing hormone–releasing hormone. GnRH neurons in the preoptic area project to the contact zone of the median eminence, ending on the hypophyseal-portal vessels. The GnRH neurons are responsive to estrogen in the female brain but not in the male brain, perhaps accounting for the cyclic secretion of FSH and LH in females. The ventromedial (VM) nucleus of the hypothalamus appears to control some aspects of sexual behavior; VM neurons respond to progesterone via receptors in the female brain but not the male brain. The male brain responds behaviorally to circulating androgens but not to estrogen. Anatomically, preoptic and VM neurons show male-female differences in morphological and synaptic features. A specialized portion of the preoptic area, the sexually dimorphic nucleus, is considerably larger in the male brain than in the female brain, apparently triggered by developmental hormonal exposure.

Sections through Hypothalamus III

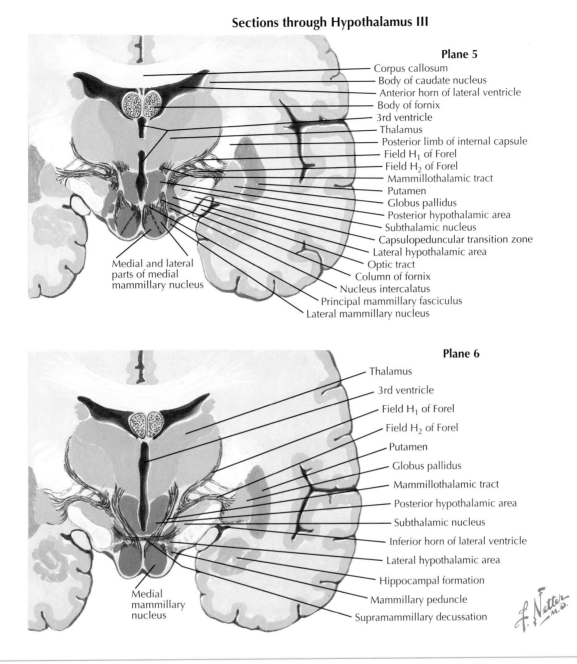

Plane 5

- Corpus callosum
- Body of caudate nucleus
- Anterior horn of lateral ventricle
- Body of fornix
- 3rd ventricle
- Thalamus
- Posterior limb of internal capsule
- Field H_1 of Forel
- Field H_2 of Forel
- Mammillothalamic tract
- Putamen
- Globus pallidus
- Posterior hypothalamic area
- Subthalamic nucleus
- Capsulopeduncular transition zone
- Lateral hypothalamic area
- Optic tract
- Column of fornix
- Nucleus intercalatus
- Principal mammillary fasciculus
- Lateral mammillary nucleus

Medial and lateral parts of medial mammillary nucleus

Plane 6

- Thalamus
- 3rd ventricle
- Field H_1 of Forel
- Field H_2 of Forel
- Putamen
- Globus pallidus
- Mammillothalamic tract
- Posterior hypothalamic area
- Subthalamic nucleus
- Inferior horn of lateral ventricle
- Lateral hypothalamic area
- Hippocampal formation
- Mammillary peduncle
- Supramammillary decussation

Medial mammillary nucleus

16.5 SECTIONS THROUGH THE HYPOTHALAMUS: MAMMILLARY ZONE

The major nuclei in the mammillary zone include the medial and lateral mammillary nuclei, the posterior hypothalamic area, and the LHA. The LHA extends throughout most of the length of the hypothalamus and shows neuronal characteristics seen in the brain stem reticular formation.

CLINICAL POINT

In the 1930s, James Papez proposed a brain circuit that was viewed as a substrate for control of emotional behavior and later as a substrate for memory, especially for consolidation of immediate and short-term memory into long-term memory. This circuit includes hippocampal formation (especially the subiculum) via the fornix to the mammillary nuclei (especially medial nuclei); via the mammillothalamic tract to the anterior thalamic nuclei; via the internal capsule to the anterior cingulate cortex; via polysynaptic connections in the cingulum to the entorhinal cortex, subiculum, and hippocampus. This circuit is proposed as a site of major damage in Wernicke-Korsakoff syndrome, a disorder that is commonly seen in chronic alcoholic patients with a vitamin B_1 (thiamine) deficiency. This syndrome includes Wernicke's encephalopathy and the memory dysfunction of Korsakoff's syndrome. Wernicke's encephalopathy involves a confused and psychotic state involving confabulation (made-up stories derived from a host of confused past memories or experiences), cerebellar ataxia, extraocular and gaze palsies, and nystagmus. Korsakoff amnestic syndrome involves the inability to consolidate immediate and short-term memory into long-term traces (anterograde amnesia) as well as long-term memory loss concerning events that have occurred since the onset of the disease. Degeneration has been described in the mammillary bodies, fornix, hippocampal formation, and anterior and medial dorsal thalamus. However, the extent to which the mammillary nuclei themselves play a role in consolidation of memory traces remains to be shown. Thiamine administration may help to reverse some of the symptoms, but the amnesias may persist. Administration of glucose (carbohydrate loading) without thiamine may cause death as the result of nutritional cardiomyopathy.

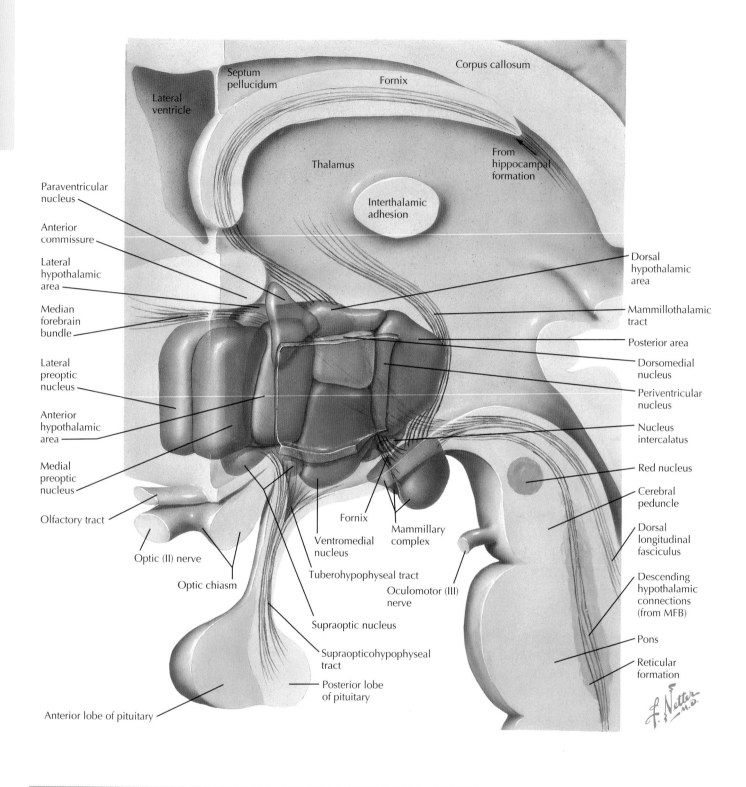

16.6 SCHEMATIC RECONSTRUCTION OF THE HYPOTHALAMUS

A schematic three-dimensional reconstruction of the hypothalamus in sagittal section shows the nuclei, areas, and zones that occupy this small, compact region of the diencephalon. Many pathways are represented in this schematic reconstruction, including the fornix, the mammillothalamic tract, the median forebrain bundle (MFB), the supraopticohypophyseal tract, the tuberohypophyseal (tuberoinfundibular) tract, and brain stem connections with the hypothalamus via the dorsal longitudinal fasciculus, the descending median forebrain bundle, the mammillotegmental tract, and descending connections from the PVN to preganglionic autonomic nuclei.

16.7 FOREBRAIN REGIONS ASSOCIATED WITH THE HYPOTHALAMUS

Numerous forebrain regions are intimately connected with the hypothalamus, some through direct fiber projections and others through indirect connections. The important regions of the cerebral cortex include the prefrontal cortex, orbitofrontal cortex, cingulate cortex, insular cortex, parahippocampal cortex, and periamygdaloid cortex. The important subcortical regions of the limbic forebrain include the hippocampal formation, amygdaloid nuclei, and septal nuclei. Important thalamic connections include the medial dorsal and anterior nuclei. Important olfactory connections include the olfactory tract, nuclei, and cortex.

Stria medullaris thalami

Habenula

Cingulate gyrus

Corpus callosum

Medial dorsal and
Anterior nuclei of thalamus

Septal nuclei

From septal, subcallosal,
preoptic, and frontotemporal areas

Prefontal cortex

Hypothalamic nuclei

Olfactory bulb

Stria
terminalis

Orbitofrontal cortex projections

Hippocampal formation

Reticular
formation

Hypophysis

Ventral amygdalofugal pathway

Amygdala

Interpeduncular nucleus

Mammillotegmental tract

Dorsal longitudinal fasciculus

Median forebrain bundle (descending)

Medullary cardiovascular centers

Vagus (X) nerve

Arrows represent afferent and efferent pathways.

16.8 AFFERENT AND EFFERENT PATHWAYS ASSOCIATED WITH THE HYPOTHALAMUS

Hypothalamic connections are numerous and complex. Some regions of the cerebral cortex (prefrontal, orbitofrontal) and thalamus (anterior) send axonal projections directly to the hypothalamus. Diverse afferent pathways arise from the hippocampal formation and the subiculum (fornix), amygdaloid nuclei (stria terminalis, ventral amygdalofugal pathway), and habenula (fasciculus retroflexus). The retina sends direct retinohypothalamic fibers to the suprachiasmatic nucleus of the hypothalamus. Numerous brain stem projections, some compact and some diffuse, ascend to the hypothalamus by multiple pathways (not shown here). Efferent connections from the hypothalamus include those to the median eminence (from multiple nuclei), the posterior pituitary (supraopticohypophyseal tract), the septal nuclei and the anterior perforated substance (median forebrain bundle), the thalamus (mammillothalamic tract), and many brain stem and spinal cord sites (dorsal longitudinal fasciculus, median forebrain bundle, mammillotegmental tract, direct connections from PVN to preganglionic neurons, and others).

CLINICAL POINT

The hypothalamus receives inputs from the hippocampal formation and subiculum, amygdaloid nuclei, habenula, retina, some cortical areas, and many brain stem regions; a good number of these inputs are limbic forebrain and brain stem connections. The role of the hypothalamus is to regulate the visceral milieu and neuroendocrine secretion, particularly via the anterior and posterior pituitary. The efferents of the hypothalamus reflect this role and are directed to the posterior pituitary and contact zone of the median eminence, some limbic forebrain structures, and widespread areas of the brain stem and spinal cord that are involved in autonomic and visceral regulation. These connections help to coordinate appropriate behavioral responses to external and internal inputs and perceived challenges in the environment. The posterior and lateral hypothalamic regions are particularly involved in sympathetic drive and activational responses, such as the acquisition of food and water, the increase of core body temperature, sympathetic arousal, activities involved in aggressive interactions with the environment, and wakefulness states. Many of these activities are coordinated through connections in the median forebrain bundle. In contrast, the anterior and medial hypothalamic regions are particularly involved in parasympathetic functions, such as satiation, decreased core body temperature, quiet and reparative homeostatis-related activities, and sleep. Many of these activities are coordinated through connections in the dorsal longitudinal fasciculus and other descending pathways.

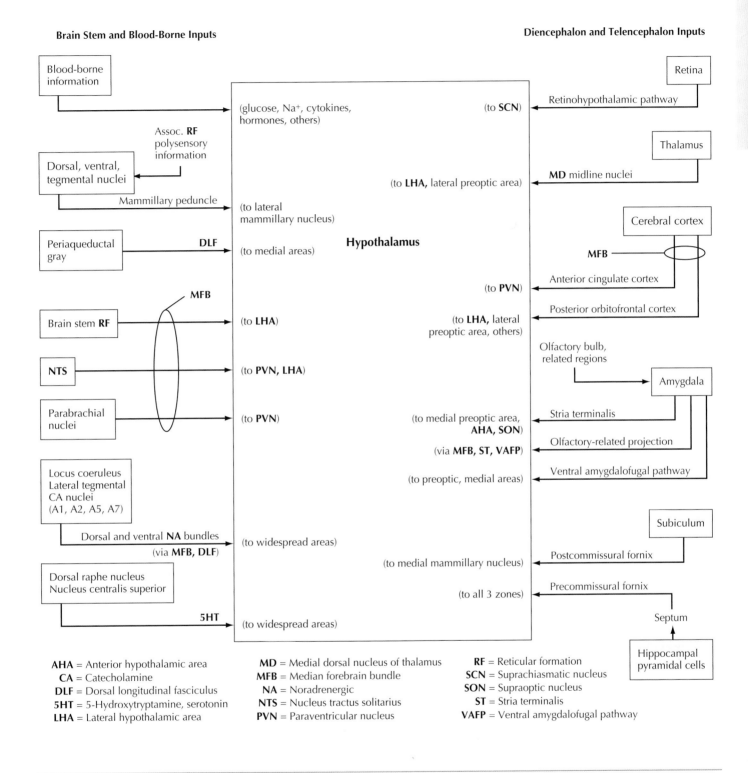

Brain Stem and Blood-Borne Inputs

Diencephalon and Telencephalon Inputs

Blood-borne information

(glucose, Na⁺, cytokines, hormones, others) (to **SCN**)

Retinohypothalamic pathway — Retina

Assoc. **RF** polysensory information

Dorsal, ventral, tegmental nuclei

(to **LHA**, lateral preoptic area) **MD** midline nuclei — Thalamus

Mammillary peduncle (to lateral mammillary nucleus)

Hypothalamus

Periaqueductal gray **DLF** (to medial areas)

Cerebral cortex

MFB

Anterior cingulate cortex

MFB (to **PVN**)

Posterior orbitofrontal cortex

Brain stem **RF** (to **LHA**)

(to **LHA,** lateral preoptic area, others)

NTS (to **PVN, LHA**)

Olfactory bulb, related regions

Parabrachial nuclei (to **PVN**)

Amygdala

(to medial preoptic area, **AHA, SON**) Stria terminalis

(via **MFB, ST, VAFP**) Olfactory-related projection

Locus coeruleus Lateral tegmental CA nuclei (A1, A2, A5, A7)

(to preoptic, medial areas) Ventral amygdalofugal pathway

Dorsal and ventral **NA** bundles (via **MFB, DLF**) (to widespread areas)

Subiculum

(to medial mammillary nucleus) Postcommissural fornix

Dorsal raphe nucleus Nucleus centralis superior

(to all 3 zones) Precommissural fornix

Septum

5HT (to widespread areas)

Hippocampal pyramidal cells

AHA = Anterior hypothalamic area
CA = Catecholamine
DLF = Dorsal longitudinal fasciculus
5HT = 5-Hydroxytryptamine, serotonin
LHA = Lateral hypothalamic area

MD = Medial dorsal nucleus of thalamus
MFB = Median forebrain bundle
NA = Noradrenergic
NTS = Nucleus tractus solitarius
PVN = Paraventricular nucleus

RF = Reticular formation
SCN = Suprachiasmatic nucleus
SON = Supraoptic nucleus
ST = Stria terminalis
VAFP = Ventral amygdalofugal pathway

16.9 SCHEMATIC DIAGRAM OF MAJOR HYPOTHALAMIC AFFERENT PATHWAYS

The hypothalamus receives extensive input from many regions of the CNS. Descending inputs arrive from limbic forebrain structures (hippocampal formation, subiculum, amygdaloid nuclei), the cerebral cortex (anterior cingulate, orbitofrontal, prefrontal), and the thalamus (medial dorsal). Ascending inputs arrive from extensive areas of the autonomic brain stem (tegmental nuclei, periaqueductal gray, parabrachial nuclei, nucleus tractus solitarius, locus coeruleus and tegmental catecholamine nuclei, raphe serotonergic nuclei) and from the brain stem reticular formation. The retina sends input directly to the suprachiasmatic nucleus, a nucleus of the hypothalamus that modulates diurnal rhythms. Blood-borne substances (cytokines, hormones, glucose, Na⁺, others) influence the hypothalamus via numerous routes and mechanisms.

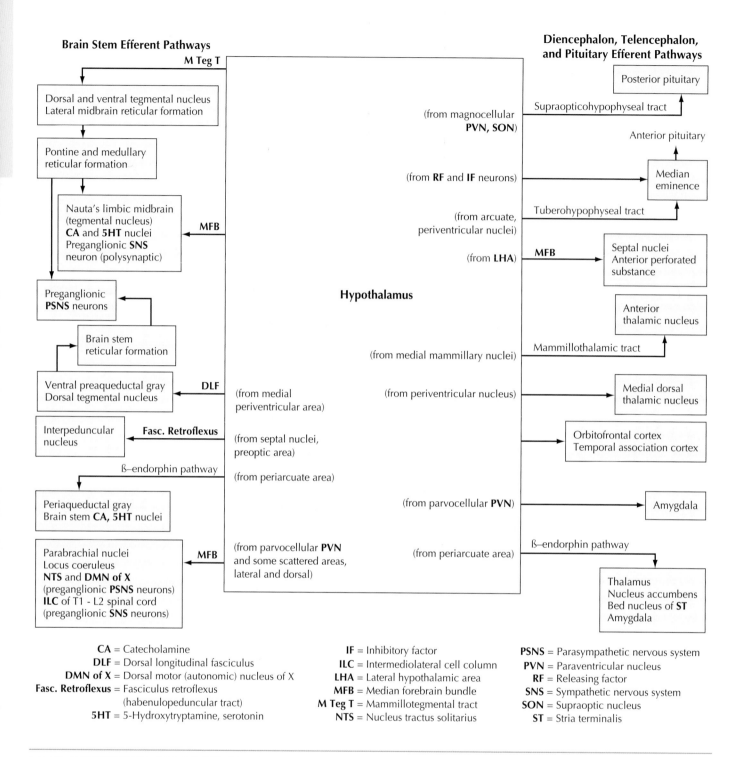

Brain Stem Efferent Pathways

M Teg T

Dorsal and ventral tegmental nucleus
Lateral midbrain reticular formation

Pontine and medullary
reticular formation

Nauta's limbic midbrain
(tegmental nucleus)
CA and **5HT** nuclei
Preganglionic **SNS**
neuron (polysynaptic)

MFB

Preganglionic
PSNS neurons

Brain stem
reticular formation

Ventral preaqueductal gray
Dorsal tegmental nucleus

DLF

Interpeduncular
nucleus

Fasc. Retroflexus

ß–endorphin pathway

Periaqueductal gray
Brain stem **CA, 5HT** nuclei

Parabrachial nuclei
Locus coeruleus
NTS and **DMN of X**
(preganglionic **PSNS** neurons)
ILC of T1 - L2 spinal cord
(preganglionic **SNS** neurons)

MFB

(from medial
periventricular area)

(from septal nuclei,
preoptic area)

(from periarcuate area)

(from parvocellular **PVN**
and some scattered areas,
lateral and dorsal)

Hypothalamus

**Diencephalon, Telencephalon,
and Pituitary Efferent Pathways**

Posterior pituitary

(from magnocellular
PVN, SON)

Supraopticohypophyseal tract

Anterior pituitary

(from **RF** and **IF** neurons)

Median
eminence

(from arcuate,
periventricular nuclei)

Tuberohypophyseal tract

(from **LHA**)

MFB

Septal nuclei
Anterior perforated
substance

Anterior
thalamic nucleus

(from medial mammillary nuclei)

Mammillothalamic tract

(from periventricular nucleus)

Medial dorsal
thalamic nucleus

Orbitofrontal cortex
Temporal association cortex

(from parvocellular **PVN**)

Amygdala

(from periarcuate area)

ß–endorphin pathway

Thalamus
Nucleus accumbens
Bed nucleus of **ST**
Amygdala

CA = Catecholamine	**IF** = Inhibitory factor	**PSNS** = Parasympathetic nervous system
DLF = Dorsal longitudinal fasciculus	**ILC** = Intermediolateral cell column	**PVN** = Paraventricular nucleus
DMN of X = Dorsal motor (autonomic) nucleus of X	**LHA** = Lateral hypothalamic area	**RF** = Releasing factor
Fasc. Retroflexus = Fasciculus retroflexus	**MFB** = Median forebrain bundle	**SNS** = Sympathetic nervous system
(habenulopeduncular tract)	**M Teg T** = Mammillotegmental tract	**SON** = Supraoptic nucleus
5HT = 5-Hydroxytryptamine, serotonin	**NTS** = Nucleus tractus solitarius	**ST** = Stria terminalis

16.10 SCHEMATIC DIAGRAM OF MAJOR HYPOTHALAMIC EFFERENT PATHWAYS

The hypothalamus gives rise to extensive efferent projections to many regions of the CNS. Ascending efferents are sent to limbic forebrain structures (amygdaloid nuclei, septal nuclei, the anterior perforated substance), the cerebral cortex (orbitofrontal cortex and temporal association cortex), and the thalamus (medial dorsal, anterior). Extensive projections are sent to the median eminence (releasing and inhibitory factors for control of anterior pituitary hormones, dopamine projections from the arcuate nucleus and periventricular nucleus)

and to the posterior pituitary. Additional efferent projections are sent directly and indirectly to the preganglionic neurons of the sympathetic and the parasympathetic nervous systems (median forebrain bundle, dorsal longitudinal fasciculus, mammillotegmental tract, and direct projections from the paraventricular nucleus); to widespread autonomic and visceral nuclei (noradrenergic neurons, serotonergic neurons, parabrachial nuclei, nucleus tractus solitarius, periaqueductal gray, tegmental nuclei, interpeduncular nucleus); and to the brain stem reticular formation.

DLF = Dorsal longitudinal fasciculus
FX = Fornix
MD = Medial dorsal nucleus of thalamus
MFB = Median forebrain bundle

MTT = Mammillothalamic tract
SNS = Sympathetic nervous system
ST = Stria terminalis
VAFP = Ventral amygdalofugal pathway

16.11 SUMMARY OF GENERAL HYPOTHALAMIC CONNECTIONS

The lateral, medial, and periventricular zones of the hypothalamus have specific connections with the cerebral cortex, limbic forebrain structures, thalamus, and widespread areas of the brain stem. Extensive efferent projections of the hypothalamus are directed toward regulation of preganglionic sympathetic and parasympathetic neurons and toward release and regulation of hormones of the anterior and posterior pituitary. The anterior pituitary hormones regulate hormonal secretion and functional activities of many target structures throughout the body.

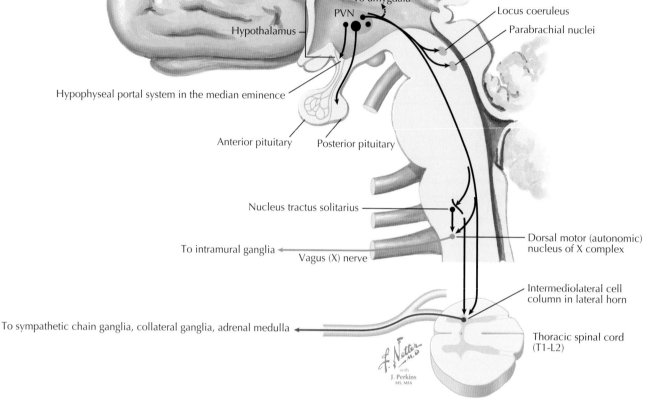

16.12 PARAVENTRICULAR NUCLEUS OF THE HYPOTHALAMUS: REGULATION OF PITUITARY NEUROHORMONAL OUTFLOW, AUTONOMIC PREGANGLIONIC OUTFLOW, AND LIMBIC ACTIVITY

The PVN has many projections that help to coordinate pituitary neurohormonal outflow, autonomic preganglionic outflow, and limbic activity. Magnocellular neurons send axons to the posterior pituitary, releasing oxytocin and vasopressin into the general circulation. Corticotropin-releasing factor (CRF) neurons and some vasopressin neurons send axons to the median eminence; these axons release their hormones into the hypophyseal portal system, influencing the release of ACTH. PVN parvocellular neurons send direct descending projections to preganglionic neurons for the parasympathetics (dorsal motor nucleus of CN X) and sympathetics (intermediolateral cell column in the T1–L2 lateral horn of the spinal cord) and to the nucleus tractus solitarius. PVN parvocellular neurons also send axons to several important limbic-related structures, such as the amygdaloid nuclei, parabrachial nuclei, and locus coeruleus.

CLINICAL POINT

The PVN of the hypothalamus is a small region along the upper borders of the third ventricle in the dorsal hypothalamus. It contains a remarkable array of chemically specific neural populations. The magnocellular neurons produce oxytocin and vasopressin along with neurophysins and project to the median eminence. Some parvocellular neurons synthesize corticotropin-releasing hormone and send axons to the contact zone of the median eminence, where corticotropin-releasing hormone is released into the hypophyseal portal vessels. Parvocellular neurons also send descending projections to the brain stem (particularly the nucleus solitarius) and the intermediolateral cell column of the thoracolumbar spinal cord, where activation of the SNS can occur. The PVN therefore can coordinate the activation of both the neuroendocrine components (hypothalamic-pituitary-adrenal axis and cortisol secretion) and the autonomic components (sympathetic activation, diminished parasympathetic activity) of a stress response or activational response. The PVN receives inputs from many limbic regions and from brain stem sites (parabrachial nuclei, brain stem noradrenergic nuclei, nucleus tractus solitarius) that provide visceral information to the PVN. In addition, the PVN receives a variety of inputs that help it to monitor inflammatory mediators (IL-1beta, IL-6, tumor necrosis factor [TNF]-alpha, prostaglandin E_2 [PGE$_2$]), and other small molecules (nitric oxide) that reflect the outside chemical milieu. This information is received through the hypothalamus and circumventricular organs, and some of it through the vagus nerve afferents and nucleus tractus solitarius. Thus, PVN is a key regulatory site for behavioral responses that require autonomic reactivity.

Behaviors Influenced by Cytokines:
Illness behavior
Affective behavior
Cognitive behavior
Autonomic and neuroendocrine
regulation

Cerebral vasculature with
blood-brain barrier (BBB)

C = **Interleukin-1β (IL-1β)**
Other cytokines acting on brain:
IL-6 (interleukin-6)
TNF-α (tumor necrosis factor-α)
IL-2 (interleukin-2)

Organum vascularum of
the lamina terminalis (OVLT)

Vasculature to hypothalamus

① Cytokines transported directly across the BBB

② Cytokines crossing into cerebrospinal fluid at
OVLT or acting on cells that release PGE₂ or
neurons that project to visceral-autonomic
structures

③ Cytokine-stimulated release of small molecules
(such as nitric oxide) that directly cross into
the brain and act as mediators

④ Cytokine stimulation of vagal afferents (through
paraneurons) that modulate activity in nucleus
tractus solitarius, influencing the multiple
activities of the paraventricular nucleus
and many other sites

⑤ Cytokine activation of other afferents that modulate
dorsal horn sensory processing to many sites

⑥ Cytokine modulation of norepinephrine release from
sympathetic nerve terminals

⑦ Cytokine modulation of neurotransmitter intracellular
signaling in target cells

⑧ Cytokine modulation of pituitary hormone release

Sensory
ganglion of X

Vagal afferents
in viscera

Vagal efferents to
intramural ganglia

Paraganglion cells
associated with
vagal afferents

Somatic
afferents

Peripheral nerve

Sympathetic
ganglion

Target

Nucleus tractus
solitarius

Dorsal motor
(autonomic)
nucleus of X

Dorsal root
ganglion

Dorsal horn

Spinal cord

16.13 MECHANISMS OF CYTOKINE INFLUENCES ON THE HYPOTHALAMUS AND OTHER BRAIN REGIONS AND ON BEHAVIOR

Cytokines, including IL-1beta, IL-6, TNF-alpha, and IL-2, can influence central neuronal activity and behavior. This figure illustrates IL-1beta access to the brain: (1) directly crossing the blood-brain barrier into the brain (especially in cortical regions); (2) acting on circumventricular organs (the OVLT) to release small mediators such as PGE₂; (3) acting on vascular endothelial cells to release nitric oxide, which acts in the CNS; (4) activating vagal afferents that project into the nucleus tractus solitarius via paraganglion cells; and (5) activating other afferent nerve fibers. IL-1beta can evoke illness behavior (fever, induction of slow-wave sleep, decreased appetite, lethargy, classical illness symptoms), can influence autonomic and neuroendocrine regulation, and can influence both affective and cognitive functions and behavior.

A key target of these influences is the PVN of the hypothalamus. Inflammatory cytokines can provoke a robust activation of cortisol secretion (through the hypothalamopituitary-adrenal axis) and SNS activation (via descending projections of the PVN). The consequences of prolonged stress activation include increased risk for many chronic diseases, such as cardiovascular disease and stroke, metabolic syndrome, type II diabetes, and many cancers. The cytokines can influence the PVN and other central neurons through several mechanisms, including some direct transport into the forebrain, actions on neurons of the OVLT that release PGE₂ and signal the PVN, release of nitric oxide from vascular endothelial cells, and activation of vagal afferents and other afferents that send neural signals to PVN. Inflammatory cytokines also can stimulate the release of some hormones from pituitary cells, can alter neurotransmitter release in both the CNS and the autonomic nervous system (especially sympathetic norepinephrine), and can interact with neurotransmitter effects on target cells of autonomic innervation. Other cytokines such as IL-2 also appear to have central effects; the infusion of IL-2 in immunotherapy for some cancers was curtailed because of adverse effects of IL-2 on the brain, including depression and suicidal behavior.

CLINICAL POINT
There is a widespread influence of cytokines, especially inflammatory cytokines (IL-1beta, IL-6, TNF-alpha), on the nervous system.

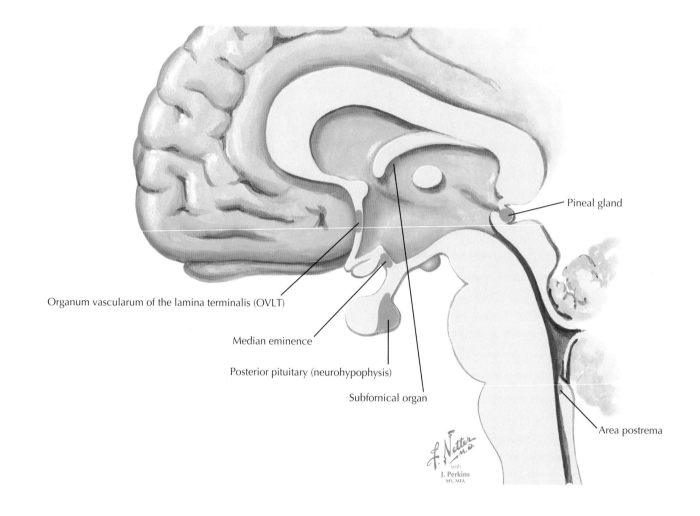

Organum vascularum of the lamina terminalis (OVLT)

Median eminence

Posterior pituitary (neurohypophysis)

Subfornical organ

Pineal gland

Area postrema

16.14 CIRCUMVENTRICULAR ORGANS

Circumventricular organs are "windows on the brain" that are devoid of the usual tight-junction endothelial appositions and instead have fenestrated vasculature. Thus, the circumventricular organs have no blood-brain barrier. Some of these organs (the OVLT, the subfornical organ, and the area postrema) have associated neurons that project to the hypothalamic and other visceral structures. They also have cells that can release small molecules such as PGE_2 into the cerebrospinal fluid, thus affecting target structures at a distance. The neurohypophysis is a site of axonal release (from PVN and SON magnocellular neurons) of oxytocin and arginine vasopressin into the general circulation. The median eminence is a zone of neuroendocrine transduction for the secretion of releasing factors and inhibitory factors into the hypophyseal portal vasculature; these factors influence the release of anterior pituitary hormones. The pineal gland synthesizes and releases the hormone melatonin.

CLINICAL POINT

The CNS is protected from damage caused by many potentially harmful substances by the blood-brain barrier. The CNS capillary endothelial cells contain tight junctions as well as specific transport mechanisms for the uptake of certain important substances (such as amino acids needed for neurotransmitter synthesis, glucose). Brain capillaries also can actively pump some substances out of the brain. Some regions of the brain contain fenestrated capillaries, and this permits the sampling of circulating substances. These are the circumventricular organs. The area postrema contains neurons that project to the nucleus tractus solitarius and activate the vomiting reflex. The subfornical organ contains neurons that respond to salt content in the blood and elicit protective neuroendocrine responses. The OVLT contains neurons that help to regulate blood pressure through an angiotensin II mechanism; these neurons also regulate PGE_2 availability to the PVN and other central areas to regulate activation of the hypothalamo-pituitary-adrenal axis and the SNS. The OVLT and subfornical organ also respond to pyrogens and help to regulate hypothalamic responses for control of body temperature. At the median eminence, circulating hormones and other substances can interact with the projecting axonal terminals that secrete releasing hormones and inhibitory hormones at the contact zone for regulation of anterior pituitary hormonal secretion. The posterior pituitary and the pineal gland also have fenestrated capillaries, perhaps enabling their secretion of hormones directly into the systemic circulation.

Blood Supply of Hypothalamus and Pituitary Gland

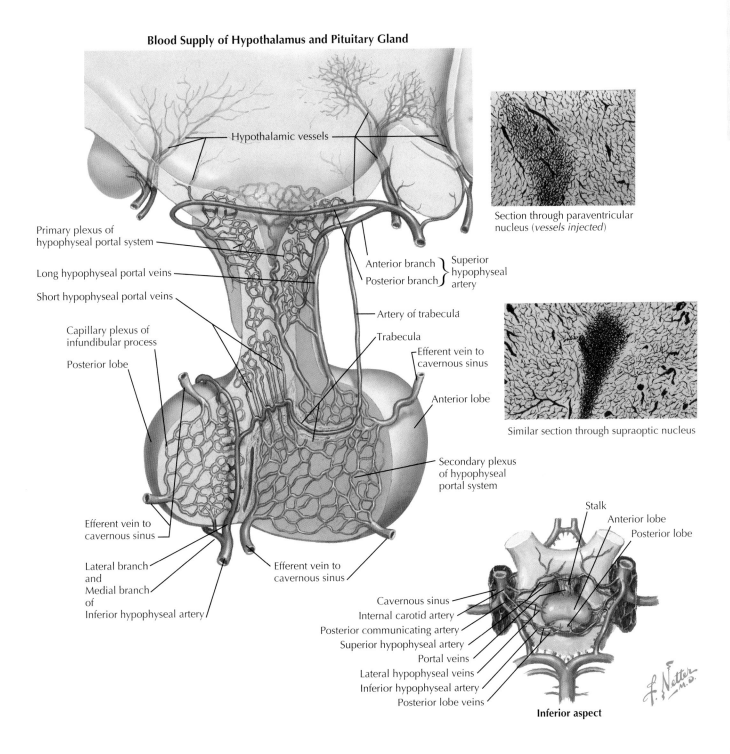

Hypothalamic vessels

Primary plexus of hypophyseal portal system

Long hypophyseal portal veins

Short hypophyseal portal veins

Capillary plexus of infundibular process

Posterior lobe

Efferent vein to cavernous sinus

Lateral branch and Medial branch of Inferior hypophyseal artery

Efferent vein to cavernous sinus

Anterior branch
Posterior branch
} Superior hypophyseal artery

Artery of trabecula

Trabecula

Efferent vein to cavernous sinus

Anterior lobe

Secondary plexus of hypophyseal portal system

Section through paraventricular nucleus (*vessels injected*)

Similar section through supraoptic nucleus

Stalk
Anterior lobe
Posterior lobe

Cavernous sinus
Internal carotid artery
Posterior communicating artery
Superior hypophyseal artery
Portal veins
Lateral hypophyseal veins
Inferior hypophyseal artery
Posterior lobe veins

Inferior aspect

16.15 THE HYPOPHYSEAL PORTAL VASCULATURE

The hypophyseal portal vascular system derives from arterioles coming into the median eminence at the base of the hypothalamus. The primary capillary plexus is a site where releasing and inhibitory factors that influence the secretion of anterior pituitary hormones are released from axons (neurocrine secretion) whose neurons reside in the hypothalamus and other CNS sites. These releasing and inhibitory factors then travel through venules into the secondary capillary plexus in very high concentrations and act directly on anterior pituitary cells that synthesize and secrete the hormones of the anterior pituitary.

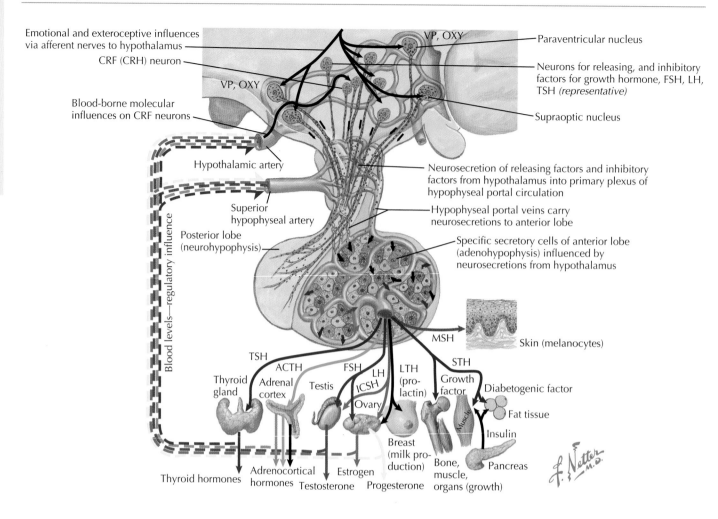

Emotional and exteroceptive influences via afferent nerves to hypothalamus
CRF (CRH) neuron
Blood-borne molecular influences on CRF neurons
VP, OXY
Hypothalamic artery
Superior hypophyseal artery
Posterior lobe (neurohypophysis)
Blood levels—regulatory influence

VP, OXY
Paraventricular nucleus
Neurons for releasing, and inhibitory factors for growth hormone, FSH, LH, TSH (representative)
Supraoptic nucleus
Neurosecretion of releasing factors and inhibitory factors from hypothalamus into primary plexus of hypophyseal portal circulation
Hypophyseal portal veins carry neurosecretions to anterior lobe
Specific secretory cells of anterior lobe (adenohypophysis) influenced by neurosecretions from hypothalamus

MSH — Skin (melanocytes)

TSH
ACTH
FSH
LH
ICSH
LTH (prolactin)
STH
Growth factor
Thyroid gland
Adrenal cortex
Testis
Ovary
Breast (milk production)
Diabetogenic factor
Fat tissue
Insulin
Bone, muscle, organs (growth)
Pancreas

Thyroid hormones
Adrenocortical hormones
Testosterone
Estrogen
Progesterone

16.16 REGULATION OF ANTERIOR PITUITARY HORMONE SECRETION

Neurons that synthesize releasing and inhibitory factors for control of anterior pituitary hormones send axons that terminate on the primary plexus of the hypophyseal portal system (the zone of neuroendocrine transduction) and release these factors into the hypophyseal portal blood. These factors then flow into the secondary hypophyseal portal plexus and regulate the release of anterior pituitary hormones. The major anterior pituitary hormones are thyroid-stimulating hormone (TSH), adrenal corticotropic hormone (ACTH), follicle-stimulating hormone (FSH), leuteinizing hormone (LH), prolactin (LTH), growth hormone (somatotropic hormone; STH), and melanocyte-stimulating hormone (MSH). These anterior pituitary hormones act on peripheral target organs to effect release of target organ hormones or to influence metabolic and functional activities. For example, CRF neurons release CRF (CRH, corticotropin-releasing hormone) into the hypophyseal portal blood, regulating the release of ACTH, which in turn regulates the release of cortisol from the adrenal cortex. Magnocellular neurons of the PVN and SON send axons directly to the posterior pituitary and release oxytocin and arginine vasopressin directly into the systemic circulation.

CLINICAL POINT

The term *hypopituitarism* refers to the deficiency or absence of one or more anterior pituitary hormones. The process of pituitary dysfunction can be very slow in onset because of the great reserve; more than 75% of the anterior pituitary must be destroyed before symptoms become evident. Pituitary damage may result from tumors, ischemia and infarction, infiltrative lesions (e.g., sarcoidosis), head injury, immunological damage during pregnancy, or other causes. With some tumors such as pituitary adenomas initial symptoms may occur because of disruption of releasing hormones, such as GnRH, leading to elevated secretion of prolactin, FSH, LH, and ACTH and cortisol, producing gonadal dysfunction. With progressive pituitary insufficiency, the first hormones to markedly fall are growth hormone (GH), which is highly conspicuous in children whose growth is impaired, and gonadotropins, causing amenorrhea in women and impotence or sexual dysfunction in men. At a later stage, impairment of TSH, ACTH, prolactin, and other hormones occurs; hormonal replacement therapy is necessary. Diabetes insipidus caused by posterior pituitary damage also may accompany pituitary insufficiency.

Many pituitary tumors secrete anterior pituitary hormones, leading to symptoms of pituitary hypersecretion. Prolactinomas (adenomas) result in excess prolactin secretion, gonadal dysfunction, and galactorrhea. GH-secreting adenomas result in gigantism if they are present before the epiphyseal plates of the long bones are closed and in acromegaly in adults, with soft tissue enlargement, enlarged hands and feet, and coarse facial features. ACTH-secreting adenomas lead to Cushing's disease. Pituitary tumors commonly impinge on the optic chiasm and produce bitemporal visual field defects (bitemporal hemianopia), usually starting in the upper outer fields.

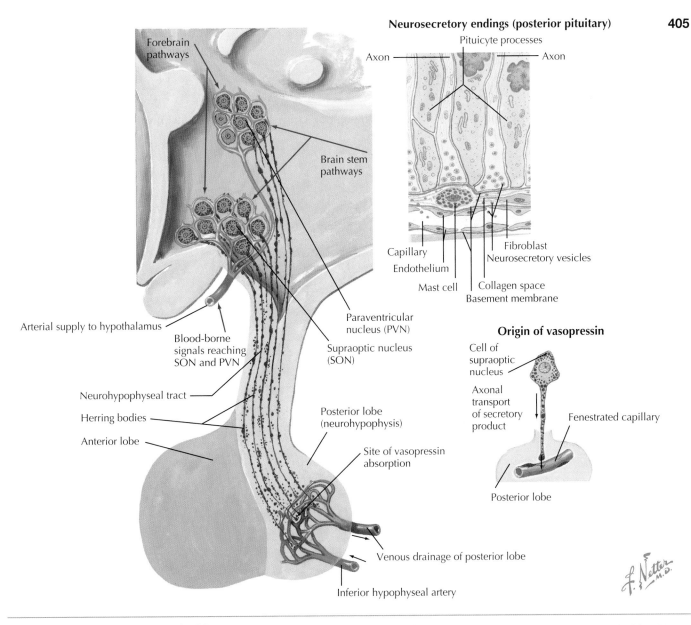

Forebrain pathways

Pituicyte processes

Axon

Axon

Brain stem pathways

Capillary

Endothelium

Mast cell

Fibroblast

Neurosecretory vesicles

Collagen space

Basement membrane

Arterial supply to hypothalamus

Blood-borne signals reaching SON and PVN

Paraventricular nucleus (PVN)

Supraoptic nucleus (SON)

Neurohypophyseal tract

Herring bodies

Anterior lobe

Posterior lobe (neurohypophysis)

Site of vasopressin absorption

Origin of vasopressin

Cell of supraoptic nucleus

Axonal transport of secretory product

Fenestrated capillary

Posterior lobe

Venous drainage of posterior lobe

Inferior hypophyseal artery

16.17 POSTERIOR PITUITARY (NEUROHYPOPHYSEAL) HORMONES: OXYTOCIN AND VASOPRESSIN

Magnocellular neurons in the PVN and SON send axons directly through the infundibular region and the pituitary stalk to terminate on the vasculature in the posterior pituitary. Neurons from both nuclei synthesize and release oxytocin and arginine vasopressin into the systemic vasculature. Brain stem and forebrain pathways terminate on the magnocellular neurons and regulate their secretion of oxytocin and vasopressin. These magnocellular neurons possess extensive protein synthesis capacity and transport the vesicles in which their hormones are packaged to the axon terminals with very fast axoplasmic transport. The hormones are released from the terminals and diffuse through the fenestrated capillaries directly into the systemic vasculature (see inset of neurosecretory efferent endings from magnocellular neurons in PVN and SON).

CLINICAL POINT

The SON and magnocellular neurons of the PVN of the hypothalamus synthesize and secrete both oxytocin and arginine vasopressin (antidiuretic hormone, or ADH), along with their neurophysin carrier proteins. A majority of vasopressin comes from the SON, and a majority of oxytocin comes from magnocellular PVN. These neuronal groups send axons (the supraopticohypophyseal tract) into the posterior pituitary, where they terminate on fenestrated capillaries and secrete their hormones directly into the systemic circulation. These neurons are called neuroendocrine transducer cells. Oxytocin cells respond to estrogen and to afferent signals caused by suckling, and they stimulate milk let-down (milk ejection reflex) and uterine contraction in pregnancy. Vasopressin neurons respond to changes in blood osmolarity, secreting vasopressin in the presence of high osmolarity. This causes the collecting tubules in the kidney to increase water resorption and prevent diuresis. If the supraopticohypophyseal tract or associated neurons (seen in congenital disorders) are damaged, as happens with pituitary stalk sectioning, diabetes insipidus results. Diabetes insipidus involves the loss of vasopressin secretion and the production of huge amounts (10+ liters per day) of dilute urine, provoking marked polydipsia. Vasopressin replacement therapy is necessary. Alcohol consumption, some antiseizure drugs (phenytoin), and anticholinergic agents may also inhibit vasopressin secretion. Excessive vasopressin secretion (called inappropriate secretion of ADH, or SIADH) may occur because of partial damage to the hypothalamus, a vasopressin-secreting tumor in the periphery (e.g., lung carcinoma), or as the result of treatment by chemotherapeutic and other pharmacological agents. SIADH results in hypo-osmolar serum, hyponatremia, and high urine osmolarity.

Mechanism of Antidiuretic Hormone in Regulating Urine Volume and Concentration

ADH is produced in supraoptic and paraventricular nuclei of the hypothalamus and descends along nerve fibers to the neurohypophysis, where it is stored for subsequent release.

Blood osmolality and volume are modified by fluid intake (oral or parenteral); water and electrolyte exchange with tissues, normal or pathological (edema); loss via gut (vomiting, diarrhea); loss into body cavities (ascites, effusion); or loss externally (hemorrhage, sweat).

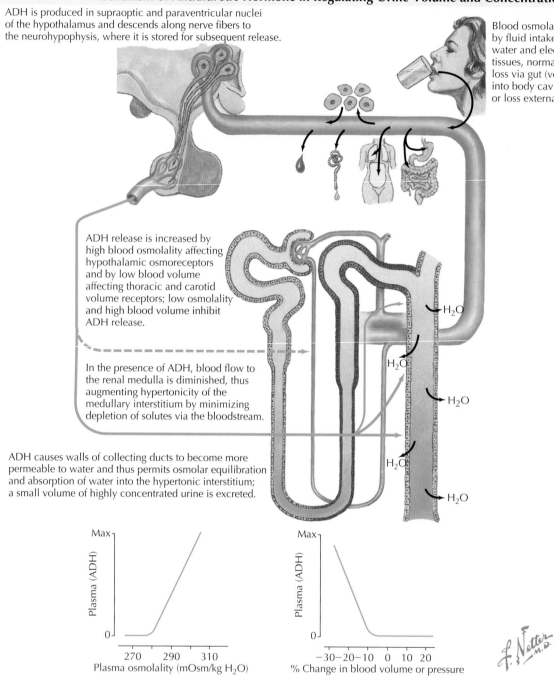

ADH release is increased by high blood osmolality affecting hypothalamic osmoreceptors and by low blood volume affecting thoracic and carotid volume receptors; low osmolality and high blood volume inhibit ADH release.

In the presence of ADH, blood flow to the renal medulla is diminished, thus augmenting hypertonicity of the medullary interstitium by minimizing depletion of solutes via the bloodstream.

ADH causes walls of collecting ducts to become more permeable to water and thus permits osmolar equilibration and absorption of water into the hypertonic interstitium; a small volume of highly concentrated urine is excreted.

Plasma (ADH) — Max — 0
270 290 310
Plasma osmolality (mOsm/kg H_2O)

Plasma (ADH) — Max — 0
−30 −20 −10 0 10 20
% Change in blood volume or pressure

16.18 VASOPRESSIN (ANTIDIURETIC HORMONE) REGULATION OF WATER BALANCE AND FLUID OSMOLALITY

Vasopressin regulates the volume of water secreted by the kidneys. Its secretion is regulated by the osmolality of body fluids and by blood volume and pressure. Changes in body fluid osmolality of a small percentage are sufficient to significantly alter vasopressin secretion. Decreases in blood volume and pressure of 10% to 15% or more are needed to affect vasopressin secretion. The blood volume and pressure sensors are found in the large pulmonary vessels, the carotid sinus, and the aortic arch. These baroreceptors respond to the stretching of the vessel wall, which is dependent on blood volume and pressure. The figure shows the mechanisms of action of vasopressin on the kidney, with resultant effects on urine volume and concentration.

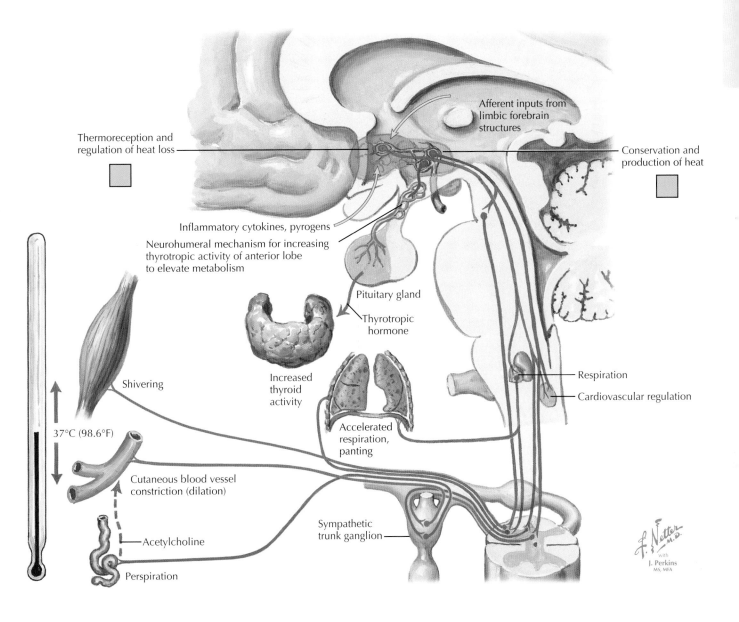

Afferent inputs from limbic forebrain structures

Thermoreception and regulation of heat loss

Conservation and production of heat

Inflammatory cytokines, pyrogens

Neurohumeral mechanism for increasing thyrotropic activity of anterior lobe to elevate metabolism

Pituitary gland

Thyrotropic hormone

Shivering

Increased thyroid activity

Respiration

Cardiovascular regulation

37°C (98.6°F)

Accelerated respiration, panting

Cutaneous blood vessel constriction (dilation)

Acetylcholine

Sympathetic trunk ganglion

Perspiration

16.19 THE HYPOTHALAMUS AND THERMOREGULATION

The preoptic area of the hypothalamus contains heat-sensitive neurons, and the posterior hypothalamic area contains cold-sensitive neurons. The preoptic area and the anterior hypothalamic area initiate neuronal responses for heat dissipation (parasympathetic); the posterior hypothalamic area initiates neuronal responses for heat generation (sympathetic). Neuronal pathways arising from the brain stem and limbic forebrain areas can modulate the activity of these thermoregulatory systems. The preoptic area is responsive to pyrogens and the inflammatory cytokine IL-1beta; this area can generate an increased set point for temperature regulation, thus initiating a disease-associated fever. Extensive hypothalamic connections with the brain stem and spinal cord are used to initiate appropriate heat-dissipation or heat-generation responses. Appropriate behavioral responses also are initiated to optimize thermoregulation (e.g., going to a warmer or cooler location).

16.20 SHORT-TERM REGULATION OF BLOOD PRESSURE

Both the sympathetic and parasympathetic divisions of the autonomic nervous system are involved in maintaining blood pressure on a second-by-second basis. Numerous descending pathways from the brain stem (including the nucleus tractus solitarius, tegmental catecholamine nuclei, locus coeruleus, raphe nuclei, rostral ventrolateral medulla and other medullary reticular regions, parabrachial nuclei, angiotensin II–containing neurons, and many other sites) and the hypothalamus regulate the outflow autonomic preganglionic neurons associated with short-term blood pressure regulation. The hypothalamus and the nucleus tractus solitarius are key sites integrating limbic forebrain and cortical influences over these brain stem regions that regulate blood pressure. The brain stem sites have extensive interconnections with each other. The example of blood pressure regulation in this figure is based on change in posture. (ACh, acetylcholine; AV, atrioventricular node; E, epinephrine; MAP, mean arterial pressure; NE, norepinephrine; SA, sinoatrial node.)

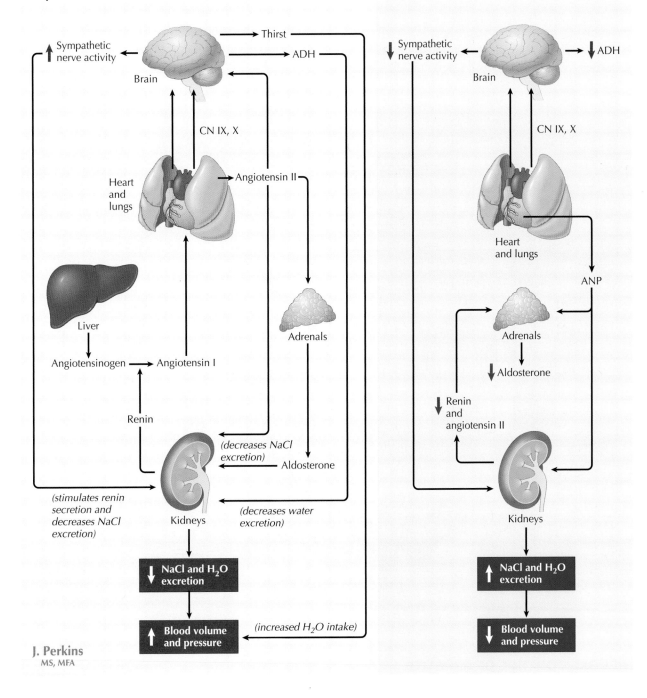

Response to Decreased Blood Volume and Pressure

Response to Increased Blood Volume and Pressure

J. Perkins
MS, MFA

16.21 LONG-TERM REGULATION OF BLOOD PRESSURE

When blood volume and blood pressure change, the kidneys respond by either retaining NaCl and water or excreting NaCl and water in order to restore blood volume to its normal homeostatic state. With increased sympathetic activation, norepinephrine and epinephrine secretion from sympathetic nerve terminals and the adrenal medulla increase in the circulation and act on the kidneys to reduce NaCl excretion. (ADH = antidiuretic hormone [also called vasopressin]; ANP = atrial natriuretic peptide.)

Smell of food

Ventromedial hypothalamic area (inhibitory: "satiety center")

Lateral hypothalamic area (facilitative: "appetite center")

Thalamus

Sight of food

Calcarine fissure

I

II

Touch (sucking reflex)

Memory and/or fantasy

Geniculate bodies (schematic)

V

VII

Chorda tympani

Dorsal nucleus of vagus

Taste of food

VIII

Nucleus of solitary tract

IX

Hearing (sounds of food preparation, call to dinner, bell, etc.)

X

Decreased levels of CCK, GLP-1, and leptin

Vagus nerve

Thoracic sympathetic ganglionic chain

Dorsal root ganglion

T6

Depletion of body nutrient stores

Myenteric and submucous plexuses

T7

T8

Mode of inducing hunger contractions unknown

Thoracic splanchnic nerves

T9

T10

KEY
— Sympathetic efferents
— Parasympathetic efferents
— Afferents (and CNS connections)
---- Indefinite paths

Hunger contractions in stomach

Celiac ganglion

16.22 NEURAL CONTROL OF APPETITE AND HUNGER

The sensations of hunger and satiety are complex and include multiple neural pathways and circulating hormones. This figure depicts pathways involved in the sensation of hunger. Although our understanding is incomplete, the hypothalamus is known to play a critical role in controlling appetite and food intake. When food is ingested, cholecystokinin (CCK) and glucagon-like peptide (GLP-1) are released from neuroendocrine cells in the intestine. These hormones suppress appetite and give the sensation of satiety. In the absence of food, the levels of these hormones are low. Long-term regulation of food intake involves the hormone leptin, which is produced by fat cells. When fat stores are high, leptin is released and appears to act on the hypothalamus to suppress appetite. When body nutrient stores are depleted, leptin levels are low. Other hormones such as ghrelins also are involved with control of hunger and satiety. Both the cerebral cortex and limbic forebrain structures have regulatory connections with this hypothalamic circuitry, permitting cognitive and emotional factors to influence appetite and eating behavior.

Neural, Neuroendocrine and Systemic Components of Rage Reaction

Rage pattern released and directed by cortex and limbic forebrain

Fornix (from hippocampal formation)

Mammillothalamic tract

Hypothalamus (blue: parasympathetic; red: sympathetic)

Dorsal longitudinal fasciculus; median forebrain bundle, and other descending pathways

Corticohypothalamic pathways

Orbitofrontal cortex

Median forebrain bundle

Olfactory bulb

Thyrotropin (elevates metabolism)

III to pupils (constriction)

VII to sublingual and submaxillary glands (secretion)

IX to parotid gland (secretion)

X to heart and GI tract (depresses heart rate and intestinal motility)

To heart (elevates rate)

Thoracic part of spinal cord

Adrenocorticotropin (releases cortisol, provokes stress reaction)

To adrenal medulla (effecting rise in blood sugar and visceral vasoconstriction)

Splenic contraction (leukocytes and platelets pressed out)

To vessels of skin (contraction) and muscles (dilation)

Spinal nerve

Sympathetic trunk ganglia

To GI tract and vessels (depression of motility; vasoconstriction)

Prevertebral ganglion

Pelvic nerve (sacral parasympathetic outflow)

Sacral part of spinal cord

To lower bowel and bladder (evacuation)

16.23 NEURAL AND NEUROENDOCRINE ROLES IN THE FIGHT-OR-FLIGHT RESPONSE

The classic sympathetic fight-or-flight response, shown here as a rage response, involves the secretion of neuroendocrine "stress hormones," including cortisol from the hypothalamo-pituitary-adrenal (HPA) axis and norepinephrine and epinephrine from sympathetic nerve terminals and the adrenal medulla. Sympathetic connections with the viscera initiate physiological changes to support the integrated fight-or-flight response. These changes include diversion of blood from the viscera and skin to the muscles, increased heart rate and cardiac output and contractility, bronchodilation, pupillary dilation, decreased gastrointestinal activation, decreased renal activity, glycogenolysis from the liver with increased blood glucose for fuel, and many other actions. Inputs from limbic forebrain regions, the cerebral cortex, and the brain stem regulate the complex hypothalamic control of neuroendocrine and autonomic outflow and are key in initiating the classic fight-or-flight response. In this response, the brain stem parasympathetic neurons are inhibited.

16.24 NEUROIMMUNOMODULATION

Connections from the cerebral cortex, limbic forebrain, hypothalamus, and brain stem can exert extensive modulation of autonomic preganglionic outflow and neuroendocrine outflow. Hormones and neurotransmitters from this outflow target lymphoid organs and cells of the immune system. This circuitry provides the substrate for behavior, emotional responsiveness, chronic stressors, and positive complementary and behavioral interventions to influence immune responses. Sympathetic postganglionic noradrenergic fibers directly innervate virtually all organs of the immune system, including (1) primary lymphoid organs (bone marrow, thymus); (2) secondary lymphoid organs (spleen, lymph nodes); (3) mucosa-associated lymphoid organs (gut and lung); and (4) skin-associated lymphoid cells. Vagal postganglionic nerve fibers innervate pulmonary- and gut-associated lymphoid tissue. Pituitary hormones in the circulation (e.g., CRF, ACTH, prolactin, GH, endorphins) and their target organ hormones (cortisol, thyroid hormone) modulate immune reactivity in all lymphoid organs. Cortisol, norepinephrine, and epinephrine are particularly important in mediating chronic stress responses related to immune reactivity. Circulating and local cytokines and inflammatory mediators act on the brain and pituitary to provide feedback information from lymphoid organs (immune-neural signaling). Cytokines and other paracrine secretions (e.g., enkephalins) also can modulate immune responses. The gene expression of hormones from secretory cells, cytokines from cells of the immune system, and neurotransmitters from neurons innervating lymphoid organs can be regulated by the presence of multiple signal molecules in the local environment. Some mediators are produced by neurons, paracrine cells, and cells of the immune system and can be considered as general mediators of all of these systems. (GALT, gut-associated lymphoid tissue; MALT, mucosa-associated lymphoid tissue.)

CLINICAL POINT

The PVN of the hypothalamus is a key regulatory site for neural modulation of immune responses; it acts through both hormonal secretion and autonomic regulation. The principal neural outflow systems that act on peripheral immunocytes are the HPA axis and the SNS connections to organs of the immune system and secretion into the general circulation. Activation of the HPA and the SNS can block some immune defenses, leading to greater susceptibility to viral infections (tenfold in experimental models of murine influenza). Other anterior pituitary hormones also exert immunomodulatory effects. Chronic stressors can influence neural-immune outflow via cortical and limbic connections to the hypothalamus (especially the PVN); chronic stressors exert both HPA and SNS effects that produce diminished cell-mediated immunity and natural killer cell activity. Both immune-inhibiting and immune-enhancing responses can be classically conditioned, a process that requires forebrain involvement and subsequent neural and hormonal outflow (but not cortisol; conditioned immunosuppression occurs in adrenalectomized animals). Both circulating cytokines and endogenous brain cytokines, including IL-1beta, IL-6, and TNF-alpha, can act on the PVN and other CNS sites involved in neuroendocrine and SNS outflow to immune targets, markedly activating cortisol production and catecholamine secretion. In adults, the regulation of secretion of dangerous inflammatory mediators as well as behavioral and lifestyle influences on the HPA axis and SNS may be important components of maintaining robust antiviral and antitumor immunity and may aid in protection from many chronic diseases. These mediators are key components targeted in integrative medical treatment.

Major Limbic Forebrain Structures

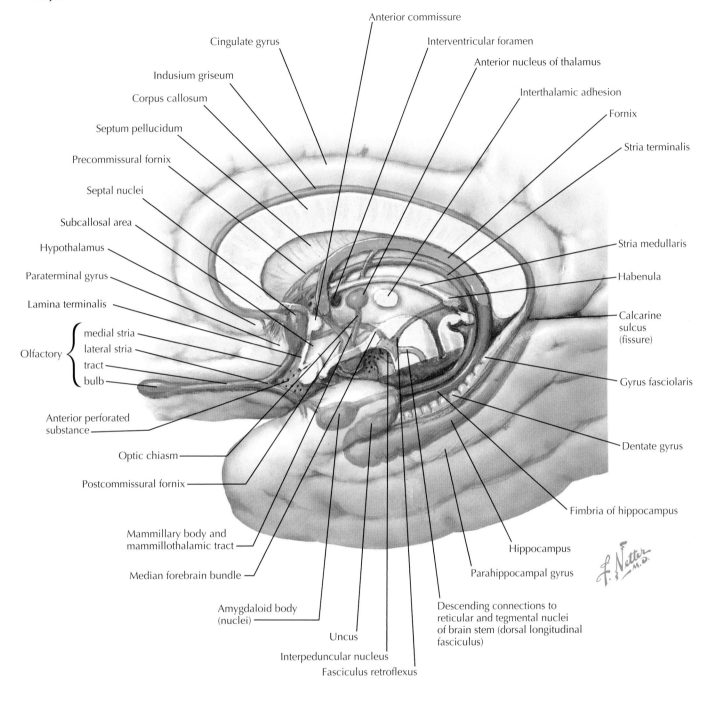

Anterior commissure

Cingulate gyrus

Interventricular foramen

Indusium griseum

Anterior nucleus of thalamus

Corpus callosum

Interthalamic adhesion

Septum pellucidum

Fornix

Precommissural fornix

Stria terminalis

Septal nuclei

Subcallosal area

Hypothalamus

Stria medullaris

Paraterminal gyrus

Habenula

Lamina terminalis

Olfactory { medial stria
            lateral stria
            tract
            bulb }

Calcarine sulcus (fissure)

Gyrus fasciolaris

Anterior perforated substance

Optic chiasm

Dentate gyrus

Postcommissural fornix

Fimbria of hippocampus

Mammillary body and mammillothalamic tract

Hippocampus

Median forebrain bundle

Parahippocampal gyrus

Amygdaloid body (nuclei)

Descending connections to reticular and tegmental nuclei of brain stem (dorsal longitudinal fasciculus)

Uncus

Interpeduncular nucleus

Fasciculus retroflexus

LIMBIC SYSTEM

16.25 ANATOMY OF THE LIMBIC FOREBRAIN

Structures of the limbic forebrain are found in a ring (limbus) that encircles the diencephalon. Two major temporal lobe structures, the hippocampal formation with its fornix and the amygdala with its stria terminalis, send C-shaped axonal projections through the forebrain, around the diencephalon, and into the hypothalamus and septal region. The amygdala also has a more direct pathway (the ventral amygdalofugal pathway) into the hypothalamus. The septal nuclei sit just rostral to the hypothalamus and send axons to the habenular nuclei via the stria medullaris thalami. The cingulate, prefrontal, orbitofrontal, entorhinal, and periamygdaloid areas of the cortex interconnect with subcortical and hippocampal components of the limbic forebrain and are often considered part of the limbic system. The limbic system is thought to be a major substrate for regulation of emotional responsiveness and behavior, for individualized reactivity to sensory stimuli and internal stimuli, and for integrated memory tasks.

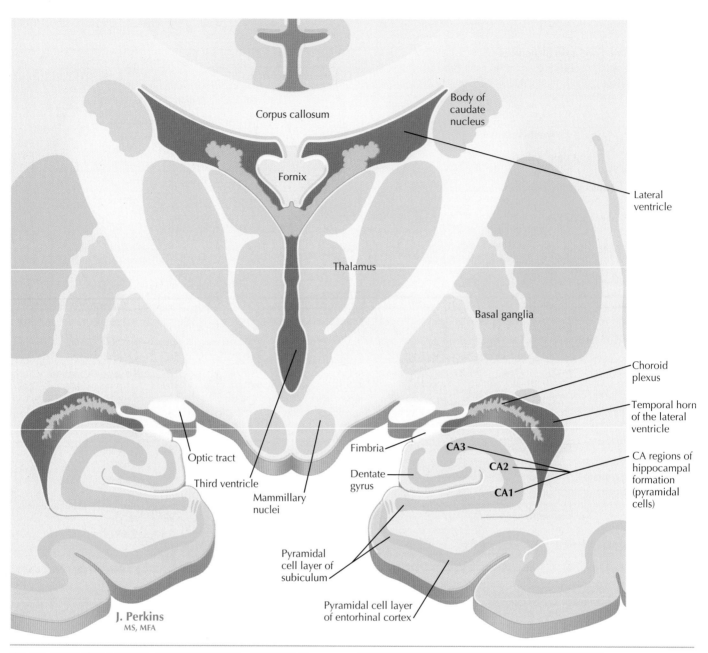

J. Perkins
MS, MFA

16.26 HIPPOCAMPAL FORMATION: GENERAL ANATOMY

The hippocampal formation consists of the dentate gyrus, the hippocampus proper (cornu ammonis [CA] regions), and the subiculum. These structures are intimately interconnected with the adjacent entorhinal cortex. The hippocampus is a seahorse-shaped structure found in the medial portion of the anterior temporal lobe. It bulges laterally into the temporal horn of the lateral ventricle. The hippocampus is divided into several zones of pyramidal cells, called CA regions (CA1–CA4). The dentate gyrus and hippocampus are three-layered cortical regions. Granule cells populate the dentate gyrus, and pyramidal cells are the main neurons in the CA regions of the hippocampus. The hippocampal formation has extensive interconnections with cortical association areas and with limbic forebrain structures, such as the septal nuclei and the cingulate gyrus. The hippocampal formation is involved with consolidation of short-term memory into long-term traces, in conjunction with extensive regions of neocortex.

CLINICAL POINT

Pyramidal cells in the CA1 region of the hippocampus are particularly vulnerable to apoptosis resulting from ischemia. Following a heart attack with delayed resuscitation, an episode of cerebral ischemia, or multi-infarct problems, or after increasingly poor blood flow in the anterior circulation to the brain, destruction of CA1 neurons (Sommer's sector) can result in loss of short-term memory and in spatial disorientation. CA3 pyramidal neurons are particularly vulnerable to high or persistently elevated levels of cortisol (or synthetic glucocorticoids), resulting in similar functional deficits. The combination of cerebral ischemia and high cortisol is particularly damaging to the hippocampus. This combination of relative ischemia and high circulating glucocorticoids may occur in older individuals with atherosclerosis and compromised cerebral blood flow (but still free of symptoms) who experience a highly stressful experience (e.g., hospitalization or institutionalization) in which they are exposed to nosocomial organisms and generate cytokine responses, further exacerbating cortisol secretion. This situation may help to precipitate hippocampal damage that leads to consolidation problems relating to immediate and short-term memory and confusion and produces disorientation, conditions frequently encountered in hospitalized or institutionalized elderly patients.

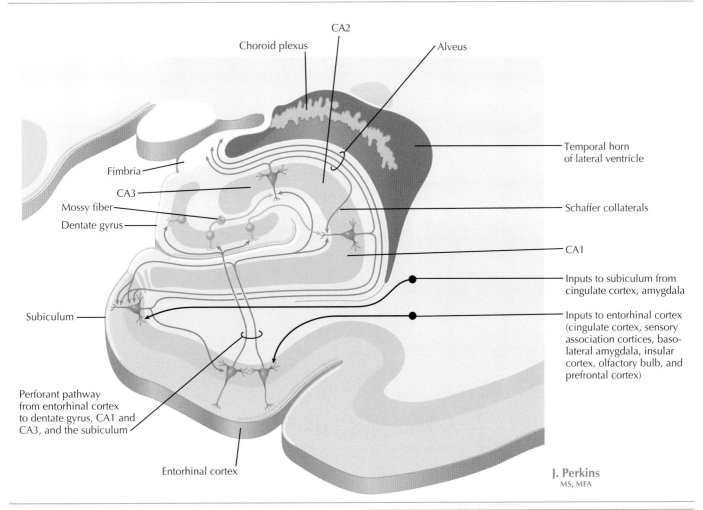

16.27 NEURONAL CONNECTIONS IN THE HIPPOCAMPAL FORMATION

The hippocampal formation has an internal circuitry that is interconnected with the entorhinal cortex. Pyramidal neurons of the entorhinal cortex send axons to granule cell dendrites in the dentate gyrus. These granule cell axons (mossy fibers) synapse on pyramidal cell dendrites in CA3. Pyramidal cells in CA3 project to pyramidal cell dendrites in CA1 (Schaffer collaterals) and CA2. CA1 pyramidal axons project to pyramidal neurons in the subiculum. The subiculum sends axonal projections back to the pyramidal neurons of the entorhinal cortex. This information flow represents an internal circuit. Superimposed on this circuitry is a host of interconnections with association regions of the neocortex and other limbic forebrain structures. Neurons of the subiculum and pyramidal neurons of CA1 and CA3 send axons into the fornix as efferent projections to target structures. The subiculum also sends axons to the amygdala and association areas of the temporal lobe.

CLINICAL POINT

Many temporal lobe structures are associated with the flow of information through the hippocampal formation, including the hippocampus, subiculum, entorhinal cortex, and associated cortical areas of the temporal lobe. Many of these cortical regions are particularly susceptible to neuronal degeneration in Alzheimer's disease (AD), a neurodegenerative disease that damages and destroys neurons in the cerebral cortex and higher centers of the brain and is accompanied by marked cognitive deficits. Disruption of hippocampal circuitry leads to the inability to consolidate immediate and short-term memory into long-term traces. Temporal lobe damage and disruption of connections with the basal forebrain, cingulate cortex, frontal cortex, and other forebrain structures also affected by AD contribute to the marked cognitive decline in patients with AD. In AD, the brain shows extensive neuronal loss, impaired functioning of synaptic connections, and damage to important neurotransmitter systems that participate in functions such as memory. AD is characterized by the accumulation of altered and aberrant proteins inside neurons, called neurofibrillary tangles, and outside of neurons, called senile plaques. However, severe cognitive decline may occur in the absence of neurofibrillary tangles and senile plaques, and the presence of these proteins in the brain is not always predictive of cognitive dysfunction. Proposed causes of AD include the accumulation of beta-amyloid protein and its precursor protein and/or excessive phosphorylation of an important protein (tau) that helps to give neurons their structural integrity. A form of apolipoprotein E (epsilon 4) is linked with excessive production of free radicals that may kill neurons. Inflammatory molecules (e.g., IL-1beta) also may cause neuronal damage. At present, there is no common agreement on a specific sequence of events or cascade of pathology in AD.

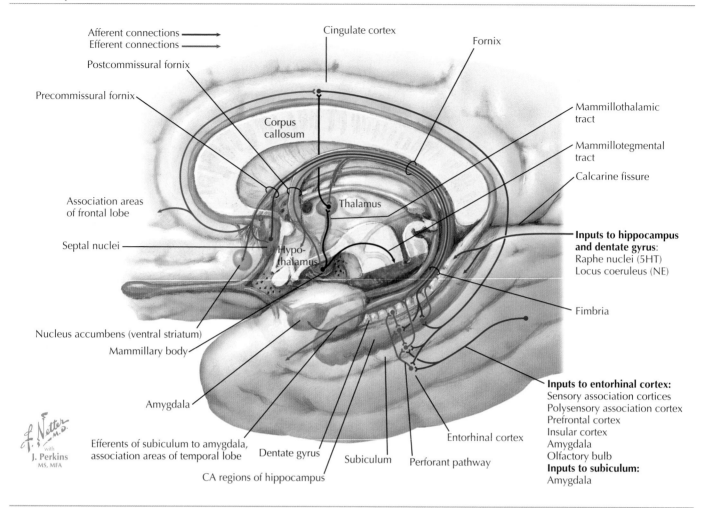

Afferent connections ⟶
Efferent connections ⟹

Postcommissural fornix
Precommissural fornix
Corpus callosum
Cingulate cortex
Fornix
Mammillothalamic tract
Mammillotegmental tract
Calcarine fissure
Association areas of frontal lobe
Thalamus
Inputs to hippocampus and dentate gyrus:
Raphe nuclei (5HT)
Locus coeruleus (NE)
Septal nuclei
Hypo-thalamus
Fimbria
Nucleus accumbens (ventral striatum)
Mammillary body
Amygdala
Inputs to entorhinal cortex:
Sensory association cortices
Polysensory association cortex
Prefrontal cortex
Insular cortex
Amygdala
Olfactory bulb
Inputs to subiculum:
Amygdala
Efferents of subiculum to amygdala, association areas of temporal lobe
Entorhinal cortex
Dentate gyrus
Subiculum
Perforant pathway
CA regions of hippocampus

16.28 MAJOR AFFERENT AND EFFERENT CONNECTIONS OF THE HIPPOCAMPAL FORMATION

Pyramidal neurons in the subiculum and hippocampal regions CA1 and CA3 give rise to the efferent fornix. The subiculum projects axons to hypothalamic nuclei (especially mammillary nuclei) and thalamic nuclei via the postcommissural fornix. CA1 and CA3 of the hippocampus send axons to the septal nuclei, the nucleus accumbens, the preoptic and anterior hypothalamic regions, the cingulate cortex, and association areas of the frontal lobe. Afferent cholinergic axons from septal nuclei traverse the fornix to supply the dentate gyrus and hippocampal CA regions. Massive inputs arrive in the hippocampal formation from sensory association cortices, polysensory association cortices, the prefrontal cortex, the insular cortex, the amygdaloid nuclei, and the olfactory bulb via projections to the entorhinal cortex. The entorhinal cortex is fully integrated into the internal circuitry of the hippocampal formation. The subiculum is connected reciprocally with the amygdala and also sends axons to cortical association areas of the temporal lobe. (5HT, 5-hydroxytryptamine [serotonin]; NE, norepinephrine.)

information about which cognitive assessment takes place. Explicit memory involves structures in the medial temporal lobe, including the hippocampal formation. Implicit memory is the process of learning how to perform tasks or acquire skills that are not recallable by conscious processes; this form of memory depends upon other brain circuitry and is not lost in classic cases of hippocampal lesions. Explicit memory recall depends upon reassembly of information stored in the brain and involves reconstruction that depends upon sensory perceptions. It is not a video record of the precise external events and can be markedly different from reality, which raises serious questions about the accuracy of "recovered memory" of past events. Explicit memory requires the formation of new synaptic connections and gene expression for new sets of neuronal proteins. The consolidation of immediate and short-term explicit memory into long-term traces involves a process of long-term potentiation, which involves a burst of activity in a specific temporal pattern from an incoming axon; that enhances the likelihood that the target neuron will be activated by this same input and other incoming inputs, providing an increased response to the same magnitude of excitation. Thus, a brief, sustained pattern of input makes it more likely that future synaptic activity will occur. Long-term potentiation occurs in dentate granule cells, CA1 neurons, and CA3 neurons. In the former two neurons, it requires N-methyl-D-aspartate receptor activation, depolarization, Ca^{++} influx, and communication between pre- and post-synaptic elements. In CA3 neurons, long-term potentiation depends on presynaptic Ca^{++} influx and subsequent cyclic adenosine monophosphate–dependent protein kinase production.

CLINICAL POINT

Explicit memory is acquisition of information about objects, stimuli, and information that is consciously noted and recallable, and it includes information about personal events, factual knowledge, and

Thalamus

Bed nucleus of the stria terminalis

Cingulate cortex

Intralaminar nuclei

Medial dorsal nucleus

Stria terminalis

Brain stem inputs:
Parabrachial nuclei
Periaqueductal gray
Ventral tegmental area (DA)
Raphe nuclei (5HT)
Locus coeruleus (NE)
Nucleus tractus solitarius

Anterior commissure

Corpus callosum

Septal nuclei

Prefrontal cortex

Hypo-thalamus

Olfactory bulb

Hypothalamic inputs:
Lateral hypothalamic area
Ventromedial nucleus

Corticomedial nuclei of the amygdala

Basolateral nuclei of the amygdala

Subiculum (hippocampal formation)

Sensory association inputs:
Temporal lobe sensory association cortex
Entorhinal cortex
Insular cortex
Medial frontal lobe

16.29 MAJOR AFFERENT CONNECTIONS OF THE AMYGDALA

The amygdala is an almond-shaped collection of nuclei in the medial portion of the anterior temporal lobe. It is involved in the emotional interpretation of external sensory information and internal states. It provides individual-specific behavioral and emotional responses, particularly those involving fear and aversive responses. The amygdala is subdivided into corticomedial nuclei and basolateral nuclei (which receive afferents and project axons to target structures) and the central nucleus, which provides mainly efferent projections to the brain stem. Afferents to the corticomedial nuclei arrive primarily from subcortical limbic sources, including the olfactory bulb, septal nuclei, and hypothalamic nuclei (VM, LHA); the thalamus (intralaminar nuclei); the bed nucleus of the stria terminalis; and extensive numbers of autonomic nuclei and monoamine nuclei of the brain stem. Afferents to the basolateral nuclei arrive mainly from cortical areas, including extensive sensory association cortices, the prefrontal cortex, the cingulate cortex, and the subiculum. (5HT, 5-hydroxytryptamine [serotonin]; NE, norepinephrine.)

CLINICAL POINT

The amygdala is a subcortical collection of nuclei in the medial anterior temporal lobe. It is involved in the emotional interpretation and "flavoring" of external sensory information and internal states. Afferents to corticomedial nuclei come from subcortical limbic structures, and afferents to basolateral nuclei derive mainly from cortical structures. Most cases in humans of bilateral destruction of the amygdala occur with trauma or temporal lobe surgery for seizures, and they involve destruction of more than just amygdaloid nuclei. On the basis of primate studies and observations in humans, it appears that amygdaloid lesions result in placid behavior, lack of fear even when confronted with normally fear-provoking stimuli, and withdrawal from social contacts. The normal integration of emotional reactive and cognitive processing is disrupted. Studies have found that patients with bilateral amygdaloid damage cannot recognize facial expressions in others that indicate fear and do not learn or remember events with strong emotional context better than those without such emotional context, as is normally the case. In patients with bilateral temporal lobe damage involving extensive cortical and subcortical neuronal destruction, the Klüver-Bucy syndrome can occur. This syndrome is characterized by placid behavior, loss of fear of potentially dangerous objects, compulsive exploration of the environment (particularly orally), visual agnosias, inappropriately directed hyperphagia (of nonedible items), and hypersexuality. In some cases, loss of consolidation of memory (hippocampal involvement) and cognitive deficits are also seen.

Bed nucleus of the stria terminalis

Stria terminalis

To brain stem:
Nucleus tractus solitarius
Dorsal motor nucleus of X
Raphe nuclei (5HT)
Locus coeruleus (NE)
Parabrachial nuclei
Periaqueductal gray
Reticular formation

Striatum (rostral areas)
Caudate nucleus
Putamen

Corpus callosum

Th
M

Frontal lobe regions:
Frontal cortex
Prefrontal cortex

Septal nuclei

H

Nucleus accumbens

Substantia innominata (with nucleus basalis ACh neurons)

Ventral amygdalofugal pathway

Corticomedial nuclei of the amygdala

Basolateral nuclei of the amygdala

Central nucleus of the amygdala

Entorhinal cortex

Subiculum

To cingulate cortex

Inferior temporal cortex (e.g., visual areas)

H = Hypothalamus:
Preoptic area
Anterior hypothalamic area
Ventromedial nucleus
Lateral hypothalamic area
Paraventricular nucleus

Th = Thalamus:
Medial dorsal nucleus

M = Midline thalamic nuclei

16.30 MAJOR EFFERENT CONNECTIONS OF THE AMYGDALA

Efferents from the corticomedial nuclei project through the stria terminalis and are directed mainly toward subcortical nuclei, such as septal nuclei, the mediodorsal nucleus of the thalamus, the hypothalamic nuclei, the bed nucleus of the stria terminalis, the nucleus accumbens, and the rostral striatum. Efferents from the basolateral nuclei project through the ventral amygdalofugal pathway to extensive cortical regions, including the frontal cortex, the cingulate cortex, the inferior temporal cortex, the subiculum, and the entorhinal cortex; and to subcortical limbic regions, including hypothalamic nuclei, septal nuclei, and the cholinergic nucleus basalis in substantia innominata. The central amygdaloid receives input mainly from internal amygdaloid connections and sends extensive efferents through the ventral amygdalofugal pathway to extensive autonomic nuclei and monoaminergic nuclei of the brain stem, the midline thalamic nuclei, the bed nucleus of the stria terminalis, and the cholinergic nucleus basalis.

CLINICAL POINT

Efferents from the corticomedial nuclei are directed mainly to subcortical limbic nuclei. Efferents from the basolateral nuclei are directed through the ventral amygdalofugal pathway to extensive cortical regions and subcortical structures. The central amygdaloid nucleus sends extensive efferents to brain stem nuclei associated with the machinery of emotional responsiveness provoked by amygdaloid activation. This central nucleus receives its input mainly from other amygdaloid nuclei. Amygdaloid stimulation has been performed in humans (for epilepsy surgery) and in experimental animals. Corticomedial stimulation produces a freezing response (cessation of voluntary movement), automated gestures (lip smacking), and parasympathetic activation that leads to voiding and defecation. Basolateral stimulation produces the vigilance responses of becoming alert and scanning the environment. These responses most likely reflect the outflow of the amygdala to brain stem circuitry that coordinates behavior appropriate to the emotional context of the stimuli. Conditioned fear responses and reactions to stressors require coordinated interaction of neuroendocrine outflow, autonomic reactivity, and behavioral activity. In humans, amygdaloid stimulation results in feelings associated with fear and anxiety. (5HT, 5-hydroxytryptamine [serotonin]; NE, norepinephrine.)

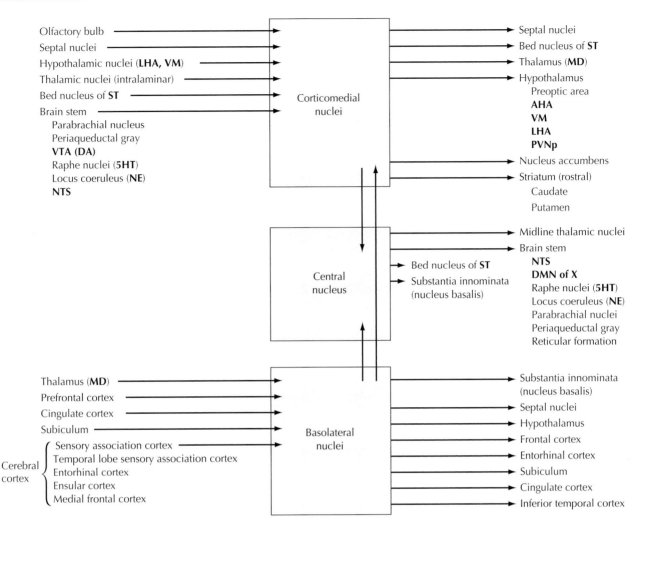

AHA = Anterior hypothalamic area
DA = Dopamine
DMN of X = Dorsal motor (autonomic) nucleus of X
5HT = 5-Hydroxytryptamine (serotonin)
LHA = Lateral hypothalamic area
MD = Medial dorsal nucleus of thalamus

NE = Norepinephrine
NTS = Nucleus tractus solitarius
PVNp = Paraventricular nucleus, parvocellular
ST = Stria terminalis
VM = Ventromedial
VTA = Ventral tegmental area

16.31 SUMMARY OF MAJOR AFFERENTS, EFFERENTS, AND INTERCONNECTIONS OF THE AMYGDALA

The corticomedial amygdala is connected reciprocally mainly with subcortical limbic forebrain structures and receives extensive additional inputs from brain stem autonomic and monoaminergic nuclei. The basolateral amygdala is connected reciprocally with extensive regions of limbic and association cortex and has additional efferents to subcortical limbic forebrain regions. Both the corticomedial and basolateral nuclei send axons to the central nucleus of the amygdala. The central nucleus has massive descending efferents to extensive autonomic and monoaminergic nuclei of the brain stem as well as to some subcortical limbic forebrain regions. These interconnections with extensive regions of the cortex, the limbic forebrain regions, and the autonomic/limbic brain stem nuclei provide the integrated circuitry that permits analysis of both external and internal information and provides an emotional and interpretive context for the initiation and control of appropriate behavioral and emotional responses.

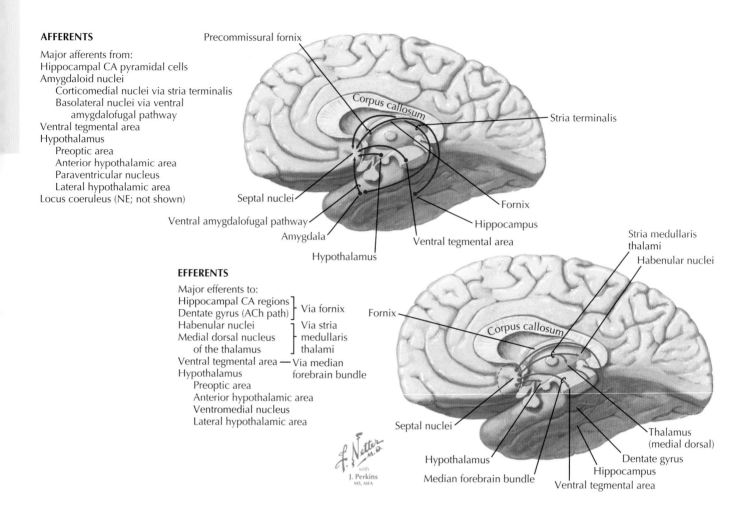

AFFERENTS

Major afferents from:
Hippocampal CA pyramidal cells
Amygdaloid nuclei
    Corticomedial nuclei via stria terminalis
    Basolateral nuclei via ventral
        amygdalofugal pathway
Ventral tegmental area
Hypothalamus
    Preoptic area
    Anterior hypothalamic area
    Paraventricular nucleus
    Lateral hypothalamic area
Locus coeruleus (NE; not shown)

Precommissural fornix
Corpus callosum
Stria terminalis
Septal nuclei
Fornix
Ventral amygdalofugal pathway
Hippocampus
Amygdala
Ventral tegmental area
Hypothalamus

EFFERENTS

Major efferents to:
Hippocampal CA regions ⎤
Dentate gyrus (ACh path) ⎦ Via fornix
Habenular nuclei ⎤ Via stria
Medial dorsal nucleus ⎬ medullaris
    of the thalamus ⎦ thalami
Ventral tegmental area — Via median
Hypothalamus   forebrain bundle
    Preoptic area
    Anterior hypothalamic area
    Ventromedial nucleus
    Lateral hypothalamic area

Fornix
Corpus callosum
Stria medullaris thalami
Habenular nuclei
Septal nuclei
Thalamus (medial dorsal)
Hypothalamus
Dentate gyrus
Median forebrain bundle
Hippocampus
Ventral tegmental area

16.32 MAJOR AFFERENT AND EFFERENT CONNECTIONS OF THE SEPTAL NUCLEI

The septal nuclei are subcortical nuclei initially implicated in early ablation and stimulation studies in the regulation of emotional responsiveness such as rage behavior. In experimental studies, the septal nuclei appear to play a role in emotional behaviors, sexual behavior, aggressive behavior, modulation of autonomic functions, and attention and memory functions (from the cholinergic neurons). Afferents to the septal nuclei arrive mainly from the hippocampus, the corticomedial and basolateral amygdala, the ventral tegmental nucleus in the midbrain, and several hypothalamic nuclei. Efferents from the septal nuclei distribute mainly to the hippocampus and dentate gyrus (via the fornix); the habenular nuclei (via the stria medullaris thalami); the medial dorsal nucleus of the thalamus (via the stria medullaris thalami); the ventral tegmental area (via the median forebrain bundle); and several hypothalamic nuclei.

CLINICAL POINT

In some humans with ischemic damage involving the septal area, rage behavior has been observed. This is consistent with early experimental studies in rodents in which septal lesions resulted in exaggerated

reactivity to both appropriate and innocuous stimuli (sham rage). In contrast, implanted electrodes in the septal nuclei for electrical self-stimulation studies resulted in prolonged and repeated stimulation, indicative of pleasurable responses.

Efferent connections to the habenula and, via its efferent pathways to the brain stem such as the fasciculus retroflexus (habenulopeduncular tract), and connections to the hypothalamus and brain stem through the descending median forebrain bundle, represent the descending regulatory circuitry from the septal nuclei through which some of the associated behaviors are accomplished. The recent findings that a cholinergic cell group in the septum, along with the bed nucleus of the stria terminalis, sends axons via the fornix to the hippocampal formation, and that these are commonly found to have degenerated in the brains of patients with AD, raises the possibility that these cholinergic neurons are contributors to the process of consolidation of immediate and short-term memory into long-term traces. Damage to the entire collection of cholinergic neurons (including nucleus basalis of Meynert) produces such memory deficits, but experimental studies of selective lesions of cholinergic neurons in the septal nucleus and bed nucleus of the stria terminalis did not result in profound loss of such memory function. It is likely that the cholinergic projections to the hippocampal formation and the cerebral cortex function as a distributive system and affect memory function through an influence on the entire circuitry involved in cognitive and memory functions.

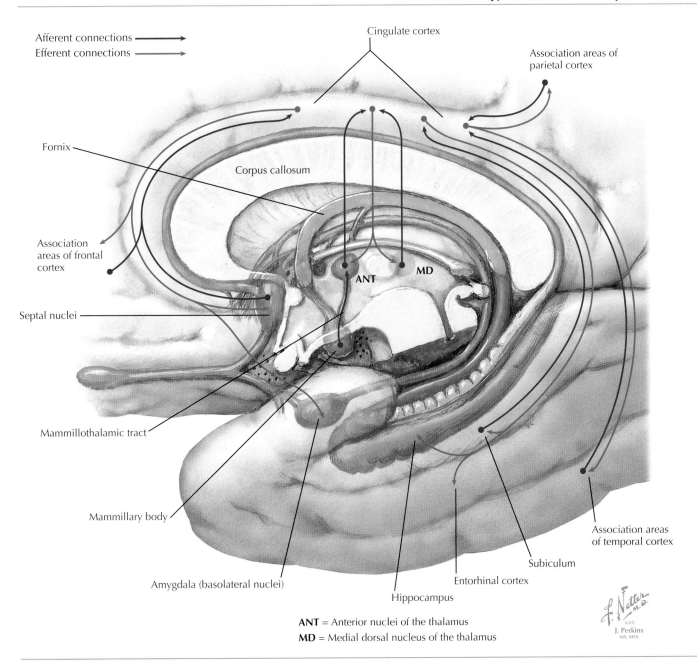

Afferent connections ⟶
Efferent connections ⟶

Cingulate cortex

Association areas of parietal cortex

Fornix

Corpus callosum

Association areas of frontal cortex

Septal nuclei

ANT   MD

Mammillothalamic tract

Mammillary body

Association areas of temporal cortex

Amygdala (basolateral nuclei)

Subiculum

Entorhinal cortex

Hippocampus

ANT = Anterior nuclei of the thalamus
MD = Medial dorsal nucleus of the thalamus

16.33 MAJOR CONNECTIONS OF THE CINGULATE CORTEX

The cingulate cortex is located above the corpus callosum. This cortical region is involved in the regulation of autonomic functions (respiratory, digestive, cardiovascular, pupillary); some somatic functions (motor tone, ongoing movements); and emotional responsiveness and behavior. Lesions in the cingulate cortex, like lesions in the orbitofrontal cortex, result in indifference to pain and other sensations that have emotional connotations and in social indifference. Afferents to the cingulate cortex arrive from association areas of the frontal, parietal, and temporal lobes, the subiculum, the septal nuclei, and the thalamic nuclei (mediodorsal, anterior). Efferents from the cingulate cortex project to association areas of frontal, parietal, and temporal lobes and to limbic forebrain regions, such as the hippocampus, the subiculum, the entorhinal cortex, the amygdala, and septal nuclei. These limbic forebrain regions send extensive projections to the hypothalamus for regulation of autonomic and somatic regions of the brain stem and spinal cord.

CLINICAL POINT

The anterior cingulate cortex may participate in selecting appropriate responses to conflicting stimuli. Inputs to the cingulate cortex derive from many regions of frontal, parietal, and temporal cortex, the subiculum, the septal nuclei, and the medial dorsal thalamus (prefrontal connections). Efferent connections project back to many of these same regions as well as to the amygdala, subiculum, and entorhinal cortex. Through these efferent connections, circuitry to the brain stem can coordinate appropriate autonomic and somatic functions. Lesions in the cingulate cortex result in indifference to pain and other sensations that have strong emotional connotations; they produce social indifference and apathy, eliminate emotional intonation in speech, and cause personality changes. Bilateral anterior cingulate lesions, or cingulotomies, have been done as "psychosurgery" to alleviate intractable pain and to incapacitate anxiety, obsessive-compulsive behavior, and intractable depression. Lesions in the posterior cingulate cortex result in diminished ability to perform spatial navigation.

A. Distribution of olfactory epithelium (blue area)

Olfactory Receptors

Olfactory bulb

Lateral nasal wall

B. Schema of section through olfactory mucosa

Cribriform plate
of ethmoid bone

Septum

Cribriform plate

Schwann cell

Olfactory gland

Unmyelinated olfactory axons

Basement membrane

Sustentacular cells

Endoplasmic reticulum

Nucleus

Olfactory cells

Dendrites

Terminal bars (desmosomes)

Olfactory rod (vesicle)

Villi

Cilia

Mucus

OLFACTORY SYSTEM

16.34 OLFACTORY RECEPTORS

Olfactory receptors are found in a patch of olfactory epithelium that lines the medial and lateral walls of the roof of the nasal cavity. Olfactory receptor cells are primitive, specialized, bipolar neurons whose nuclei are in the base of the epithelium. A dendritic process extends toward the epithelial surface, widening into a rod with 10 to 30 motile cilia that extend into the mucous cover. Odorants act on receptors (G-protein coupled) on these cilia and bring about a slow, depolarizing generator potential. Odorant interactions with receptors are complex, often requiring odorant-binding proteins to carry the odorant through the mucus. The bipolar neurons of the olfactory epithelium are CNS neurons; they are unusual because they undergo continuous replacement and turnover from basal stem cells in the epithelium. The unmyelinated olfactory axons cluster together in groups (collectively enwrapped by a single Schwann cell sheath) before passing through the cribriform plate. Injuries to the cribriform plate can tear these axons and result in anosmia.

CLINICAL POINT

Anosmia, the loss of smell, may not be obvious to a patient; it may present with a blunting of the taste of food. The most common cause of anosmia is a cold, followed by allergic rhinitis. Unilateral anosmia not attributable to local nasal problems suggests involvement of the olfactory nerves, bulb, or tracts and stria. Trauma causing injury to the cribriform plate is the most common cause of olfactory nerve damage. Impairment of olfactory discrimination but with intact ability to detect odors points to possible involvement of forebrain structures, such as limbic circuitry in Wernicke-Korsakoff syndrome, in the prefrontal cortex, in cortical areas damaged by neurodegenerative conditions such as AD, or in thalamic regions.

Efferent fibers

Afferent fibers

Granule cell (excited by and inhibiting to mitral and tufted cells)

Mitral cell

Recurrent process

Tufted cell

Periglomerular cell

Glomerulus

Olfactory nerve fibers

Subcallosal (parolfactory) area

Septal area and nuclei

Fibers from contralateral olfactory bulb

Fibers to contralateral olfactory bulb

Anterior commissure

Medial olfactory stria

Olfactory trigone and olfactory tubercle

Anterior perforated substance

Habenula

Lateral olfactory stria

Lateral olfactory tract nucleus

Piriform lobe

Hippocampal fimbria

Dentate gyrus

Uncus

Parahippocampal gyrus

Amygdala (in phantom)

Entorhinal area

Olfactory epithelium

Olfactory nerves

Olfactory bulb

Olfactory tract

Anterior olfactory nucleus

Cribriform plate of ethmoid bone

16.35 OLFACTORY PATHWAYS

Primary sensory axons from bipolar neurons pass through the cribriform plate and synapse in the olfactory glomeruli in the glomerular layer of the olfactory bulb. The glomeruli are the functional units for processing specific odor information. The olfactory nerve fibers synapse on the dendrites of the tufted and mitral cells, the secondary sensory neurons that give rise to the olfactory tract projections. Periglomerular cells are interneurons that interconnect the glomeruli. Granule cells modulate the excitability of tufted and mitral cells. Centrifugal connections (from serotonergic raphe nuclei and the noradrenergic locus coeruleus) modulate activity in the glomeruli and periglomerular cells. The olfactory tract bypasses the thalamus and projects to the anterior olfactory nucleus, the nucleus accumbens, the primary olfactory cortex (in the uncus), the amygdala, the periamygdaloid cortex, and the lateral entorhinal cortex. The olfactory cortex has interconnections with the orbitofrontal cortex, the insular cortex, the hippocampus, and the lateral hypothalamus.

CLINICAL POINT

The olfactory bulb and tract can be damaged by meningiomas of the olfactory groove or, less commonly, of the sphenoid ridge. These tumors produce Foster-Kennedy syndrome, which consists of ipsilateral anosmia, ipsilateral optic atrophy resulting from direct pressure, and papilledema caused by increased intracranial pressure. If the ipsilateral optic nerve is completely atrophic, papilledema will not be observed on that side. The olfactory bulb and tract also can be damaged by tumors of the frontal bone, pituitary tumors with frontal extension, frontal tumors such as gliomas that act as mass lesions, aneurysms at the circle of Willis, and meningitis. These conditions are distinguished from the olfactory groove meningiomas by the additional symptoms they cause.

Index

Page numbers followed by b indicate box (Clinical Point).